# Plant Diseases-Current Threats and Management Trends

*Edited by Snježana Topolovec-Pintarić*

Published in London, United Kingdom

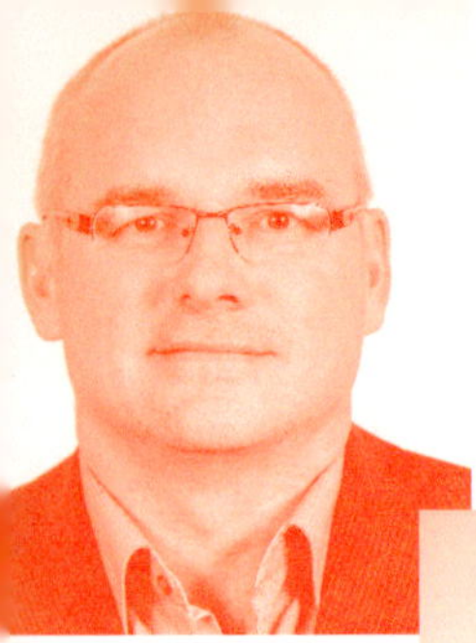
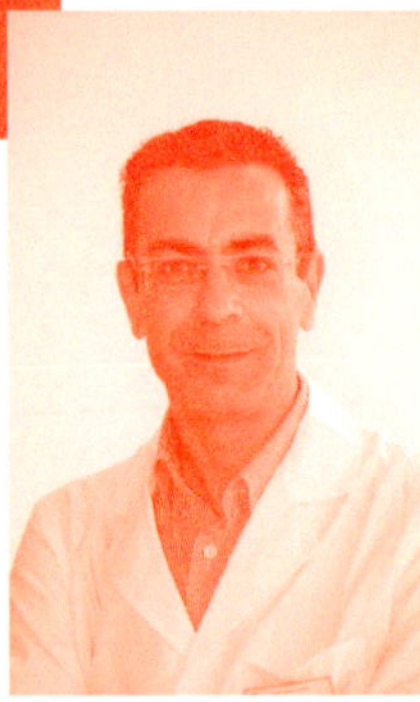
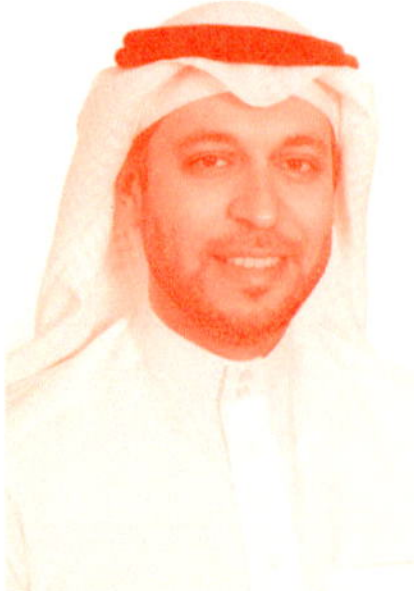
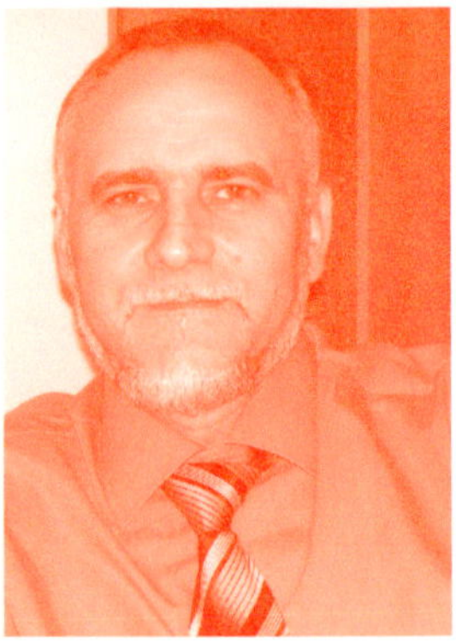
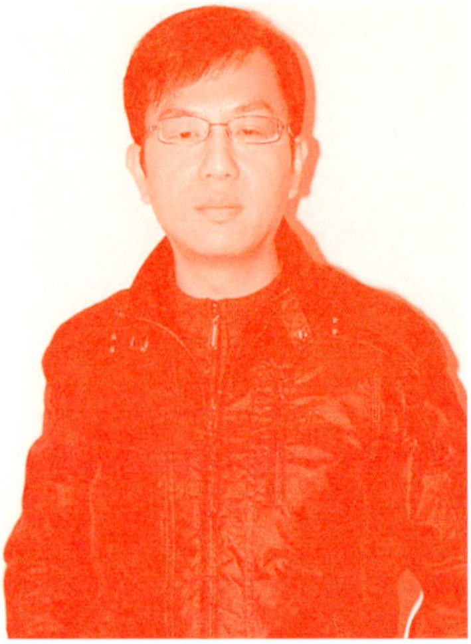
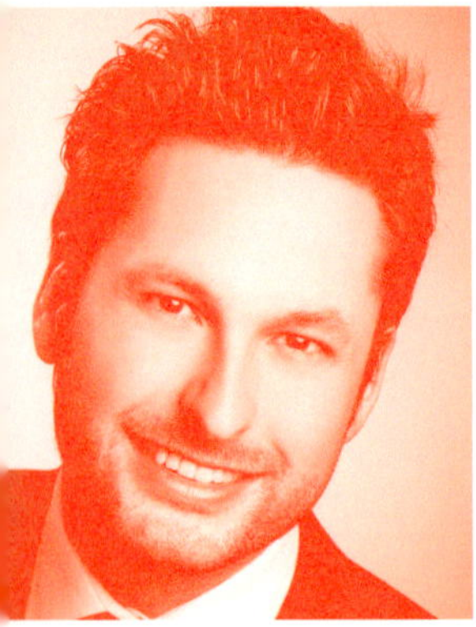
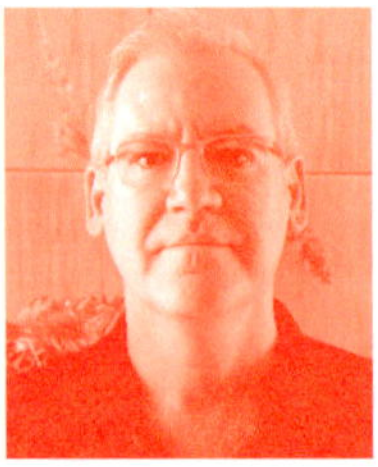

IntechOpen

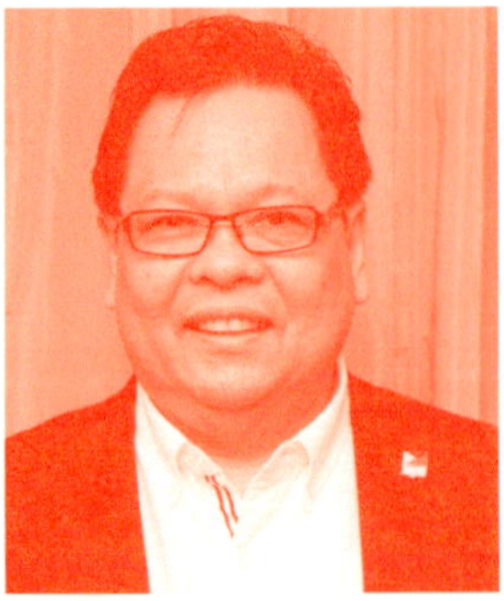
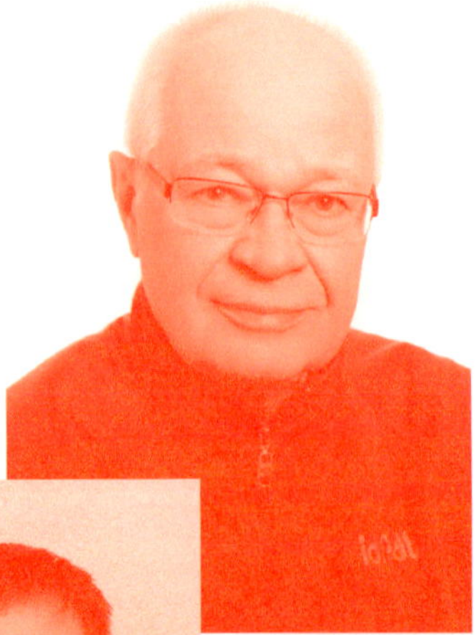
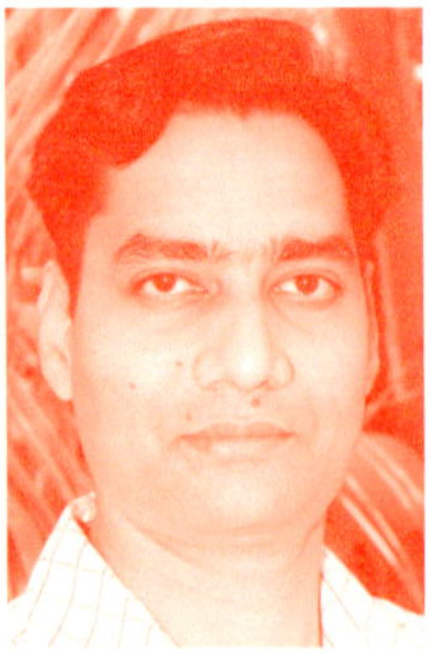
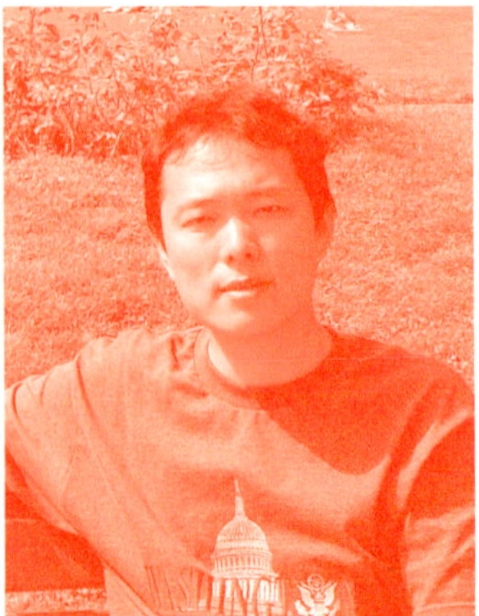
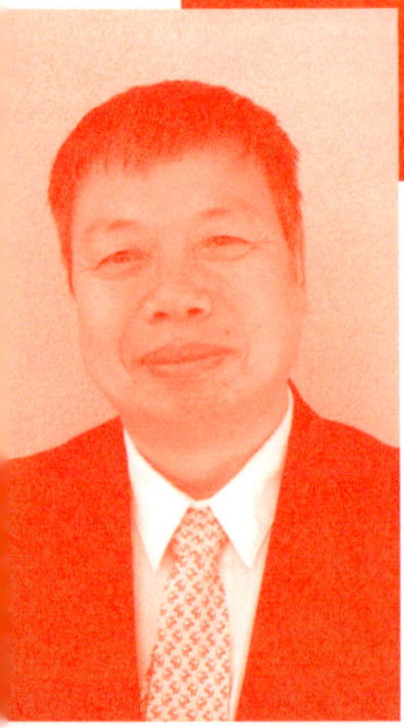
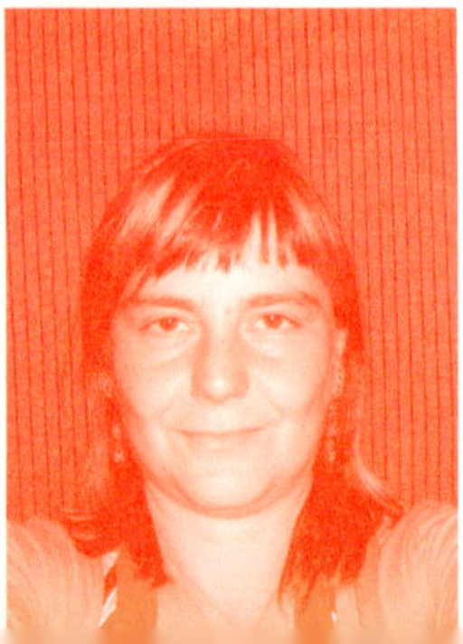

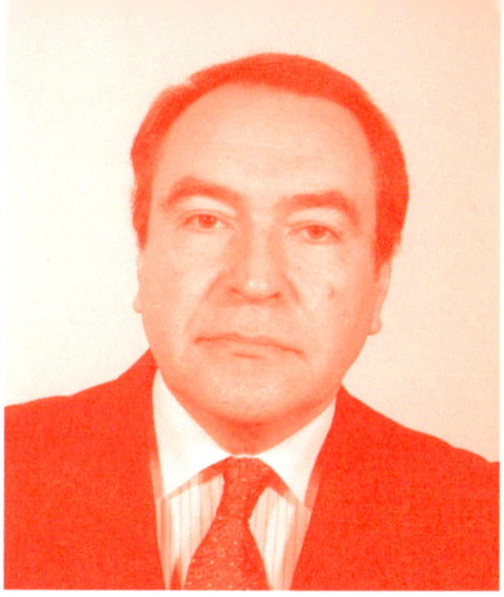

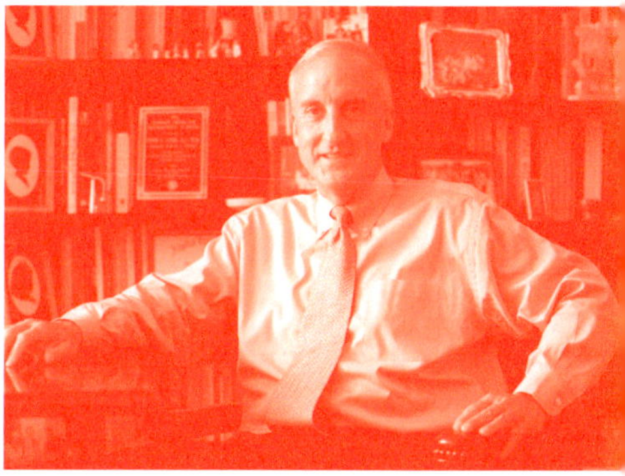

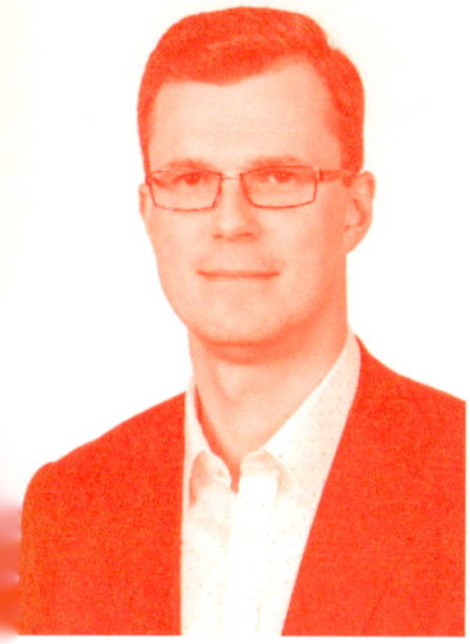

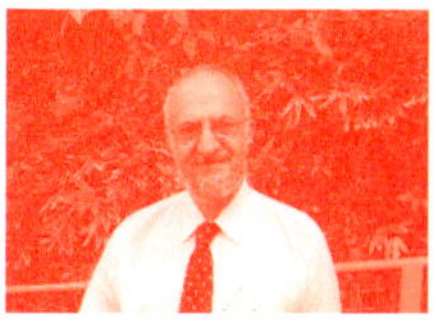

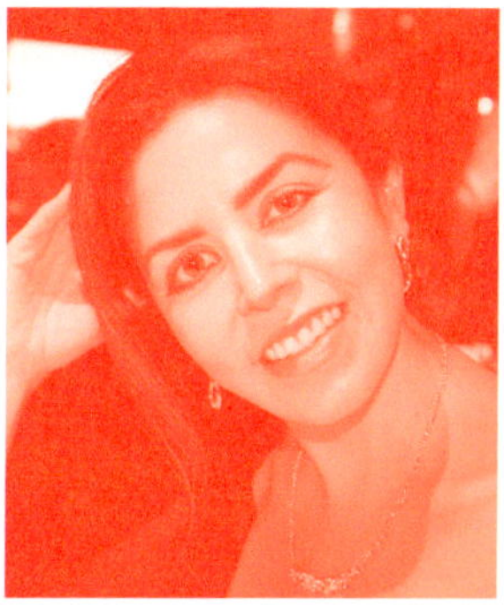

*Supporting open minds since 2005*

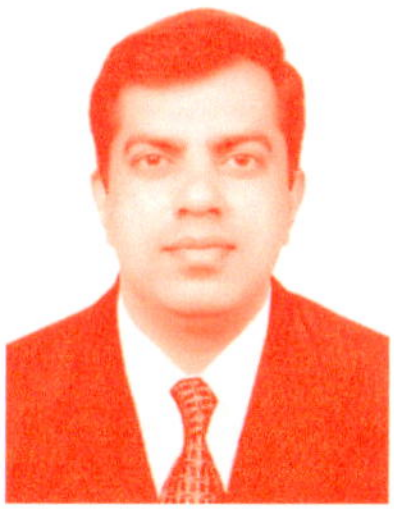

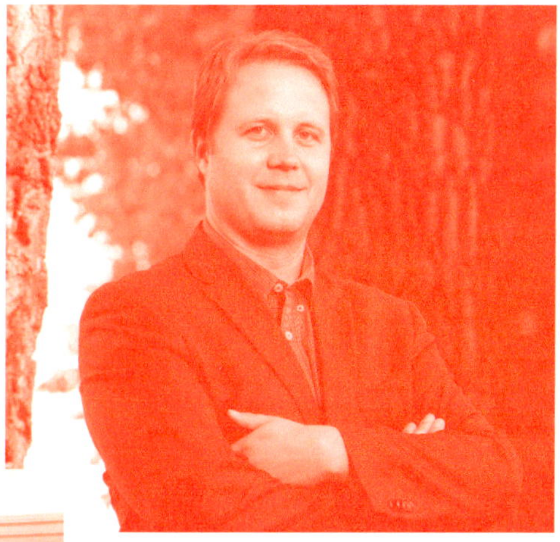

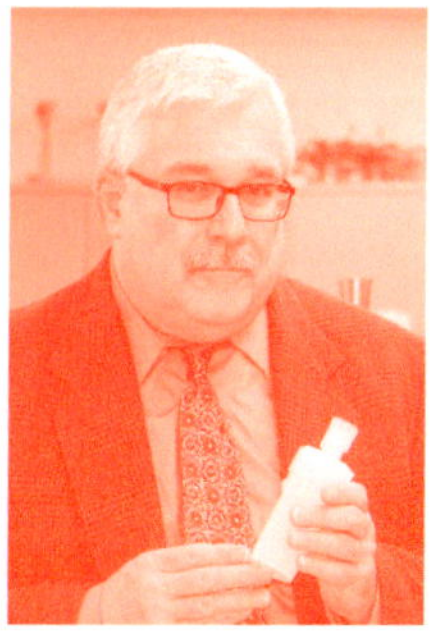

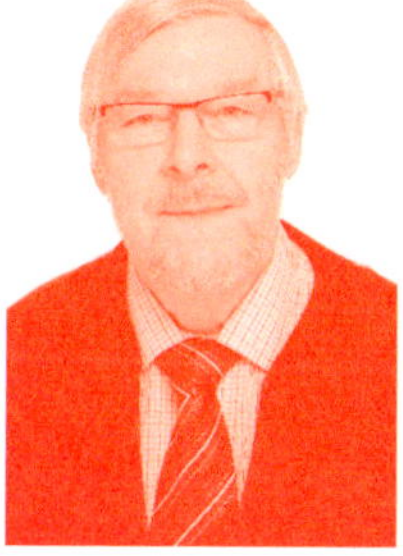

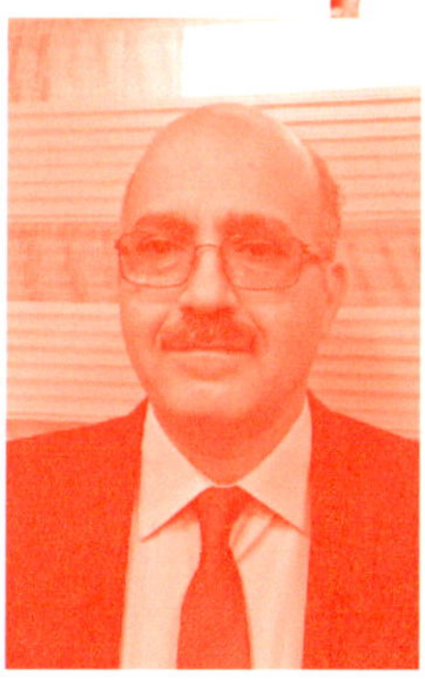

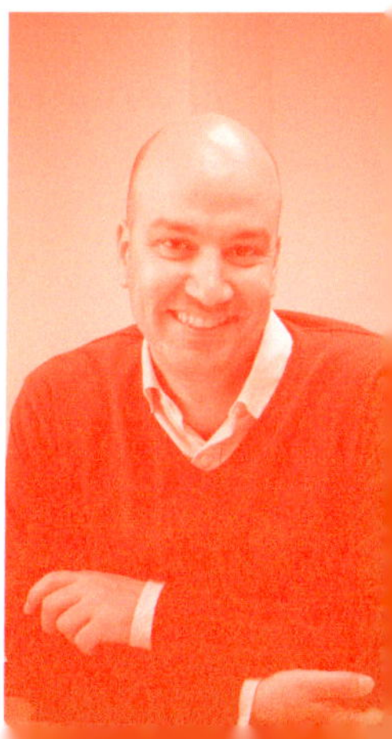

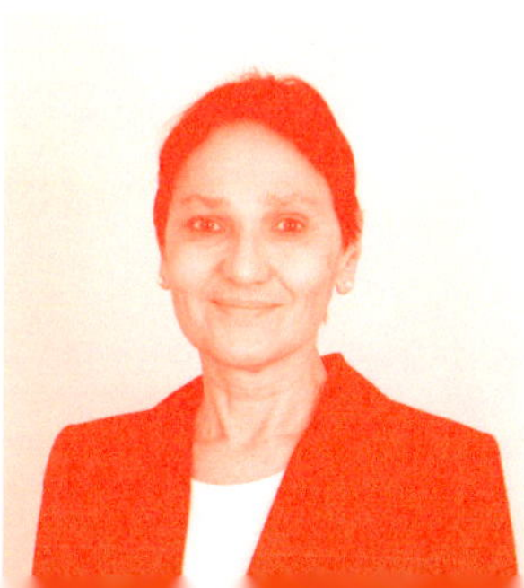

Plant Diseases-Current Threats and Management Trends
http://dx.doi.org/10.5772/intechopen.80762
Edited by Snježana Topolovec-Pintarić

Contributors
Aviv Dombrovsky, Elisheva Smith, Rajarshi Kumar Gaur, Avinash Marwal, Sahar Zayan, George Akumfi Ameyaw, Muqing Zhang, Muralidharan Govindaraju, Yisha Li, Jorge De Souza, Valter Cruz-Magalhaes, Jackeline Andrade, Yasmim Figueiredo, Phellippe Marbach, Srđan Aćimović, Danielle Martin, Richard Turcotte, Christopher Meredith, Isabel Munck, Juan Carlos Caicedo, Sonia Villamizar, Philip Donkersley, Farley William Souza Silva, Murilo Alves, Claudine Carvalho, Simon Elliot, Abdullah M. Al-Sadi, Xochitl Sofía Ramírez-Gómez, Vicente Beltran Campos, Sandra Neli Jimenez Garcia, María De Lourdes García Campos, Nobuya Tashiro, Mizuho Nita, Youichi Ide, Mayumi Noguchi, Hisayoshi Watanabe, Snježana Topolovec-Pintaric, Katarina Martinko



First published in London, United Kingdom, 2020 by IntechOpen
IntechOpen is the global imprint of INTECHOPEN LIMITED, registered in England and Wales, registration number: 11086078, 7th floor, 10 Lower Thames Street, London, EC3R 6AF, United Kingdom
Printed in Croatia

British Library Cataloguing-in-Publication Data
A catalogue record for this book is available from the British Library

Additional hard and PDF copies can be obtained from orders@intechopen.com

Plant Diseases-Current Threats and Management Trends
Edited by Snježana Topolovec-Pintarić
p. cm.
Print ISBN 978-1-78985-115-1
Online ISBN 978-1-78985-116-8
eBook (PDF) ISBN 978-1-78984-698-0

For EU product safety concerns:
IN TECH d.o.o., Prolaz Marije Krucifikse Kozulić 3, 51000 Rijeka, Croatia, info@intechopen.com or visit our website at intechopen.com.

# Meet the editor

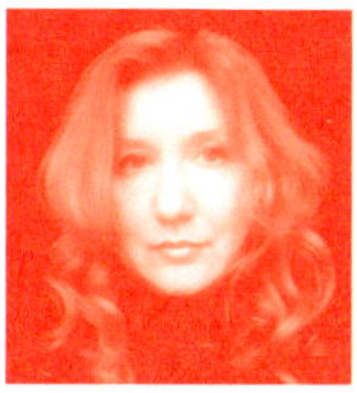

Snježana Topolovec-Pintarić is an associate professor at the University of Zagreb Faculty of Agriculture, Department of Plant Pathology. Her main research activities are in plant pathology, mycology, and plant protection. She has been involved in 7 projects with chemical industries on the evaluation of fungicidal efficacy and 2 US projects on biological control of weeds. Since 2005, she has investigated biological control of plant pathogenic fungi with indigenous *Trichoderma* species as well as *Trichoderma* effects on plant growth. She was involved in 2 projects on the investigation possibilities of *Trichoderma* encapsulation. For six years she was in the Organization Committee for the annual national Symposium of Plant Protection and was the secretary of the Croatian Plant Protection Society and on the Governing Board. She contributed as lecturer and organizer in 2 workshops on seed pathology. She is trained as an instructional designer for e-learning and online courses. She likes to use her artistic skills in educational purposes by creating videos and art exhibitions to educate people about phytopathogenic fungi.

# Contents

# Preface

The science of plant diseases (plant pathology or phytopathology) has become like a child of needfulness. Plant diseases have caused concern throughout history since the first crop plants were domesticated during the transition to agriculture between 2,000 to 12,000 years B.C. The first record of plant disease symptoms was found in Vedas (Rugveda, Athavaeda) as early as 1,200 B.C. Control of a disease was mentioned in "VRIKSHAYURVED" by Surapal in ancient India. Mention of plant disease has been made in Buddhist literature in 500 B.C. The Greek philosopher Aristotle wrote about plant diseases in 350 B.C. Theophrastus also wrote about cereal disease and even suggested some remedies to control them (in 300 B.C). In the Medieval Ages, the writings of the Arabian Ibn-al-Awam (10th Century, Seville, Spain) described symptoms and control measures for some plant diseases. There are references in the Old Testament of the Bible to blights, blasts, and mildews (6th century B.C.). Following the above-mentioned references, we can begin to understand that with domestication of crop species, their pathogens have also developed.

Since ancient times, plant pathogens, as the causal agents of plant diseases, have challenged farmers because agriculture was crucial in supporting growing human populations. The need for the study of plant pathogens gave rise to the development of new sciences, new technologies for plant breeding, and the agrochemical industry for pesticide development. Yet, all our actions and efforts to suppress or eradicate these diseases has constantly pressured these various organisms to evolve and adapt for survival. This ability is a natural phenomenon or evolution. For the pathogens in modern agro-ecosystems, the selection pressures are provided by human. Pathogens constantly find new ways to adapt to conditions that humans create and keep existing. Is it possible that with the cultivation of plants, we have also cultivated pathogens?

Plant diseases today are diseases of high standards because all agricultural techniques and pest management methods implemented in modern agricultural crop production to cherish the crop simultaneously provide ideal homogenous environments for their pathogens. In particular, large areas under monoculture production of genetically uniform plant population, fertilization, and irrigation creates an environment with fewer factors that could reduce populations or even extermination of pathogens. Moreover, the co-evolution of pathogens and their plant host may occur even faster in agricultural ecosystems (agro-ecosystems) than in natural ecosystems. Because of the implementation of agricultural techniques and pest management, the agricultural field is less prone to environmental fluctuations. Therefore, it is important to understand the evolutionary processes especially because speciation may occur more rapidly for plant pathogens than for other organisms. In the 21st century, the principles of evolutionary biology are implemented in phytopathology because of the understanding of the evolutionary processes that leading to the emergence of new pathogens. Understanding that the nature of the agro-ecosystems has played and continues to play a critical role in the emergence and spread of pathogens is essential to assessing the risks posed by potential future pathogens. When it is possible to predict the occurrence and spread of the pathogen, the control strategies can be developed.

New discoveries and insights into the plant-pathogen interaction and their coevolution are requiring revisions to existing knowledge about familiar plant pathogens. For instance, Common Barberry (*Berberis vulgaris*) is a major alternative host for the stem rust pathogen (*Puccinia graminis f. sp. tritici*) and was recently found in China to be an alternative host for the stripe rust pathogen (*P. striiformis f. sp. tritici*) although their associations have not been found in US Pacific Northwest. The new liberibacter species *Candidatus Liberibacter solanacearum* was first identified in 2008, simultaneously in the United States and New Zealand in tomato and pepper and then in potato, as well as several other solanaceous species. Recently, this species of liberibacter has also been documented in Northern Europe on carrot (*Daucus carota* L.) and the Mediterranean Region on celery (*Apium graveolens*). In August 2012, it was identified in France in two commercial carrot fields infested with its insect vector, the psyllid *Trioza apicalis*. Their introduction in the region is not clear and they are currently under eradication. Recently, downy mildew of Basil (*Ocimum basilicum*) has become one of the most destructive diseases of Sweet Basil, which is grown as a specialty crop in greenhouses. The problem is especially pronounced in eco-grown plants because of the limited fungicide use. Once infected, Basil plants are no longer marketable. Another, new downy mildew disease, caused by *Peronospora aquilegia*, has recently devastated and rapidly spread throughout numerous gardens and nurseries of the ornamental *Aquilegia* in the UK, but so far does not seem to have reached continental Europe.

This book is a response to the increasing interest in some plant pathogens that arise as new threats to modern plant production worldwide. The table of contents provides a descriptive feel about the topics which seize the attention and concern of phytopathologists today. The book is composed of three sections. The number of literature citations was not restricted and this constitutes a strength of the book.

Section I - *Host-pathogen coevolution* delivers an overview of new insights on existing pathogens that have begun to show a new face as a result of adapting to their host's existing production conditions. Here the readers can read about: i) the threat of rapid global spread of devastating downy mildew on Basil; ii) the difficulties of monitoring asymptomatic infections using PCR based methods especially of monitoring asymptomatic infections caused by the pathogen of Witches Broom disease of lime, and iii) leaf scald of sugarcane recently found in China and now becoming a serious threats to sugar industries.

Section II - *Novel approaches to plant disease* has the most chapters as much of the progress in plant pathology has been in the areas of how plants defend themselves against pathogens, how pathogens can be suppressed by other beneficial organisms, and the near future applicable methods exploiting discoveries in molecular genetics. Here the reader will read about: i) expanding prospects of nanotechnology in plant pathology; ii) the safe and effective alternative to control various phytopathogens by phytochemicals derived from secondary metabolism of medicinal plants, iii) two different approaches for biological control of *Xanthomonas citri* subsp. *citri* the possible bio-agent of *Pseudomonas* bacteria and inhibitors of quorum quenching; and iv) near-future management strategies in the production of major cultivated vegetable crops from *Solanaceae* and *Cucurbitaceae* family such as genome editing, engineering rootstocks for tobamovirus resistance, and implementation of cross- protection approach.

Section III - *Management of plant diseases* also gives insight into novelties in the area of fungicide-resistance and new application techniques. Here the reader will read about: i) new threats of resistance to stroubilurines of strobilurin-quinone resistant strains of *Colletotrichum gloeosporioides,* the causal agent of Japanese pear anthracnose; ii) current research efforts and strategies aimed at minimizing of cacao swollen shoot virus (CSSV) disease continuous spread and devastation on Ghana's cocoa production, new techniques for delivering the chemicals; and iii) possibilities to control *Venturia inaequalis* and *Erwinia amylovora* by trunk injection of fungicides used for *Diplodia corticola*.

This book is not only an interesting mix of all the topics discussed above but a compilation of the recent methods and knowledge about plant pathogens that are at the present time found to be of most concern. There is no doubt that the future will introduce some new plant pathogens and new concerns and problems will arise with them. Due to the simultaneous co-evolution of plants and their pathogens, all of our present-day knowledge will change in the future. In recent times, several plant pathogenic fungi have been reported as pathogenic to humans posing serious health challenges in both relatively healthy individuals as well as in those with serious underlying medical conditions. Since the 1980s at least 100 fungi not previously connected with disease in humans, have been identified as pathogenic. Some plant pathogenic fungi implicated in human diseases are *Mucor mucedo*, *Penicillium chrysogenum*, *Alternaria tenuis*, *Aspergillus flavus*, *Curvularia lunata*, *Fusarium culmorum*, *Botryodiplodia theobromae*, *Trichoderma hazianum* and *Bipolaris* sp. These fungi are melanized and melanin is considered as one of their major virulence factors. Plant-attacking mycoflora capable of causing human mycoses has stirred up public health concerns. This has imposed new challenges to scientists, among them phytopathologists, and they need to join forces to combat and find novel user-friendly antifungal compounds to maintain human health.

Phytopathology has experienced a major increase in attention and in an atmosphere of constant evolutionary change, we must ask: *Quo vadis* Phytopathology? If we draw a parallel with historical development, we can predict that phytopathology will retain the image of necessity and will extend into new science fields. Like Alice in Wonderland said, *"If we wish to go anywhere we must run twice as fast as that"* so we need to constantly broaden our knowledge.

I would like to express my appreciation to all the authors and co-authors that collaborated on this book. They are all recognized authorities in their field of expertise and this book is based on their research.

I am especially grateful to Mrs. Lucija Tomičić Dromgool, Commissioning Editor of IntechOpen who contacted me and encouraged me to become the editor of this book and for the kind empathy in my loss.

I would also like to thank Mr. Gordan Tot, Author Service Manager of IntechOpen for his assistance and kind understanding during the publication process.

Finally, completion of this undertaking could not have been possible without IntechOpen staff and their contribution is gratefully acknowledged.

**Snježana Topolovec-Pintaric**
Professor,
Faculty of Agriculture,
University of Zagreb,
Croatia

## Section 1

# Novel Approaches to Plant Disease

Chapter 1

# Downy Mildew of Basil: A New Destructive Disease Worldwide

*Snježana Topolovec-Pintarić and Katarina Martinko*

## Abstract

Oomycete pseudofungus (*Peronospora belbahrii*) is a causal of devastating basil downy mildew disease because once infected basil plants are no longer marketable. The host range is limited to basil and hyssop. Coleus was previously considered as host as well, but pathogen causing downy mildew on coleus has been shown genetically different and specified as *P. belbahrii sensu lato*. Therefore, *P. belbahrii* is described as a complex species, likely defined by plant host. The *P. belbahrii* is air-borne and seed-borne pathogen and it does not need a vector for dispersal. The disease was firstly reported from Africa where it is assumed to have originated on sweet basil and 70 years later it was reported from Europe. Currently, basil downy mildew is of pandemic occurrence and the pathogen is present in almost all areas around the world where basil is cultivated. Since the pathogen is transmitted by the seed, there is a high risk of the pathogen spread by the seed trade.

**Keywords:** *Agastache*, downy mildew, *Lamiaceae*, *Ocimum*, *Peronospora*

## 1. Introduction

Downy mildew caused by *Peronospora belbahrii* Thines is one of the most destructive diseases of sweet basil (*Ocimum basilicum*) of the family *Lamiaceae* Lindl. (alternatively *Labiaceae* Dulac) which except field farming is also grown as a specialty crop in greenhouses. Downy mildew of basil was first reported in 1932 from Uganda, Africa as *Peronospora* spp. and again in 1937 as *P. lamii* from where it is assumed to have originated on sweet basil [1, 2].

First report from Europe was in 2001 from Switzerland where it was observed in greenhouses [3]. After that, the disease was detected in Italy in 2003 on sweet basil in several greenhouses located in Liguria region (Northern Italy). In 2004, it was found in France on some basil crops near Saint Tropez (Southern France) [4]. In the same year, it was found in Belgium, but there are no data about the first detection.

After those first European reports, the pathogen was rapidly spread through Europe. In summer 2009, it was detected in United Kingdom in *Agastache* (hyssop) plants (*Agastache mexicana* and *Agastache* sp.) at Wisley gardens (Surrey) and on the summer of 2010 in protected basil plants in south-east England [5, 6]. In 2010, a significant incidence of downy mildew was reported in Hungary at two plant stands at Budapest-Soroksár and Tordasal though a similar disease had been observed in 2003 in a greenhouse at Albertirsa [7]. It was reported from Czech Republic in 2012 as well as from Cyprus [8]. In 2014, it was found again in United Kingdom but in several plants of coleus (*Solenostemon scutellarioides* cv. 'Chocolate Mint') but in 2016 has been shown that the pathogen causing coleus downy mildew is *P. belbahrii sensu lato* [9]. In 2016, it has been reported from Spain on basil collected from the island of Tenerife (Islas Canarias) and afterwards was also noted that has been causing severe symptoms and economic losses in Almería, Andalucía [10].

In the United States, downy mildew of basil is considered as relatively new disease but the pathogen has been detected in October 2007 in South Florida [11]. Since its first detection in the United States, it has been observed on basil in at least 42 states [11, 12]. Interesting is founding in 2008 on basil plants produced in various nurseries in Sebastopol, Sonoma County because trace-back investigation revealed that the seeds had originated from Italy. This disease was also reported in Argentina in February 2008 [13] and Canada in 2011 [14]. In 2011, it was reported in Hawaii for the first time and in Mexico in 2015 [15].

First report in Asia was in Iran, where a severe outbreak of downy mildew was observed in sweet basil fields in 2006 [16]. A year later, in April 2007, it has been found in Japan on coleus plants cultivated in a greenhouse in Chiba Prefecture (Honshu) [17]. In the spring of 2009, it has been found in Taiwan in the field of Nantu and Yunlin [18]. In Israel, it was firstly found in December 2011 near Bet She'an, and in 2012 the disease has been spread throughout the country to all basil-growing areas [19]. Recently, it has been found in China in July 2014 on basil on the island of Hainan in Sanya City and in 2016 in the Shunyi and Daxing districts of Beijing which is concerned as first report in mainland China [20, 21]. Last Asian report is from Korea, where it has been first observed in November 2015 on sweet basil plants growing in plastic greenhouses in Gwangmyeong [22].

Until 2017, the disease was considered exotic to Australia, when it has been reported from South-east Queensland. Within 6 months, the disease was present along the eastern seaboard from north Queensland to Victoria, South Australia and the Northern Territory. In the scientific literature, Australia has been listed as a host country as early as 2015; however, no records of detections could be traced [23].

Finally, the first report of *P. belbahrii sensu lato* detection on coleus (*Plectranthus* spp.) in Brazil was reported in 2019 [24].

The first official report for Croatia was done in 2015 by Croatian Agency for Agriculture and Food based on symptoms and morphological characteristic not confirmed by molecular diagnostic [25]. In October 2015, as part of regular reporting reviews conducted by the Advisory Service, infected plants were found in greenhouses in the Varaždin County. The disease was spread soon after that founding on areas of four more counties (Krapina-Zagorje, Međimurje, Split-Dalmatian and Zagreb). Interestingly, in Dubrovnik-Neretva County, the disease was found on pot-plants imported from Italy. Up to date in Croatia, downy mildew is recorded only in production of basil in greenhouses. This chapter authors are currently investigating the occurrence on basil in the greenhouse 'Green friends' of eco-grower of culinary herbs and spices, situated in Rakovica in the Zagreb County. We confirmed determination of the *P. belbahrii* by molecular diagnostic (PCR sequence comparison of the ITS rDNA sequences and Cox2 region) (unpublished).

## 2. Disease symptoms

The first symptoms can be spotted on lower leaves, where infection starts and progresses upwards. The most noticeable symptom is yellowing (slightly chlorotic) of the leaves with the veins remaining green. The initial yellowing can be misinterpreted as a nutritional deficiency and so disease can go unrecognised. With time on upper surface of leaves, large chlorotic lesions with soft margins are developing. Chlorosis often involved the entire leaf surface. Since the pathogen is a biotroph, it causes dying of cells from which it absorbed nutrients and therefore necrotisation

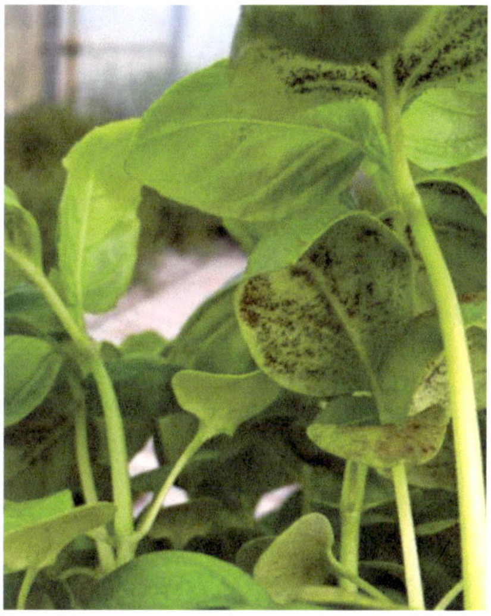

**Figure 1.**
*Brown growth of* Peronospora belbahrii *on abaxial side of basil leaf.*

occur after chlorosis and the central portion of a chlorotic lesion become necrotic. This can lead to slight curvature of leaves. Necrotic spots are variable in size and of irregular shape as they are limited by the main veins. In some cases, entire area of the leaf surface is affected. In humid conditions, necrotic regions can become dark brown to black in colour. On abaxial leaf surfaces, both in chlorotic and necrotic regions, a typical greyish to brown, furry or downy moulds could be observed giving the leaves a dirty appearance (**Figure 1**). Parasitisation results in shrinkage of leaf and premature leaf fall.

Disease can go asymptomatic under cool and dry conditions [26] and sometimes plants not showing symptoms at harvest can develop symptoms during transport [27]. In report from Taiwan, it was noted that the pathogen caused chlorosis and leaf shrinkage on basil in the field, but did not cause any symptom on coleus, Pai-tsai Chinese cabbage (*Brassica rapa*), leaf lettuce (*Lactuca sativa*) and melon (*Cucumis melo*) [18].

## 3. Hosts range

Sweet basil is the natural host of *P. belbahrii* and the majority of *P. belbahrii* findings have been on sweet basil. In 2009, Thines et al. concluded that coleus is also the natural host of this pathogen [28]. They also investigated the downy mildew of sage, but were unable to confirm that it is caused by *P. belbahrii* so did not considered sage as natural host. Coleus has been confirmed as host of *P. belbahrii* in Japan, United States, United Kingdom and Germany [29]. Species concept has been refined recently and pathogen causal of coleus downy mildew was specified as *P. belbahrii sensu lato* [9]. Moreover, an unidentified species of *Peronospora* sp. infects coleus in Israel [30]. Interestingly, Israeli isolates of *P. belbahrii* from sweet basil do not infect coleus although infects other *Lamiaceae* species: rosemary (*Rosmarinus officinalis*) Nepeta (*Nepeta curviflora*), Clinopodium (*Micromeria fruticosa*) and two species of sage (*Salvia pinnata* and *S. fruticosa*) [30]. Further, the conidia from mentioned species failed to infect sweet basil and therefore the role of these species in the epidemiology of basil downy mildew in Israel is unknown [30]. The *Peronospora* sp. on coleus was reported in 2005 Louisiana, New York and Florida in U.S. [31, 32]. In 2015, *Peronospora* sp. on coleus was reported in Tennessee, and the morphological and molecular characteristics were consistent with Thines description of P. *belbahrii sensu lato* [9, 28]. So, Rivera et al. concluded that *P. belbahrii* can be described as complex of species likely defined by plant host [9]. Recently, coleus downy mildew causal pathogen is confirmed as *P. belbahrii sensu lato* host based on pathogenicity test in Brazil, and this is the first such report for the South America [24].

In 2009, the *Agastache* species (*Lamiaceae*) was also named as the new *P. belbahrii* host by Henricot et al. [6]. The host range is today broadened and as alternative hosts are considered culinary and ornamental varieties related to basil and coleus from *Lamiaceae* family and here are mint (*Mentha* spp.) and sage (*Salvia* spp.). All cultivars of sweet basil are hosts and as highly susceptible ones are cv. Genovese Nufar, Italian Large Leaf, Queenette, Superbo, Poppy Joe's and Milita [27]. Some of the exotic, spice and ornamental basils cultivars such as red types (*O. basilicum purpurescens* cv. Red Rubin, Red leaf), lemon basil (*O. citridiorum* cv. Lemon std., Mrs. Burn's Lemon, Lemona & Lime) and lime basil (*O. americanum* cv. Blue Spice, Spice & Blue Spice F1) have been found less susceptible or even resistant to downy mildew [9, 28, 33]. This chapter's authors detected downy mildew on spice cultivars of basil, and *P. belbahrii* was confirmed as causal pathogen by molecular analysis (unpublished).

## 4. Description of pathogen

The causal pathogen of basil's downy mildew is pseudofungus *Peronospora belbahrii* Thines and has been formally introduced under name *P. belbahrii* by Thines et al. in 2009 as dedication to Lassaard Belbahrii who first suggested that the pathogen on basil might be a distinct undescribed species and distinguished it from a different closely related species that parasitizes sage (*Salvia officinalis*) [28]. It is assumed that *P. belbahrii* is of African origin, as its host basil is native to this continent [28]. As oomycete it is classified in *Chromysta*, *Oomycota*, *Oomycetes*, *Peronosporales* and *Peronosporaceae*. The pathogen was molecularly determined in 2005 by Belbahri et al. [3] and showed through ITS sequencing that it is a newly occurring species on basil that differs from *P. lamii*, the only previously reported downy mildew on sweet basil and also differs from *Peronospora* species that is affecting lamiaceous hosts worldwide [1, 2]. Perhaps, previous findings of *Peronospora* sp. on sweet basil and coleus may be *P. belbahrii* but have been misidentified as *P. lamii* before sequence identification was carried out and before it was first described as a new species *P. belbahrii*. Confusion between species is likely to occur without sequence data; therefore, samples must be submitted to a competent testing laboratory for identification. Using morphological comparison and molecular phylogenetic reconstructions, Thines et al. also confirmed that *P. belbahrii* is not identical to *P. swingleii* on *Salvia reflexa* [28]. *P. belbahrii* on basil and coleus seems to be closely related yet; it has been shown that they are morphologically and genetically different [28]. Limited potential to infect basil has been reported for the isolates from coleus, as it was described earlier [30]. The significance of differences between causal pathogen of downy mildew on basil and coleus needs to be investigated further; but for now, the pathogen on coleus is determined as *P. belbahrii sensu lato.*

The growths on the underside of the symptomatic leaves in a form of a brown downy mould are asexual organs, sporangia bearing sporangiophores which emerge from leaf stomata. Microscopic observations will show that they are consistent with the characteristics of a genus *Peronospora*. The first descriptions of sporangia and sporangiophores on basil and coleus that were confirmed by molecular determination were provided by Thines et al. in 2009 [28]. The sporangia of genus *Peronospora* are spore-like structures and they act as conidia and germinate into a germ-tube when they are near a leaf stoma. Therefore, the use of synonym conidia, or simply spore, has become commonplace for sporangia.

Conidia are dark brown to olive in colour and pedicel is absent. They are rounded and egg-shaped with a length 24–29–30.8–33–36 μm on basil and 26–29–31.3–33–37 μm on coleus. They width are 20–23–24–26–29 μm on basil and 20–23–24.5–26–29 μm on coleus. Ratio of length and width is 1.1–1.2–1.29–1.4–1.5 on basil and 1.1–1.2–1.28–1.4–1.5 on coleus [28].

Sporangiophores are colourless (hyaline) with a long, straight trunk and monopodially with a length 270–300–400–520–680 μm on basil and 330–380–466–570–650 μm on coleus [28]. Numbers of ramifications were 3–4–4.9–5–7 per sporophore on basil and 4–5–5.2–6–7 μm on coleus. Ultimate branchlets were in pairs, curved, longer one in length 13–18–20.6–26–31 μm on basil and 12–13–18–22–31 μm on coleus while the shorter one in length 3.8–7.7–9.80–10–15 μm on basil and 5.1–7.7–10.7–13–17 μm on coleus. Ratio of longer to shorter branches is 1.3–1.8–2.25–2.7–4 on basil and 1.1–1.6–1.71–1.9–2.5 on coleus. Ultimate branches end dichotomically and tips (sterigmata) are acute to subacute on both, basil and coleus. Tips are bearing single sporangia.

The shortest sporangiophores were reported in Iran and were 130–290 μm (avg. 194 μm) long and branched two to five times [16]. The longest sporangiophores were recorded in Hungary, and they were in length of 416–784 μm (avg. 572 μm) and monopodially branched five to seven times [7].

There are two oospore detections published up to date, both from Israel, found in leaves of susceptible sweet basil cultivar 'Peri'. In 2013, Cohen et al. identified and described oospores as thick-walled, brown in colour, measuring of 46.2 ± 2.8 μm in diameter [34]. Oospores never occurred on the infected leaf surface, but inside the mesophyll [30]. In 2016, in walk-in tunnel experiments that simulated commercial production conditions, oospores were observed attached to the leaf surface, to older parts of the infection area, and also found to water washes of the leaf surface by Elad et al. [35]. Discovery of oospores suggests the potential for sexual reproduction, but little is known on *P. belbahrii* oospore formation or is it homothallic or heterothallic. Currently, only one mating type has been found [22], although it is already presumed that it is heterothallic [26, 36, 37]. The pathogenicity of oospores is investigated, but without positive infections [30, 38], and their role in the basil downy mildew epidemiology is not known.

## 5. Disease cycle and dispersal

The *P. belbahrii* thrives in warm, humid conditions and produce conidia that can infect in temperatures as low as 15°C (59°F) [26]. For example, downy mildew is present in Israeli basil-cropping regions where in the cooler season temperatures may reach minimum of 5–10°C at night and a maximum of 10–25°C during the day [35]. This corroborates with our observations. Pathogen can tolerate cold weather (10–15°C) but, like its host basil, cannot survive freezing winter temperatures at continental climate. Conidia cannot survive harsh winters and as pathogen is biotroph it needs living host. Therefore, in climates with harsh winters and with just one mating type of the *P. belbahrii* it can survive only on living plants in greenhouse production operations that produce basil year round. In mild winters and in warm, temperate regions where the host, basil will not freeze, the second overwintering inoculum are mycelium and conidia in infected plant buds, plant stems, leaf tissue and shoots. Congruently, the most devastating damage is often seen in warm and humid conditions, late summer and in greenhouses.

Most of *Peronospora* species can reside in soil as soil-borne oospores that are formed in leaf tissue and may overwinter in leaf litter or may be released into the soil as leaves decay and considered as soil-borne inoculum. Any movement of soil particles with soil-borne oospores inoculum can spread it from infected plants to non-infected ones. Although *Peronospora* species are biotrophs, they can survive without host as oil-borne oospores because they are in dormancy and can be viable for few years depending on species. Until now, there are no reports about *P. belbahrii* soil-borne oospores even in cases when oospores were detected inside the mesophyll of the leaves [30, 35]. Large-scale experiments were conducted to elucidate the pathogenicity of oospores to basil plants. Soil was infested with oospores (10 oospores/5 g of soil/well) and three to four basil seeds were planted in each well. Plants were grown until the four-leaf stage, but none of the 2000 plants that developed showed symptoms of downy mildew or sporulation of *P. belbahrii* [30]. Also, the experiments conducted in the Israeli walk-in tunnels lead to a conclusion that oospores are minimally affected by high temperature, and therefore the high temperature presumably did not affect pathogen survival [35].

The life cycle of *P. belbahrii* is initiated as abundantly produced air-borne conidia which can readily be spread by moist wind [37]. The conidia can be carried by rain drops, by wind, and can be splashed by rain to wet leaves near the ground. It does not need a vector for dispersal. Survivability of conidia, contrary to oospores, are strongly affected by temperature and duration of exposure so, a longer exposure period and higher temperature weakened the infection capacity of the conidia. Wetted-dried conidia lost their activity after 55 h at 25°C, 20 h at 30°C and 9 h at 40°C [30]. Therefore, conidia are short lived and viable just for few days so, they will endanger only susceptible host within the conidia dispersal area. McGrath conducted an experiment with field-grown basil at the Long Island Horticultural Research and Extension Center (LIHREC) in Riverhead, NY and considered the primary source of initial inoculum in this area to be long-distance wind dispersed conidia from affected plants [39] although the distance is not specified. The possibility to use frozen conidia as inoculum was also tested and those collected from infected leaves frozen for 3 months at −20°C or 2 years at −80°C retain high germination capability [30]. In other trial, frozen conidia germinated at 25% in contrast to nearly 90% germination rate of freshly harvested conidia [40]. Their germination was favoured between 5 and 15°C on water agar *in vitro*. Inoculation of basil plants with frozen or fresh conidia ($3 \times 10^4$ $mL^{-1}$) resulted in high disease severity 14 days post inoculation [40].

Sporulation occurs in moisture saturated atmosphere at an appropriate temperature and often during the night, in the dark and in chlorotic lesions 5–15 days old [41]. In controlled greenhouse experiments, sporulation occurs 6–7 days post inoculations [37]. The sporulation starts when pathogen biomass in the leaf mesophyll reached a certain threshold and complete within 8–12 h from onset of darkness in optimal conditions (saturated atmosphere at 18°C). During the first 6 h, hyaline sporophores are formed and as they emerge from stomata gradually become dichotomously. In the subsequent 5 h, dark spores are produced on the tips of the sporophore branchlets (sterigmata) [41]. The light strongly inhibits spore formation, but not sporophore development and emergence through leaf stomata. Yet, sporophores formed under the light are abnormal and unable to form spores. Cohen et al. in 2013 discovered that lightning during the second half of the night inhibits spore formation, and narrow band led illumination showed that red light ($\lambda$max 625 nm) was most inhibitory to spore formation comparing to blue light ($\lambda$max 440 nm) while in other oomycetes is quite the opposite [41]. They speculate that probably *P. belbahrii* has a different photoreceptor sensitive to red light. The sporulation is greater when the portion of carbohydrates in the leaf is higher [41].

The carbohydrates accumulating during the day are hydrolysed to hexoses during the first half of the night which pathogen uses for formation of conidia during the rest of the night [41]. Therefore, the greater the accumulation of carbohydrates in infected leaves during the daytime contributes to the greater sporulation in the following dark, wet period of the night. This all suggests that the sporulation terminates with necrosis of leaf which obstructs assimilation as plant cells die because of pathogen absorbed all nutrients from it.

Conidia germinate in 3–5 days into one or two germ tubes and infect plant tissues via a germ-tube which penetrates through leaf stomata [28, 36] and it takes 3 h [35]. Germ tubes rarely form an appressoria-like structures prior infection. Developing hypha grows into intercellular spaces within the leaf mesophyll, proliferate and eventually invaginate the host cell plant cells through special globuse structures called haustoria (a hallmark oomycete structure) for nutrient acquisition [37]. Further branching and spreading of this initial hypha lead to forming of a cushion of intercellular mycelia just below the stomata. From this cushion, sporangiophores arise and emerge through stomata on sterigmata bearing sporangia. Conidia are produced simultaneously and are carried by wind and rain to new infection sites of the same or different plant. Leaf wetness of at least 6 h is required for conidial infection [42, 43]. Under favourable conditions, sporulation progresses in the polycyclic disease cycle leading to an epidemic of downy mildew disease.

*P. belbahrii* is also a seed-borne pathogen. Detection of *P. belbahrii* in several commercially produced basil seed batches confirmed that the pathogen is seed-borne [3, 28, 44]. It is considered that infected seed act as primary inoculum source in basil production, and is so far considered to be the most important way of this pathogen spreading as it can explain the rapid global spread of *P. belbahrii*. Great example for the spreading of *P. belbahrii* with seed transport and seed-marketing to long distances is that the biotype that was detected for the first time in US in 2007 was genetically identical to the one reported in Switzerland in 2001 [27]. Also, the disease occurrence in US Sonoma County in 2008 was connected with the origin of the used seed that was introduced from Italy. Investigation conducted by Farahani-Kofoet and Römer detected *P. belbahrii* on 80–90% of randomly selected commercial seed stocks [45] and assumed that *P. belbahrii* can be spread by transport and marketing of seed stocks.

On contaminated seeds, *P. belbahrii* has been found in form of conidia and oospore [38, 45]. Until now, *P. belbahrii* was not reported inside the basil seed or embryo. Based on their observations, Farahani-Kofoet and Römer concluded that *P. belbahrii* is able to survive for several years on seeds [45]. Generally, oospores of *Peronospora* species can also be formed on seeds and infect the emerging seedling. Their oospores germinate in a way similar to that described for conidia and the infection process is similar. Investigation of *P. belbahrii* oospore infection of basil seeds was conducted, but plants developed from seeds planted in soil infested with oospores were symptomless and sporulation characteristic for *P. belbahrii* did not occur [30].

It has not yet been clarified whether the pathogen infects the seed deeply and systematically or is just a contaminant. In some European investigations, systemic infections in seeds and in different plant parts (leaves, stems) even in a symptomless plant have been detected [44, 45]. Novel investigation of seed transmission conducted in Israel showed that *P. belbahrii* is seed-borne but not seed-transmitted, as seeds produced by infected plants in the field can be externally contaminated with conidia that were embedded in the surface, but not entirely [46]. Further, plants grown in growth chambers until 5–6 leaf stage from contaminated seeds did not show any symptom of downy mildew and did not carry latent infection. Also, systemic infections were rarely seen in the field. They confirmed systemic spread of mycelium in the basil plants which corroborated with previous finding [45]. Systemically infected plants remained stunt and produced no seeds. Therefore, the Israeli investigators postulated that seed infections and seed transmission may occur in Europe, as it was reported [44, 45], and other locations with wetter summers, especially under prolonged wetness periods at the flowering and seed production.

Both investigations, European and Israeli, confirmed that contaminated seeds can be harvested from symptomless, latently infected plants and also, that contaminated seeds can give symptomless, latently infected plants [44–46].

*Peronospora belbahrii* can also be spread through vegetative materials like contaminated plant cuttings, transplants and fresh leaves. Novel Israeli investigation showed that *P. belbahrii* is spread systematically in basil plants [46]. Mycelium has been found to grow acropetally to the stem apex and basipetally to the cotyledons and hypocotyl and laterally to the axillar buds but, mycelium has never reached the roots. Especially in young basil plants, this pathogen systemically runs through tissue and causes plant stunt and fail to produce seeds.

## 6. Management of basil downy mildew

The control methods of the downy mildew pathogen today involve fungicides, seed treatment and breeding for resistance. In the greenhouses, they can be augmented with physical measures: nocturnal illumination, ventilation and daytime solar heating. The last one is also suitable for net-houses [47].

Current control measures rely mainly on fungicide application. In conventionally produced basil, it can be controlled in a preventive program with conventional foliar fungicides. The efficient once are based on mefenoxam, azoxystrobin, cyazofamid, mandipropamid, fluopicolide and fenamidone [11, 12, 26, 34, 38]. There are also phosphorous acid fungicides which are in most cases labelled and allowed in greenhouses. The best control of 98% was achieved with preventive fungicide application, before symptoms occurred, on a weekly schedule [38].

The *P. belbahrii* developed mefenoxam-resistance within 1 year of use in Israel and was reported in 2013 [34]. It was also detected in Italy were mefenoxam (metalaxyl-M) plus copper has been the most widely used and effective product against *P. belbahrii*, since its registration on basil in Italy in 2004 [48]. As the systemic fungicides are prone to the resistance development, ingredients with different modes of action are needed [32]. The novel fungicides with extremely high efficacy against oomycete including *P. belbahrii* are oxathiapiprolin [30] and valifenalate [49]. Oxathiapiprolin acts at multiple stages of the pathogen's asexual life cycle at extremely low concentrations and due to translaminar and acropetally systemic movement, it protects treated leaves and new leaves as they emerge and grow. In *P. belbahrii*, it inhibits sporangia germination and curatively, it stops mycelial growth within the host plant before visible lesions occur and inhibits further lesion expansion, offering protection at 1 and 2 days post-infection [50]. It was found to be effective against mefenoxam-resistant biotypes as well [30]. But, as it is a single-site inhibitor and its target is the oxysterol binding protein, the resistance to oxathiapiprolin assume to be medium to high and resistance management is required [51]. The soil application of mixture of oxathiapiprolin and benthiavalicarb or their single application against *P. belbahrii* was tested. Application to the root of 1 mg active ingredient per plant in the field experiment provided durable protection of up to 4 weeks against *P. belbahrii* [52]. The mixture performed better than single applications of those two compounds suggesting a synergistic interaction between them. The valifenalate is also a single-site inhibitor and acts as the inhibitor of cellulose synthesis in the Oomycete plant pathogens [49]. The resistance to valifenalate is assumed to be low to medium risk [51].

In organic farming, conventional fungicides are not allowed, so neem oil, potassium bicarbonate and hydrogen dioxide can be used for protection only, but they do not give satisfied protection [38]. Organic fungicides are contacts and do not go into plant tissue where is the pathogen and they are not able to translocate to abaxial side of leaves where sporulation occur. Therefore, their performance is not commercially acceptable and as they provide limited to no control, including when applied twice weekly on a preventive schedule to a moderately resistant variety [12, 38, 39]. As alternative, there are some bio-products based on *Bacillus amyloliquefaciens*, *Streptomyces lydicus* and the extract of *Reynoutria sachalinensis* [38]. Organic production should be in protected conditions and better transplanting then seeding as pathogen-free seed is not available. In greenhouse, it is important to prevent favourable conditions for disease development.

Certain cultural practices which create less optimal conditions for the pathogen can be helpful in reducing the amount of infection. Such practices include providing good soil drainage and good air circulation among plants. Increasing plant spacing in the field or greenhouse prevents the creation of high-humidity conditions on plant surfaces and can inhibit infection as *P. belbahrii* requires humidity for sporulation as well as free leaf moisture for infection. The humidity should be keeping below 85% and this is crucial. In the greenhouse, the use of plastic mulch and drip irrigation is recommended instead of bare ground and overhead irrigation. Effective measure for reducing ambient relative humidity and avoids vapour deposition of leaves surface is ventilation [47]. In some experiments, combining daytime solar heating with nocturnal illumination without fungicide applications showed to be an effective control in organic farming [30, 47]. High temperature is detrimental to the *P. belbahrii* and exposure of infected plant of 35–45°C for 6–9 h suppressed survival of conidia and mycelia [47]. Subsequently, solar heating has been used to cure plants. In Israel, solar energy was captured by closing greenhouse windows or covering the house with a transparent IR polyethylene sheet during sunny hours of the days: best is to use three consecutive daily exposures of 3–4 h starting at 8 am [47]. Solar heating should be conducted cautiously to avoid plant heat damage [47]. Ensuring light during the night, especially red light should prevent sporulation. The protective effect of nocturnal illumination was determined in laboratory and greenhouse trials; but in Israel, field trials (net-houses) also demonstrated that light can be successfully used to supress downy mildew in field-grown basil [41]. The inhibitory effect of incandescent or CW fluorescent light of 3.5 or 6 μmoles.$m^2$.$s^{-1}$ on sporulation was 100% on lower leaf surface even when only the upper leaf surface was exposed to light [41].

The rapid global spread of the downy mildew may be related to transmission of *P. belbahrii* by infected seeds and/or trade of basil cuttings and plants with latent infection [3, 38, 45, 46]. Infested seeds are a great risk for spreading the pathogen by transport and seed-marketing to long distances. Implementation of seed-certification schemes to exclude seed batches infested with *P. belbahrii* from marketing would be of great value for both seed-producing companies and growers [45]. Therefore, improving seed production; developing and implementing seed testing, certification protocols, and standards for the basil seed industry and strict following of import restriction may have halted *P. belbahrii* [38, 45]. To limit the spread of the pathogen by seed shipments, it is crucial for breeders and growers to draw on an early, fast and specific detecting test [45].

Seed should be tested on the presence of *P. belbahrii* and for that purpose real-time PCR have been designed [3]. Belbahri et al. have designed a specific primer pair (Bas-F/Bas-R) based on sequences within the unique genomic ribosomal DNA

(ITS1) and the primer pair generates a single fragment of approximately 134 base pairs [3]. The PCR method proved to be very sensitive for direct detection of *P. belbahrii* on seeds and plant samples [45]. The PCR detection limit of *P. belbahrii* in artificially infested seeds corresponded to the DNA amount of a single spore per seed (3.4 pg of *P. belbahrii* genomic DNA extracted from a pure spore suspension at a density of 103 spores $ml^{-1}$ using 1 μl as a template) [45]. Further, with this PCR protocol, *P. belbahrii* can be detected with high sensitivity in leaves and stems as well and not only at seeds, even if symptoms are not evident. Finding that latent systemic infection can result in the contamination of basil seed and vice versa supported the necessity to implement PCR-based detection in a seed-certification scheme [45]. Pathogen-free seed is most important for greenhouse crops plantings not expected to be exposed to wind dispersed spores [53]. It should be emphasised that the presence of pathogen DNA in seeds does not implicate spontaneous disease outbreaks because the PCR test cannot assess the viability of spores as specific fragments can also be generated from DNA material of dead spores. Moreover, the disease inception and development depends on host-pathogen interaction and existing environmental conditions. Yet, PCR test allows the testing of high numbers of samples within a short time and rapidly gives accurate information on *P. belbahrii* presence. Considering all, it is recommendable to be admitted in seed-certification schemes for routine testing of seed materials in order to inhibit marketing of infested seeds. As the PCR test can be used for detection in different plant parts, it can also be used for evaluation of procedures to control the downy mildew pathogen.

Seed treatments and at-seedling fungicides may have the potential for the good start of basil production [38]. There are no fungicides labelled for use on seed, but the at-seedling fungicides are available although not labelled for use on basil seed. Mefenoxam can be applied at seedling into the soil in field growing basil [38]. In novel trails, the root treatment of mixture of oxathiapiprolin and benthiavalicarb given to the young seedlings, growing in the multi-cell trays in the nursery, may be effective basil downy mildew measure [52]. The only organic fungicide labelled for ground application is based on the extract of *Reynoutria sachalinensis* [38].

Novel, non-chemical basil seed treatment is steam-air treatment and USA seed companies start to implement it [53]. Steam-air treatment of basil seeds against seed-borne fungi was tested in 1997 in Australia [54]. Steam-air treatment at 54–58°C for 30 min was successful in two-cylinder configuration in the steam-air machine. They noticed that this configuration against sixth-cylinders configuration provides extra steam velocity that prevents basil seed clumping which happened because when wet basil seed easily stick together as they have very thick gelatinous coat. Therefore, basil seeds are not amenable to hot-water treatment as the seed clumping makes the seed challenging to handle [53, 54].

The cultivation of resistant sweet basil cultivars also can be efficient control strategy. Highly resistant cultivars will be especially welcome in organic farming. Earlier, some cultivars of red types, lemon and lime basil have been found less susceptible [9, 30, 31, 33, 39]. New resistant basil varieties started to be marketed in USA in 2018 [53]. The first commercially available resistant variety is Eleonora. The Rutgers University basil breeding program released Devotion, Obsession, Passion, and Thunderstruck. They are marketed by VDF Specialty Seeds. Organically produced seed is available and marketed like Prosperais (Johnny's Selected Seeds), Emma and Everleaf (aka Basil Pesto Party and M4828Z) [53].

That accurate monitoring can be of great importance in field growing as well as in protected conditions as instrumentation for optimization of plant protection measures was shown by USA monitoring programme. It started in 2009 by McGrath and augmented knowledge of basil downy mildew [38]. It is an online spreadsheet program set-up in Google Docs accessible by anyone. Until 2019, each year a spreadsheet page was set up for anyone to log and view occurrence reports [53]. In 2019, a new website was launched with a mapping program that mapped reports by county plus information about basil downy mildew. The growers need to be educated to accurately based on first symptoms recognise the diseases on time. In greenhouses, monitoring should be on daily basis as downy mildew can develop very quickly [38, 41].

## 7. Conclusion

'*One touch of nature makes the whole world kin*' Shakespeare wrote and this is so valid for the pandemic downy mildew agent like *P. belbahrii* from sweet basil. The only way to deal with this pathogen is knowledge. To fill the existing knowledge gaps research into various aspects of the pathogen will be needed. The dual identification according to the morphology and ITS sequence analysis is recognised and implemented. It would be of the most value to investigate *P. belbahrii* sexual reproduction and to identify mating types and mechanisms of their compatibility if it is heterothallic. Further, valuable will be to obtain knowledge of the *P. belbahrii* natural distribution range because its present distribution is due to human activity and trades. More research into aspects of *P. belbahrii* physiology, asymptomatic infections and oospore role in epidemiology. The seed transmission still needs to be elucidated and the question of whether the pathogen penetrates into the seed should be answered. Because it has been already spread worldwide, the *P. belbahrii* is not on the quarantine lists; although, it will be beneficial to follow the quarantine guideline, in the context of global trade with seeds.

## Author details

Snježana Topolovec-Pintarić* and Katarina Martinko
Faculty of Agriculture, Department of Plant Pathology, University of Zagreb, Zagreb, Croatia

*Address all correspondence to: tpintaric@agr.hr

## References


[1] Hansford CG. Annual report of the mycologist. Review of Applied Mycology. 1933;**12**:421-422

[2] Hansford CG. Annual report of the mycologist. Review of Applied Mycology. 1938;**17**:345-346

[3] Belbahrii L, Calmin G, Pawlowski J, Lefort F. Phylogenetic analysis and real time PCR detection of a presumably undescribed *Peronospora* species on sweet basil and sage. EPPO Mycological Research. 2005;**109**:1276-1287. DOI: 10.1017/S0953756205003928

[4] Garibaldi A, Minuto A, Gullino ML. First report of downy mildew caused by *Peronospora* sp. on basil (*Ocimum basilicum*) in France. Plant Disease. 2005;**89**(6):683. DOI: 10.1094/PD-89-0683C

[5] Webb K, Sansford C, MacLeod A, Matthews-Berry S. Rapid Assessment of the Need for a Detailed Pest Risk Analysis for *Peronospora belbahrii*. UK Risk Register Details for *Peronospora belbahrii*. London: UK Plant Health Risk Register (DEFRA); 2012. Available from: https://secure.fera.defra.gov.uk/phiw/riskRegister/downloadExternalPra.cfm?id=3901 [Accessed: 06 November 2019]

[6] Henricot B, Denton J, Scrace J, Barnes AV, Lane CR. *Peronospora belbahrii* causing downy mildew disease on *Agastache* in the UK: A new host and location for the pathogen. New Disease Reports. 2009;**20**:26. DOI: 10.1111/j.1365-3059.2010.02264.x

[7] Nagy G, Horváth A. Occurrence of downy mildew caused by *Peronospora belbahrii* on sweet basil in Hungary. Plant Disease. 2011;**95**(8):1034. DOI: 10.1094/PDIS-04-11-0329

[8] Kanetis L, Vasiliou A, Neophytou G, Samouel S, Tsaltas D. First report of downy mildew caused by *Peronospora belbahrii* on sweet basil (*Ocimum basilicum*) in Cyprus. Plant Disease. 2014;**98**:283. DOI: 10.1094/PHYTO-02-15-0032-FI

[9] Rivera Y, Salgado-Salazar C, Windham AS, Crouch JA. Downy mildew on Coleus (*Plectranthus scutellarioides*) caused by *Peronospora belbahrii* sensu lato in Tennessee. Plant Disease. 2016;**100**:655. DOI: 10.1094/PDIS-10-15-1120-PDN

[10] Gómez Tenorio MA, Lupión Rodríguez B, Boix Ruiz A, Ruiz Olmos C, Moreno Díaz A, Marín Guirao JI, et al. El mildiu nueva enfermedad de la albahaca en España. Phytoma España. 2016;**282**:48-52

[11] Zhang S, Mersha Z, Roberts PD, Raid R. Downy Mildew of Basil in South Florida. Gainesville: University of Florida, IFAS Extension; 2009. Doc. PP271. Available from: http://edis.ifas.ufl.edu/pdffiles/PP/PP27100.pdf [Accessed: 15 September 2019]

[12] McGrath MT. Expect and Prepare for Downy Mildew in Basil. Ithaca, NY: Department of Plant Pathology, Cornell University; 2019. Available from: http://vegetablemdonline.ppath.cornell.edu/NewsArticles/BasilDowny.html [Accessed: 24 November 2019]

[13] Saude C, Westerveld S, Filotas M, McDonald MR. First report of downy mildew caused by *Peronospora belbahrii* on Basil (*Ocimum* spp.) in Ontario. Plant Diseases. 2013;**97**(9):1248. DOI: 10.1094/PDIS-01-13-0026-PDN

[14] Ronco L, Rollan C, Choi YJ, Shin HD. Downy mildew of sweet basil (*Ocimum basilicum* ) caused by *Peronospora* sp. in Argentina. Plant Pathology. 2009;**58**:395. DOI: 10.1111/j.1365-3059.2008.02006.x

[15] Romero M, Amador BM, Picazo LS, Nieto-Gariby A. First report of *Peronospora belbahrii* on sweet basil in Baja California Sur Mexico. Journal of Phytopathology. 2015;**4**:1-5. DOI: 10.1111/jph.12391

[16] Khateri H, Calmin G, Moarrefzadeh N, Belbahri L, Lefort F. First report of downy mildew caused by *Peronospora sp.* on basil in Northern Iran. Journal of Plant Pathology. 2007;**89**(3):S70

[17] Ito Y, Takeuchi T, Matsushita Y, Chikuo Y, Satou M. Downy mildew of coleus caused by *Peronospora belbahrii* in Japan. Journal of General Plant Pathology. 2015;**81**(4):328-330. DOI: 10.1007/s10327-015-0601-3

[18] Chen CH, Huang JH, Hsieh TF. First report of *Peronospora belbahrii* causing downy mildew on basil in Taiwan. Plant Pathology Bulletin. 2010;**19**:177-180

[19] Cohen Y, Galperin M, Vaknin M, Ben-Naim Y, Rubin AE, Silverman D, et al. Downy mildew in basil, a new disease in Israel. Phytoparasitica. 2013;**41**(4):458

[20] Kong XY, Wang S, Wan SL, Xiao CL, Luo F, Liu Y. First report of downy mildew on basil (*Ocimum basilicum*) in China. Plant Disease. 2015;**99**:1642. DOI: 10.1094/PDIS-01-15-0077-PDN

[21] Hu B, Li Z, Hu M, Sun H, Zheng J, Diao Y. Outbreak of downy mildew caused by *Peronospora belbahrii* on *Ocimum basilicum* var. polosum in China. New Disease Reports. 2018;**37**:1. DOI: 10.5197/j.2044-0588.2018.037.001

[22] Choi YJ, Choi IY, Lee KJ, Shin H. First report of downy mildew caused by *Peronospora belbahrii* on sweet basil (*Ocimum basilicum*) in Korea. Plant Disease. 2016;**100**(11):2335. DOI: 10.1094/PDIS-05-16-0771-PDN

[23] Grice K, Sun G, Trevorrow P. Basil Downy Mildew Management Options—Is it Seedborne? Agri-Science Queensland Innovation Opportunity. Brisbane: Department of Agriculture and Fisheries; 2018. Available from: http://era.daf.qld.gov.au/id/eprint/6386/7/H%26FS%20-%20Basil%20Downy%20Mildew%20%28Grice%29%20FINAL.pdf [Accessed: 18 November 2019]

[24] Gorayeb E, Pieroni LP, Cruciol GCD, de Pieri C, Dovigo LH, Pavan M, et al. First Report of downy mildew on coleus (*Plectranthus* spp.) caused by *Peronospora belbahrii* sensu lato in Brazil. Plant Disease. 2020;**104**(1):294. DOI: 10.1094/PDIS-07-19-1551-PDN

[25] Novak A, Sever Z, Ivić D, Čajkulić AM. Plamenjača Bosiljka (*Peronospora belbahrii*)—Destruktivna bolest u proizvodnji bosiljka, Hrvatski centar za poljoprivredu, hranu i selo—Zavod za zaštitu bilja. Glasilo Biljne Zaštite. 2016;**16**(6):544-547

[26] Grabowski M. Basil Downy Mildew *Peronospora belbahrii*. Saint Paul: Regents of the University of Minnesota, University of Minnesota Extension; 2012. Available from: http://www.extension.umn.edu/garden/yard-garden/vegetables/basil-downy-mildew/docs/basil-downy-mildew-pub.pdf [Accessed: 06 September 2019]

[27] Roberts PD, Raid RN, Harmon PF, Jordan SA, Palmateer AJ. First report of Downy Mildew caused by a *Peronospora* sp. on basil in Florida and the United States. Plant Disease. 2009;**93**:199. DOI: 10.1094/PDIS-93-2-0199B

[28] Thines M, Telle S, Ploch S, Runge F. Identity of the downy mildew pathogens of basil, coleus, and sage with implications for quarantine measures. Mycological Research. 2009;**113**(5):532-540. DOI: 10.1016/j.mycres.2008.12.005

[29] Harlan BR, Hausbeck MK. Diseases of coleus. In: McGovern R, Elmer W, editors. Handbook of Florists' Crops Diseases. Handbook of Plant Disease Management. Cham: Springer; 2018. pp. 911-925. DOI: 10.1007/978-3-319-39670-5_32

[30] Cohen Y, Ben Naim Y, Falach L, Avia E. Epidemiology of basil downy mildew. Phytopathology. 2017;**107**:1149-1160. DOI: 10.1094/PHYTO-01-17-0017-FI

[31] Harlan B, Linderman S, Hyatt L, Hausbeck M. Research gives clues for preventing coleus downy mildew. Greenhouse Grower. 2015. Available from: https://www.greenhousegrower.com/production/crop-inputs/research-gives-clues-for-preventing-coleus-downy-mildew/ [Accessed: 16 October 2019]

[32] Farr DF, Rossman AY. Fungal Databases. Systematic Mycology and Microbiology Laboratory, ARS, USDA; 2015. Online Publication. Available from: http://nt.ars-grin.gov/fungaldatabases/ [Accessed: 01 October 2019]

[33] Babadoost M. Downy mildew of basil. Department of Crop Science, University of Illinois. RPD No. 1216. 2016. Available from: http://extension.cropsciences.illinois.edu/fruitveg/pdfs/1216.pdf [Accessed: 12 September 2019]

[34] Cohen Y, Vaknin M, Ben-Naim Y, Rubin AE, Galperin M, Silverman D, et al. First report of the occurrence and resistance to mefenoxam of *Peronospora belbahrii*, causal agent of downy mildew of basil (*Ocimum basilicum*) in Israel. Plant Disease. 2013;**97**(5):692. DOI: 10.1094/PDIS-12-12-1126-PDN

[35] Elad Y, Omer C, Nisan Z, Harari D, Goren H, Adler U, et al. Passive heat treatment of sweet basil crops suppresses *Peronospora belbahrii* downy mildew. The Annals of Applied Biology. 2016;**168**:373-389. DOI: 10.1111/aab.12269

[36] Zhang G, Thompson A, Schisler D, Johnson ET. Characterization of the infection process by *Peronospora belbahrii* on basil by scanning electron microscopy. Heliyon. 2019;**5**:e01117. DOI: 10.1016/j.heliyon.2019.e01117

[37] Pyne RM. Introgression of genetic resistance to downy mildew (*Peronospora belbahrii*) in a non-model plant species, sweet basil (*Ocimum basilicum*) [Thesis]. New Jersey, USA: Graduate School-New Brunswick Rutgers, The State University of New Jersey; 2017

[38] Wyenandt CA, Simon JE, Pyne RM, Homa K, McGrath MT, Zhang S, et al. Basil downy mildew (*Peronospora belbahrii*): Discoveries and challenges relative to its control. Disease Control and Pest Management. 2015;**105**(7):885-894. DOI: 10.1094/PHYTO-02-15-0032-FI

[39] McGrath MT, LaMarsh KA. Evaluation of organic and conventional fungicide programs for downy mildew in basil. Plant Disease Management Reports. 2015;**9**:V026. DOI: 10.1094/PHYTO-02-15-0032-FI

[40] Farahani-Kofoet D, Römero P, Grosch R. Selecting basil genotypes with resistance against downy mildew. Scientia Horticulturae. 2014;**179**(24):248-255. DOI: 10.1016/j.scienta.2014.09.036

[41] Cohen Y, Vaknin M, Ben-Naim Y, Rubin AE. Light suppresses sporulation and epidemics of *Peronospora belbahrii*. PLoS One. 2013;**8**(11):e81282. DOI: 10.1371/journal.pone.0081282

[42] Garibaldi A, Bertetti D, Gullino ML. Effect of leaf wetness duration

and temperature on infection of downy mildew (*Peronospora* sp.) of basil. Journal of Plant Diseases and Protection. 2007;**114**:6-8. DOI: 10.1007/BF03356196

[43] Cohen Y, Ben-Naim Y. Nocturnal fanning suppresses downy mildew epidemics in sweet basil. PLoS One. 2016;**11**:e0155330. DOI: 10.1371/journal.pone.0155330

[44] Garibaldi A, Minuto G, Bertetti D, Gullino ML. Seed transmission of *Peronospora* sp. of basil. Journal of Plant Diseases and Protection. 2004;**111**:465-469

[45] Farahani-Kofoet RD, Römer P, Grosch R. Systemic spread of downy mildew in basil plants and detection of the pathogen in seed and plant samples. Mycological Progress. 2012;**11**:961-966. DOI: 10.1007/s11557-012-0816-z

[46] Falach-Block L, Ben-Naim Y, Cohen Y. Investigation of seed transmission in *Peronospora belbahrii*: The causal agent of basil downy mildew. Agronomy. 2019;**9**(205):1-11. DOI: 10.3390/agronomy9040205

[47] Cohen Y, Rubin AE. Daytime solar heating controls downy mildew *Peronospora belbahrii* in sweet basil. PLoS One. 2015;**10**(5):e0126103. DOI: 10.1371/journal.pone.0126103

[48] Collina M, Merighi M, Turan C, Pirondi A, Minuto G, Brunelli A. First report of resistance of *Peronospora belbahrii*, causal agent of downy mildew of basil, to Mefenoxam in Italy. Plant Disease. 2016;**100**(8):1787. DOI: 10.1094/PDIS-02-16-0237-PDN

[49] Blum M, Boehler M, Randall E, Young V, Csukai M, Kraus S, et al. Mandipropamid targets the cellulose synthase-like PiCesA3 to inhibit cell wall biosynthesis in the oomycete plant pathogen, *Phytophthora infestans*. Molecular Plant Pathology. 2010;**11**(2):227-243. DOI: 10.1111/j.1364-3703.2009.00604.x

[50] Cohen Y, Rubin AE, Galperin M. Oxathiapiprolin-based fungicides provide enhanced control of tomato late blight induced by mefenoxam-insensitive *Phytophthora infestans*. PLoS One. 2018;**13**(9):e0204523. DOI: 10.1371/journal.pone.0204523

[51] FRAC Code List ©*. Fungal Control Agents Sorted by Cross Resistance Pattern and Mode of Action (Including FRAC Code Numbering). 2019. Available from: https://www.frac.info/docs/default-source/publications/frac-code-list/frac-code-list-2019-finale0af2a2c512362eb9a1eff00004acf5d.pdf?sfvrsn=7d8c489a_2 [Accessed: 25 November 2019]

[52] Cohen Y. Root treatment with oxathiapiprolin, benthiavalicarb or their mixture provides prolonged systemic protection against oomycete foliar pathogens. PLoS One. 2020;**15**(1):e0227556. DOI: 10.1371/journal.pone.0227556

[53] McGrath MT. Expect and Prepare for Downy Mildew in Basil. 2019. Available from: http://blogs.cornell.edu/livegpath/extension/basil-downy-mildew/where-in-the-usa-is-basildowny-mildew/ [Accessed: 16 December 2019]

[54] Mebalds M, Henderson B, Hepworth G. Development of Steam-Air Treatment to Control Seed-Borne Diseases of Vegetables and Flowers. HRDC Project No. NY536. Gordon, Australia: Horticultural Research and Development Corporation; 1997. Available from: https://www.greenlifeindustry.com.au/Attachment?Action=Download&Attachment_id=1773 [Accessed: 16 December 2019]

Chapter 2

# Nanophytovirology: An Emerging Field for Disease Management

*Avinash Marwal and R.K. Gaur*


## Abstract

Nanotechnology positions as a new armament in our collection against the increasing challenges in disease management and plant/human health. The application of nanotechnology in plant/human disease administration, diagnosis, and genetic transformations is still in its early stages. Apart from the scope of this chapter, there is also a mounting collection of new tools and techniques where nanoparticles are employed as delivery vehicles for genetic material in plants. Due to their nanoscale dimensions, nanoparticles may knockout virus particles and thus may open a novel arena of virus control in plants/humans. Our aim is to enlighten and enthuse researchers about the swiftly expanding prospects of nanotechnology in plant pathology i.e., "nanophytovirology."


**Keywords:** nanoparticles, plant pathology, human pathology, virology, disease diagnosis, disease management, plant protection, case study

## 1. Introduction

Food security has always been the principal apprehension for mankind [1]. Food losses because of crop infections by pathogens like bacteria, fungus and viruses are known as obstinate issues in agriculture since centuries around the globe [2]. Even countries, societies and their administrations have been facing this problem a long time. Quarantine strategies employed for crops and ornamental plants a requite effective in preventing harmful diseases and arthropod pest epidemics from being imported and getting spread in the purchasing country [3]. Plants are infected by a number bacterial, fungal and virus species [4–8]. Viruses are considered as the minutest known microbes to the mankind and yet they reason for the most significant losses in agriculture sector [9], thus putting the plants under stress [10]. Same holds true for humans as well. Many a time, the finest recognized treatment for viruses is the innate immunological resistance system of host; else, the initial prevention of viral infection is the only substitute [11]. Consequently, diagnosing host for viruses at earliest is the prime approach toward controlling and eliminating harmful virus [12, 13]. The starter of a novel class of nanoscale particles with numerous exceptional properties and functions has flashed a series of innovative applications [14]. Engineered nano-materials (nanoparticles) range from 1 to 100 nm in size [15]. Engineered nanoparticles can be synthesized to precise dimensions and intended in numerous composite arrays, making their function and efficacy applicable in many fields. Suitable sensors and good delivery systems might help infighting viruses and other crop pathogens.

 

Nanoparticles might employ an important integrity in future plant and human disease management that might range from disease diagnosis to disease treatment [16]. In recent past several nanoparticles has been synthesized across the globe by eminent scientists in various forms [17, 18]. Like quantum dots, metalloids, metallic oxides, nonmetals, carbon nanomaterials [19], dendrimers, liposomes [20], Virus-based nanoparticles (VNPs) are few examples of this category [21, 22]. Nanoparticles greatest advantage lies in their small size, greater surface area and strong reactivity: such efficient activity favors for vast application in plant and human pathology [23]. Nanoparticles can be synthesized either by chemical route or by green synthesis method taking in account the top down or bottom up approach, whichever better feasible. This can be further categorized into chemical, reduction, microemulsion, colloidal, sonochemical, electrochemical, microwave, solvothermal and microbial synthesis of nanoparticles [24]. The present study focuses and centric towards the above said aspects of nanoparticles vs. plant virology ("nanophytovirology"), thus summarizing the available scattered literature at one place for the common audience.

## 2. Pre-era of "nanophytovirology"

Earlier several methods have been given by pioneers for virus detection in the host plant (crops, ornamental plants, weeds) [25]. Therefore, techniques for recognition and detection of viruses, equally in crops and carrier vectors, participate for a decisive role in virus disease management. All of them are listed as: electron microscopy [26], symptoms determination [27, 28], biotest [29, 30], mechanical transmission [31], seed transmission [32], serological techniques [enzyme-linked immunosorbent assay, phage display, tissue blot immunoassay (TIBA), lateral flow devices, immunocapture transmission electron microscopy (ICTEM)] [33, 34], restriction fragment length polymorphism (RFLP) [35], thermostable amplification based methods [PCR and reverse transcription-polymerase chain reaction (RT-PCR), multiplex PCR/RT-PCR, immunocapture PCR (IC-PCR), immuno-precipitation PCR (IP-PCR), nested PCR, multiplex nested PCR, real time PCR (qPCR), multiplex real time PCR, Co-operational PCR (Co-PCR)] [36–39], isothermal amplification based methods [helicase dependent amplification (HDA), recombinase polymerase amplification (RPA), nucleic acid sequence base amplification (NASBA), loop-mediated isothermal amplification (LAMP), rolling circle amplification (RCA)] [40, 41], nucleic acid sequence hybridization techniques [in situ hybridization, microarray, lateral flow microarrays] [42, 43], next generation sequencing (NGS), recombinant DNA approach [44]. Accessibility of the few above-mentioned diagnostic methods endow with a superior elasticity, increased sensitivity, and specificity for quick judgment of virus diseases. The accurate and reliable detection of the associated virus pathogens therefore forms the first line of defense in management of these diseases.

Likewise, number of methods has been devised in viral disease management [45–48]. It is conceivable that destruction/killing arthropod vectors, either via biological control or with traditional methods, helpful in reducing the viral populations. *Scymnus offmanni*, *Coccinella septempunctata*, *Propylaea japonica*, *Euseius cutalis*, etc. are some natural predators of whiteflies. Chemiecological technique employs honeydews excreta of whitefly, which work as a kairomone to attract natural prey, i.e., *Encarsia formosa*. Such approach has been successfully used in the Mediterranean regions against whiteflies vector. Even plant age is also crucial in vector population controlling. Field trial has been successful where young plants were covered with plastic bag (yellow polyethylene film) or grown under green house until maturing phase, limits the contact with arthropods vectors. Similarly masking the crop with living ground covers of perennial peanuts, cinquillo and coriander plants condensed the impact of incoming whitefly adults. An old age practice helps in diminishing the virus populations by destroying the weeds growing in the near vicinity of the crop fields, or even sowing the seeds a little later when the vector populations flourishes. Both help in viral disease management [49].

Further the use of insecticides against various arthropod vectors is also helpful to a certain extent. Few of them are Neonicotinoids, Buprofezin, Thiamethoxam 70 WS, Imidacloprid 600 FS, Imidacloprid 70WS and Carbosulfan 25 DS, Triazophos, Ethion, Imidacloprid, Acephate 95 SG, Spirotetramat, Diafenthiuron, Nitroguanidines, Thiamethoxam, Ryanodine and Pymetrozine, quite lethal against whiteflies [50]. Two remarkable technology has come up as one the best solution against plant viruses, i.e., interference RNA (RNAi) and clustered regularly interspaced short palindromic repeats (CRISPR). RNAi-mediated virus resistance was reported against potato virus Y (PVY) in transgenic tobacco plants, against African cassava mosaic virus (ACMV), croton yellow vein mosaic virus (CYVMV) and many more [51–53]. RNAi is usually associated with methylation of nuclear DNA corresponding to the transcribed region of the target RNA despite transcription levels of the transgene remains unaffected [54]. CRISPR-Cas (CRISPR Associated Systems) is an adaptive immune system in many archaea and bacteria that cleaves foreign DNA based on sequence complementarity. Virus based guide RNA (gRNA) delivery system for CRISPR/Cas9 mediated plant genome editing cause mutations in target genome locations and resulted in transgenic plants showing resistance against viruses [55].

## 3. Epoch of "nanophytovirology"

"Nanophytovirology" is a front-line science which customs nanotechnology in diagnosis, detection and management of plant viral diseases and their pathogens especially arthropods at an initial phase, helping in plant protection from the epidemic diseases [56]. Among the various plant diseases, the diseases caused by viruses are the most difficult to manage [57], as one must stop the spread of the disease by the vectors. Nanotechnological-based disease diagnosis and management for virus infecting crop plants is attaining magnitude with the increased spread of viruses and threats of their epidemics [58]. Therefore, there is a demand for an improved management of viruses employed by a series of strategies [59, 60]; in-fact such practices relied on the ecology of the virus. Many approaches have been used to decrease crop losses due to viruses, only a few are effective in their management. Even understanding the plant mediated interactions between viruses and their carrier vector is quite important to tackle epidemiology of viral diseases [59, 60]. Developments in nanofabrication and nanotechnology endow a crucial part in plant viral disease detection, simplicity in handling and are cost-effective as compared to other plant viral diagnostic methods.

Earlier fluorescent dyes were used straight away for staining the viruses, now nanoparticles and quantum dots (QDs) have been developed which helps in carrying the detection tags (dyes or anti-viral antibodies) and are quite efficient in identifying the viruses, which are also helpful as labeling and imaging agents. Such fluorescent tags are easily detected in flow cytometry enabled devices. In yet another instance nano-biosensor was developed against plasmodiophoromycete *Polymyxa betae* which is responsible for the carrier of beet necrotic yellow vein virus (BNYVV) and caused the deadly disease rhizomania in sugarcane plants. The authors used specific antibodies against conjugated with Cadmium-Telluride

QDs against the glutathione-S-transferase protein's (GST). The developed nano-biosensor showed enough fluorescence resonance energy transfer (FRET) to detect the plasmodiophoromycete *Polymyxa betae*. Cadmium-Telluride QDs conjugated to antibodies were also developed against citrus tristeza virus (CTV) using the similar approach [61].

Surface plasmon resonance (SPR) is also an optical based technique which employs diagnosis of viruses by change in refractive index on a metal surface. In this gold nanoparticles are conjugated with anti-viral antibodies adsorbed on a glass substrate and are sensed by SPR. Quartz-crystal microbalance (QCM) is a well-known, commercially accessible mass sensor technique generally employed in quantitative measurement of the thickness of thin films. The principal is that the exterior part of the quartz-crystal device (microchip: dimensions in nanometer) is typically coated with anti-viral antibodies against the targeted plant viruses. Now when a virus is encountered on the quartz-crystal surface there results an increase in the mass, thereby resonant frequency decreases, the change in the frequency before and after of the chip is measured subsequently. SPR and QCM based nano-biosensor has been manufactured successfully for the detection of orchid viruses, tobacco mosaic virus (TMV), cymbidium mosaic virus (CymMV), odontoglossum ringspot virus (ORSV), etc. [62].

Microcantilevers are in the micrometer range, but their tip end is in the nanometer scale and is widely used for various biosensing applications. Microcantilevers works in two different modes, i.e., straining and resonating mode, both are helpful in identifying viruses. Resonating mode is like QCM, whereas straining mode relies on the changes in electrical resistance whenever a virus particle bound to the surface. The major limitation is the low performance of device in the liquid medium, hence the sample need drying before application. For virus particle detection nanowire employed transistors have been devised. An immuno-biosensor was developed for the detection of Plum pox virus in plum (*Prunus domestica*) and tobacco (*Nicotiana benthamiana*) leaves sap, where gold electrodes were modified with 1,6-hexanedithiol, gold nanoparticles, anti-PPV IgG polyclonal antibody and BSA. Nanowires can be engaged against the target virus, and when encountering a charged virus capsid, a depletion or gain of charge in the nanowires is thus recorded as a simple conductance change. In a similar instance a lithographically patterned nanowire electrodeposition (LPNE) technique was used to develop a label-free chemiresistive sensors based on a polypyrrole (PPy) nanoribbon conjugated with anti-viral antibodies against cucumber mosaic virus (CMV) [63].

Nanotechnology benefits agriculture sectors and diminish environmental pollution. This is carried out by manufacturing of pesticides and chemical fertilizers using nanoparticles and nano-capsules and has the capability to control or delayed the delivery and absorption of pesticides and chemical fertilizers with lower dose. "Nano-5" is a marketed product pesticide to control several plant viruses. It was found effective at dilution of 1:500 against Mosaic, ringspot, transitory yellowing, tristeza virus, exocortis viroid by spraying "Nano-5" onto the surface of leaves and apply to the roots once every 3 days. It was reported that chitosan nanoparticles have the ability to induce resistance in host crops against few viruses, for example mosaic virus of alfalfa, snuff, peanut, potato, and cucumber were targeted. Similarly, gold nanoparticles showed antiviral effects against Bean mild mosaic virus in beans, barley yellow mosaic virus in barley and tobacco necrosis virus in tobacco plants. Peoples also claimed silver nanoparticles application made the host plant resistance against sun-hemp rosette virus (infecting bean plants) and bean yellow mosaic virus (causing disease in faba bean crops) [64].

RNAi technique were also employed in coupling with nanotechnology, a remarkable study was carried out to show resistance against cucumber mosaic virus (CMV) and pepper mild mottle virus (PMMoV). In this wonderful approach dsRNA was loaded onto LDH (Layered double hydroxides) nanoparticles, called BioClay and were sprayed on the challenged plants. Plants showed resistance against the above-mentioned viruses for 20 days as compared to controlled ones [65]. It is clear from the above discussion that "nanophytovirology" represent an attractive advancement, owing to their potential advantages for the plant disease management against deadly crop viruses.

## 4. Challenges adjoining "nanophytovirology"

The application of nanoparticles, particularly in plant disease management, need specific structural and physicochemical features, and any slight variations to their planned properties can hinder the function and performance of designed nanoparticle conjugate [66]. Hence, numerous factors related to nanoparticle synthesis are quite important for the development of an effective virus detection assay. Further, the methods employed in making/synthesizing nanoparticles seem easy and quick for large scale production but getting the final product in uniformity (shape and size) remains challenging. Nanoparticles itself cannot detect the viruses solely and thus need additional biomolecule specific in sensing the pathogen. In comparison to nanoparticles, biomolecules are quite delicate to severe chemical and physical alterations (high temperature, high salt concentrations, reducing agents) which might can harmfully affect their reactivity and specificity [67]. Therefore, such procedures demand for proper optimization steps aimed at in detecting viruses.

But when employing/using nanoparticles and its conjugates for the application in virus disease management, their biosafety and toxicity on human health and environment is yet another a major challenge. For example, nano-pesticides might get inhaled by the workers during treatment process. Similarly, other nano-composites might get deposit on the leaves or flowers, can affect animals, birds, honey bees, etc. They may clog the stomatal pores and might hinder the penetration of pollen grains on stigma. If get inside the plant system, nanoparticle might affect plant metabolism and can cause similar effect on humans as well. Cellular toxicity can be induced by nanoparticles (NPs) that lead to toxic side effects such as enhanced ROS generation, disruption of redox homeostasis, lipid peroxidation, impaired mitochondrial function, and membrane damage. Due to their long persistence and greater reactivity nano-pesticides may contaminate water and soil system [68]. Regardless of these developments in nanotechnology, there are some unsolved problems concerning the detection of many plant viruses due to their low titer in the plants, their uneven distribution, the existence of latent infection and lack of validated sampling protocols.

## 5. Conclusion

Virologists need complete knowledge about viral infection and of effects on host plants so that correct control procedures can be implemented [69]. Specificity of viruses varies greatly [70]. Some of them can colonize different species and some are specific or interact to specific cell machinery. There is more focus on reduction of crop loss by controlling pathogen movement from infected plants to healthy plants rather than treating the infected plants [71]. The work on the development of nanoparticles done by the pioneers in the field is particularly significant and beneficial for the humans and to the agriculture sector which supports the lives of growing population [72, 73]. Nanoparticles affect the pathogens in a similar way as the chemical pesticides do at a very low concentration [74]. Nanomaterials have been used as carrier of active ingredients of pesticides, host defense inducing chemicals, etc. [75, 76], to target the viral pathogens. These nano-based diagnostic kits not only increase the speed of detection but also increase the power of the detection. Thus, finding nanotechnology-based solutions, will enable researchers to explore better management practices against viruses in a better way for the plants which are constantly challenged in the natural conditions.

## Conflict of interest

The authors have no conflict of action to declare.

## Author contributions

A.M. and R.K.G. drafted the manusxxcript. A.M. and R.K.G. contributed to acquisition of literature data. All authors read and approved the final version of the manuscript.


## Author details

Avinash Marwal[1] and R.K. Gaur[2]*

1 Department of Biotechnology, Mohanlal Sukhadia University, Udaipur, Rajasthan, India

2 Department of Biosciences, School of Sciences, Mody University of Science and Technology, Lakshmangarh, Sikar, Rajasthan, India

*Address all correspondence to: gaurrajarshi@hotmail.com

## References

[1] Kleve S, Booth S, Davidson ZE, Palermo C. Walking the food security tightrope—Exploring the experiences of low-to-middle income Melbourne households. International Journal of Environmental Research and Public Health. 2018;**15**:2206. DOI: 10.3390/ijerph15102206

[2] Gaur RK, Prajapat R, Marwal A, Sahu A, Rathore MS. First report of a Begomovirus infecting *Mimosa pudica* in India. Journal of Plant Pathology. 2011;**93**:S4.80. DOI: 10.4454/jpp.v93i4.2394

[3] Almeida RPP. Emerging plant disease epidemics: Biological research is key but not enough. PLoS Biology. 2018;**16**:e2007020. DOI: 10.1371/journal.pbio.2007020

[4] Marwal A, Prajapat R, Sahu A, Gaur RK. Current status of Geminivirus in India: RNAi technology, a challenging cure. Asian Journal of Biological Sciences. 2012;**5**:273-293. DOI: 10.3923/ajbs.2012.273.293

[5] Prajapat R, Marwal A, Jha PN. *Erwinia carotovora* associated with potato: A critical appraisal with respect to Indian perspective. International Journal of Current Microbiology and Applied Sciences. 2013;**2**:83-89

[6] Mahmood S, Lakra N, Marwal A, Sudheep NM, Anwar K. Crop genetic engineering: An approach to improve fungal resistance in plant system. In: Singh DP, editor. Plant-Microbe Interactions in Agro-Ecological Perspectives. Singapore: Springer; 2017. pp. 581-591. DOI: 10.1007/978-981-10-6593-4_23

[7] Sudheep NM, Marwal A, Lakra N, Anwar K, Mahmood S. Fascinating fungal endophytes role and possible applications. In: Singh DP, editor. Plant-Microbe Interactions in Agro-Ecological Perspectives. Singapore: Springer; 2017. pp. 255-273. DOI: 10.1007/978-981-10-5813-4_13

[8] Marwal A, Sahu AK, Gaur RK. Molecular characterization of begomoviruses and DNA satellites associated with a new host Spanish flag (*Lantana camara*) in India. ISRN Virology. 2013;**2013**:5. DOI: 10.5402/2013/915703

[9] Marwal A, Prajapat R, Gaur RK. First report of recombination analysis of Betasatellite and Aplhasatellite sequence isolated from an ornamental plant Marigold in India: An in silico approach. International Journal of Virology. 2016;**12**:10-17. DOI: 10.3923/ijv.2016.10.17

[10] Marwal A, Mishra M, Sekhsaria C, Gaur RK. Computational analysis and predicting ligand binding site in the rose leaf curl virus and its Betasatellite proteins: A step forward for antiviral agent designing. In: Saxena S, Tiwari AK, editors. Begomoviruses: Occurrence and Management in Asia and Africa. Singapore: Springer; 2017. pp. 157-168. DOI: 10.1007/978-981-10-5984-1_9

[11] Marwal A, Sahu A, Gaur RK. New insights in the functional genomics of plants responding to abiotic stress. In: Gaur RK, Sharma P, editors. Molecular Approaches in Plant Abiotic Stress. Boca Raton, Florida, US: CRC Press, Science Publishers, Taylor & Francis Group; 2014. pp. 158-180. DOI: 10.1201/b15538

[12] Quatrini L, Wieduwild E, Escaliere B, Filtjens J, Chasson L, Laprie C, et al. Endogenous glucocorticoids control host resistance to viral infection through the tissue-specific regulation of PD-1 expression on NK cells. Nature Immunology. 2018;**19**:54-962. DOI: 10.1038/s41590-018-0185-0

[13] Prajapat R, Marwal A, Goyal M. In silico characterization of hemagglutinin protein of influenza a virus [A/canine/Beijing/cau9/2009(H1N1)] of H1N1 subtype. Journal of Advances in Biotechnology. 2014;**1**:40-47. DOI: 10.24297/jbt.v1i1.1786

[14] Prajapat R, Marwal A, Shaikh Z, Gaur RK. Geminivirus database (GVDB): First database of family Geminiviridae and its genera Begomovirus. Pakistan Journal of Biological Sciences. 2012;**15**:702-706. DOI: 10.3923/pjbs.2012.702.706

[15] Das AK, Marwal A, Sain D, Pareek V. One-step green synthesis and characterization of plant protein-coated mercuric oxide (HgO) nanoparticles: Antimicrobial studies. International Nano Letters. 2015;**5**:125-132. DOI: 10.1007/s40089-015-0144-9

[16] Das AK, Marwal A, Sain D. One-step green synthesis and characterization of flower extract-mediated mercuric oxide (HgO) nanoparticles from Callistemon viminalis. Research and Reviews: Journal of Pharmaceutics and Nanotechnology. 2014;**2**:25-28

[17] Antonacci A, Arduini F, Moscone D, Palleschi G, Scognamiglio V. Nanostructured (bio)sensors for smart agriculture. TrAC Trends in Analytical Chemistry. 2018;**98**:95-103. DOI: 10.1016/j.trac.2017.10.022

[18] Das AK, Marwal A, Verma R. Datura inoxia leaf extract mediated one step green synthesis and characterization of magnetite ($Fe_3O_4$) nanoparticles. Research and Reviews: Journal of Pharmaceutics and Nanotechnology. 2014;**2**:21-24

[19] Das S, Debnath N, Cui Y, Unrine J, Palli SR. Chitosan, carbon quantum dot, and silica nanoparticle mediated dsRNA delivery for gene silencing in Aedes aegypti: A comparative analysis. ACS Applied Materials & Interfaces. 2015;**7**:19530-19535. DOI: 10.1021/acsami.5b05232

[20] Das AK, Marwal A, Pareek V. Nanoparticles-protein hybrid based magnetic liposome. World Academy of Science, Engineering and Technology, International Journal of Chemical, Nuclear, Materials and Metallurgical Engineering. 2015;**9**:230-233

[21] Das AK, Marwal A, Verma R. Preparation and characterization of nano-bio hybrid based magneto liposome. International Journal of Pharmaceutical Sciences and Research. 2015;**6**:367-375. DOI: 10.13040/IJPSR.0975-8232.6(1).367-75

[22] Guenther RH, Lommel SA, Opperman CH, Sit TL. Plant virus-based nanoparticles for the delivery of agronomic compounds as a suspension concentrate. Methods in Molecular Biology. 2018;**1776**:203-214. DOI: 10.1007/978-1-4939-7808-3_13

[23] Das AK, Marwal A, Sain D. One-step green synthesis and characterization of flower extract-mediated mercuric oxide (HgO) nanoparticles from *Callistemon viminalis*. In: Bhoop BS, Sharma A, Mehta SK, Tripathi SK, editors. Nanotechnology: Novel Perspectives and Prospects. New Delhi, India: Tata-McGraw Hill; 2014. pp. 466-472

[24] Das AK, Marwal A, Pareek V, Joshi Y, Apoorva. Surface Engineering of Magnetite Nanoparticles by Plant Protein: Investigation into Magnetic Properties. Nano Hybrid and Composites. Vol. 11. Trans Tech Publication; 2016. pp. 38-44. DOI: 10.4028/www.scientific.net/NHC.11.38

[25] Prajapat R, Marwal A, Sahu AK, Gaur RK. First report of Begomovirus infecting *Sonchus asper* in India. Science International. 2013;**1**:108-110. DOI: 10.5567/sciintl.2013.108.110

[26] Marwal A, Sahu AK, Prajapat R, Choudhary DK, Gaur RK. Molecular and recombinational characterization of Begomovirus infecting an ornamental plant *Alternanthera sessilis*: A new host of tomato leaf curl Kerala virus reported in India. Science International. 2013;**1**:51-56. DOI: 10.17311/sciintl.2013.51.56

[27] Marwal A, Sahu AK, Gaur RK. Evidence of the association of begomovirus and its betasatellite with the yellow vein disease of an ornamental plant *Calendula officinalis* (pot marigold) in Rajasthan, India: Molecular, sequence and recombination analysis. Journal of Advances in Biology. 2013;**1**:29-44. DOI: 10.24297/jab.v1i1.1554

[28] Prajapat R, Marwal A, Gaur RK. Datura leaf curl betasatellite associated for the first time with *Datura inoxia* leaf curl syndrome in India. Journal of Advances in Biotechnology. 2014;**1**:1-7. DOI: 10.24297/jbt.v1i1.5055

[29] Marwal A, Sahu AK, Gaur RK. Association of begomovirus and an alphasatellite with the leaf curl disease of ornamental plant *Vinca alba* in Punjab, India. Journal of Agricultural Research. 2014;**52**:339-356

[30] Marwal A, Sahu AK, Gaur RK. First report on the association of a begomovirus with *Chrysanthemum indicum* exhibiting yellowing of leaf vein disease characterized by molecular studies. Journal of Horticultural Research. 2013;**21**:17-21. DOI: 10.2478/johr-2013-0017

[31] Sahu AK, Nehra C, Marwal A, Gaur RK. First report of a begomovirus associated with betasatellites infecting new host spinach (*Spinacia oleracea*) in India. Journal of General Plant Pathology. 2015;**81**:146-150. DOI: 10.1007/s10327-014-0576-5

[32] Sahu AK, Marwal A, Nehra C, Shahid MS, Gaur RK. First report of a begomovirus and associated betasatellite in *Rosa indica* and in India. Australasian Plant Disease Notes. 2014;**9**:147

[33] Nehra C, Verma RK, Mishra M, Marwal A, Sharma P, Gaur RK. Papaya yellow leaf curl virus: A newly identified begomovirus infecting *Carica papaya* from the Indian subcontinent. The Journal of Horticultural Science & Biotechnology. 2019;**94**:475-480. DOI: 10.1080/14620316.2019.1570827

[34] Marwal A, Sahu A, Gaur RK. Molecular marker: Tools for genetic analysis. In: Verma AS, Singh A, editors. Animal Biotechnology: Models in Discovery and Translation. Waltham, MA, US: Academic Press, Elsevier; 2014. pp. 289-305. DOI: 10.1016/B978-0-12-416002-6.00016-X

[35] Chen J, Adams MJ. A universal PCR primer to detect members of the Potyviridae and its use to examine the taxonomic status of several members of the family. Archives of Virology. 2001;**146**:757-766. DOI: 10.1007/s007050170144

[36] Marwal A, Sahu AK, Gaur RK. First report of molecular characterization of begomovirus infecting an ornamental plant *Tecoma stans* and a medicinal plant *Justicia adhatoda*. Science International. 2013;**25**:837-839

[37] Nehra C, Sahu AK, Marwal A, Gaur RK. Natural occurrence of Clerodendron yellow mosaic virus on Bougainvillea in India. New Diseases Report BSPP. 2014;**30**:19. DOI: 10.5197/j.2044-0588.2014.030.019

[38] Zhang S, Ravelonandro M, Russell P, McOwen N, Briard P, Bohannon S, et al. Rapid diagnostic detection of plum pox virus in Prunus plants by isothermal AmplifyRP(®) using reverse transcription-recombinase polymerase amplification. Journal of Virological Methods. 2014;**207**:114-120. DOI: 10.1016/j.jviromet.2014.06.026

[39] Nehra C, Marwal A, Verma RK, Gaur RK. Molecular characterization of Begomoviruses DNA-A and associated beta satellites with new host *Ocimum sanctum* in India. Proceedings of the National Academy of Sciences, India Section B: Biological Sciences. 2018. DOI: 10.1007/s40011-018-1006-9

[40] Marwal A, Sahu AK, Gaur RK. Molecular characterization of a begomovirus infecting a new host Golden Duranta (*Duranta erecta*) in India. International Journal of Current Microbiology and Applied Sciences. 2013;**2**:45-48

[41] Lamptey JNL, Osei MK, Mochiah MB, Osei K, Berchie JN, Bolfrey-Arku G, et al. Serological detection of tobacco mosaic virus and cucumber mosaic virus infecting tomato (*Solanum Lycopersicum*) using a lateral flow immunoassay technique. Journal of Agricultural Studies. 2013;**1**:102-113. DOI: 10.5296/jas.v1i2.3768

[42] Elbeaino T, Digiaro M, Uppala M, Sudini H. Deep sequencing of pigeonpea sterility mosaic virus discloses five RNA segments related to emaraviruses. Virus Research. 2014;**188**:27-31. DOI: 10.1016/j.virusres.2014.03.022

[43] Marwal A, Kumar R, Khurana SMP, Gaur RK. Complete nucleotide sequence of a new geminivirus isolated from *Vitis vinifera* in India: A symptomless host of grapevine red blotch virus. Virus Disease. 2018;**30**:106-111. DOI: 10.1007/s13337-018-0477-x

[44] Boonham N, Glover R, Tomlinson J, Mumford R. Exploiting generic platform technologies for the detection and identification of plant pathogens. In: Collinge DB, Munk L, Cooke BM, editors. Sustainable Disease Management in a European Context. Dordrecht: Springer; 2008. pp. 355-363. DOI: 10.1007/978-1-4020-8780-6_15

[45] Marwal A, Prajapat R, Gaur RK. Prediction of binding site in eight protein molecules of Begomovirus and its satellite components i.e., Betasatellite and Alphasatellite isolated from infected ornamental plant. Plant Pathology Journal. 2016;**15**:1-4. DOI: 10.3923/ppj.2016.1.4

[46] Marwal A, Mishra M, Verma RK, Prajapat R, Gaur RK. In silico study of the Geminiviruses infecting ornamental plants. In: Choudhary DK, Kumar M, Prasad R, Kumar V, editors. In Silico Approach for Sustainable Agriculture. Singapore: Springer; 2018. pp. 69-90. DOI: 10.1007/978-981-13-0347-0_4

[47] Prajapat R, Marwal A, Sahu A, Gaur RK. Phylogenetics and in silico docking studies between coat protein of Mimosa yellow vein virus and whey α-lactalbumin. American Journal of Biochemistry and Molecular Biology. 2011;**1**:265-274. DOI: 10.3923/ajbmb.2011.265.274

[48] Makkouk KM. A study on tomato viruses in the Jordan valley with special emphasis on tomato yellow leaf curl. Plant Disease Report. 1978;**64**:259-262. DOI: 10.1007/BF02979527

[49] Kayser H, Kaufmann L, Schürmann F. Pymetrozine (CGA 215¢944): A novel compound for aphid and whitefly control. In: An Overview of Its Mode of Action. Proceedings of Brighton Crop Protection Conference–Pests and Diseases. Vol. 2; Brighton. 1994. pp. 737-742

[50] Sanjaya VVS, Prasad V, Kirthi N, Maiya SP, Savithri HS, Sita GL. Development of cotton transgenics with antisense AV2 gene for resistance against cotton leaf curl virus (CLCuD) via agrobacterium tumefaciens. Plant Cell, Tissue and Organ Culture. 2005;**81**:55-63. DOI: 10.1007/s11240-004-2777-7

[51] Sahu AK, Marwal A, Nehra C, Choudhary DK, Sharma P, Gaur RK. RNAi mediated gene silencing against betasatellite associated with Croton

yellow vein mosaic begomovirus. Molecular Biology Reports. 2014;**41**:7631-7638. DOI: 10.1007/s11033-014-3653-0

[52] Marwal A, Sahu AK, Prajapat R, Choudhary DK, Gaur RK. RNA silencing suppressor encoded by Betasatellite DNA associated with Croton yellow vein mosaic virus. Open Access Scientific Reports. 2012;**1**:153. DOI: 10.4172/scientificreports.153

[53] Das S, Marwal A, Choudhary DK, Gupta VK, Gaur RK. Mechanism of RNA interference (RNAi): Current concept. In: International Proceedings of Chemical, Biological and Environmental Engineering; Singapore. Vol. 9. 2011. pp. 240-245

[54] Ali Z, Abulfaraj A, Idris A, Ali S, Tashkandi M, Mahfouz MM. CRISPR/Cas9-mediated viral interference in plants. Genome Biology. 2015;**16**:238. DOI: 10.1186/s13059-015-0799-6

[55] Worrall EA, Hamid A, Mody KT, Mitter N, Pappu HR. Nanotechnology for plant disease management. Agronomy. 2018;**8**:285. DOI: 10.3390/agronomy8120285

[56] Prajapat R, Marwal A, Gaur RK. Evidence of the Association of Solanum leaf curl Lakshmangarh virus with a weed plant *Solanum nigrum* in Rajasthan, India. Science International. 2013;**1**:379-383. DOI: 10.17311/sciintl.2013.379.383

[57] Khurana SMP, Marwal A. Recent developments towards detection & diagnosis for management of plant viruses. Indian Phytopathology. 2016;**69**:30-34

[58] Marwal A, Gaur RK. Understanding functional genomics of PTGS silencing mechanisms for tobacco streak virus and other Ilarviruses mediated by RNAi and VIGS. In: Singh DP, editor. Plant-Microbe Interactions in Agro-Ecological Perspectives. Volume 1: Fundamental Mechanisms, Methods and Functions. Singapore: Springer; 2017. pp. 489-499. DOI: 10.1007/978-981-10-5813-4_24

[59] Nehra C, Marwal A, Gaur RK. Diversity and phylogeny of Begomovirus populations and their managements. Acta Microbiologica Bulgarica. 2016;**32**:108-113

[60] Vardhan H, Marwal A, Mathur P, Prajapat R. In silico characterization of hemagglutinin protein of H1N1 subtype. International Journal of Biological Technology. 2012;**3**:62-66

[61] Marwal A, Sahu A, Sharma P, Gaur RK. Transmission and host interaction of Geminivirus in weeds. In: Gaur RK, Hohn T, Sharma P, editors. Plant Virus-Host Interaction: Molecular Approaches and Viral Evolution. Waltham, MA, US: Academic Press, Elsevier; 2014. pp. 143-161. DOI: 10.1016/B978-0-12-411584-2.00007-X

[62] Shojaei TR, Salleh MAM, Sijam K, Rahim RA, Mohsenifar A, Safarnejad R, et al. Fluorometric immunoassay for detecting the plant virus Citrus tristeza using carbon nanoparticles acting as quenchers and antibodies labeled with CdTe quantum dots. Microchimica Acta. 2016;**183**:2277-2287. DOI: 10.1007/s00604-016-1867-7

[63] Hayden O, Bindeus R, Haderspock C, Mann KJ, Wirl B, Dickert FL. Mass sensitive detection of cells, viruses, and enzymes with artificial receptors. Sensors and Actuators B: Chemical. 2003;**91**:316-319. DOI: 10.1016/S0925-4005(03)00093-5

[64] Chartuprayoon N, Rheem Y, Ng JCK, Nam J, Chend W, Myung NV. Polypyrrole nanoribbon based chemiresistive immunosensors for viral plant pathogen detection. Analytical Methods. 2013;**5**:3497-3502. DOI: 10.1039/C3AY40371H

[65] Elbeshehy EKF, Elazzazy AM, Aggelis G. Silver nanoparticles synthesis

mediated by new isolates of Bacillus spp., nanoparticle characterization and their activity against bean yellow mosaic virus and human pathogens. Frontiers in Microbiology. 2015;**6**:453. DOI: 10.3389/fmicb.2015.00453

[66] Mitter N, Worrall EA, Robinson KE, Li P, Jain RG, Taochy C, et al. Clay nanosheets for topical delivery of RNAi for sustained protection against plant viruses. Nature Plants. 2017;**3**:16207. DOI: 10.1038/nplants.2016.207

[67] Spicer CD, Jumeaux C, Gupta B, Stevens MM. Peptide and protein nanoparticle conjugates: Versatile platforms for biomedical applications. Chemical Society Reviews. 2018;**47**:3574. DOI: 10.1039/C7CS00877E

[68] Jazayeri MH, Amani H, Pourfatollah AA, Toroudi HP, Sedighimoghaddam B. Various methods of gold nanoparticles (GNPs). Conjugation to antibodies. Sensing and Bio-Sensing Research. 2016;**9**:17-22. DOI: 10.1016/j.sbsr.2016.04.002

[69] McGee CF, Storey S, Clipson N, Doyle E. Soil microbial community responses to contamination with silver, aluminium oxide and silicon dioxide nanoparticles. Ecotoxicology. 2017;**26**:449-458. DOI: 10.1007/s10646-017-1776-5

[70] Marwal A, Gaur RK, Khurana SMP. Possible approaches for developing different strategies to prevent transmission of Geminiviruses to important crops. In: Gaur RK, Khurana SMP, Dorokhov Y, editors. Plant Viruses: Diversity, Interaction and Management. Boca Raton, Florida, US: CRC Press, Taylor & Francis Group; 2018. pp. 301-319

[71] Sanfaçon H. Grand challenge in plant virology: Understanding the impact of plant viruses in model plants, in agricultural crops, and in complex ecosystems. Frontiers in Microbiology. 2017;**8**:860. DOI: 10.3389/fmicb.2017.00860

[72] Marwal A, Verma RK, Khurana SMP, Gaur RK. Molecular interactions between plant viruses and their biological vectors. In: Gaur RK, Khurana SMP, Dorokhov Y, editors. Plant Viruses: Diversity, Interaction and Management. Boca Raton, Florida, US: CRC Press, Taylor & Francis Group; 2018. pp. 205-216

[73] Das AK, Marwal A, Verma R. Plant protein-mediated green synthesis and characterization of magnetite ($Fe_3O_4$) Bionano hybrid. In: Bhoop BS, Sharma A, Mehta SK, Tripathi SK, editors. Nanotechnology: Novel Perspectives and Prospects. New Delhi, India: Tata-McGraw Hill; 2014. pp. 136-143

[74] Arts JH, Hadi M, Keene AM, Kreiling R, Lyon D, Maier M, et al. A critical appraisal of existing concepts for the grouping of nanomaterials. Regulatory Toxicology and Pharmacology. 2014;**70**:492-506. DOI: 10.1016/j.yrtph.2014.07.025

[75] San Miguel K, Scott JG. The next generation of insecticides: DsRNA is stable as a foliar-applied insecticide. Pest Management Science. 2016;**72**:801-809. DOI: 10.1002/ps.4056

[76] Ghosh SKB, Hunter WB, Park AL, Gundersen-Rindal DE. Double strand RNA delivery system for plant-sap-feeding insects. PLoS ONE. 2017;**12**:e0171861. DOI: 10.1371/journal.pone.0171861

Chapter 3

# Aspects in *Tobamovirus* Management in Intensive Agriculture

*Elisheva Smith and Aviv Dombrovsky*

## Abstract

In the recent years, disease spread of old and newly evolved tobamoviruses has occurred worldwide, affecting production of various vegetable and ornamental crops. The tobamoviruses are highly stable plant viruses that could cause severe disease symptoms. The well-known tobamovirus *Cucumber green mottle mosaic virus* (CGMMV) has recently caused severe damages in the cucumber, melon, and watermelon cucurbitaceous crops, worldwide. Similarly, a recent widespread of the newly identified tobamoviruses, *Tomato mottle mosaic virus* (ToMMV) and *Tomato brown rugose fruit virus* (ToBRFV), has reduced the solanaceous crop production. The primary route of tobamoviral infection is through mechanical means. These viruses adhere to agricultural facilities, contaminate the soil, infect seeds, and spread via beneficial pollinators and irrigation water. Mechanical plant injury suffices to initiate viral infection. Practicing hygiene by plant growers and in nurseries is currently the main strategy for mitigation of tobamoviral infection. Promoting the production of solanaceous vegetable crops genetically resistant to ToMMV and ToBRFV infection is a promising approach. However, CGMMV-resistant sources of cucurbitaceous vegetable crops are scarce. Conferring resistance to rootstocks and cross-protection strategies are newly implemented approaches that could alleviate tobamovirus disease spread in both solanaceous and cucurbitaceous crops.

**Keywords:** Solanaceae, Cucurbitaceae, primary infection, secondary spread, strobilurins, resistant rootstocks, cross-protection

## 1. Introduction

In the recent years, there has been a growing concern regarding disease damages and losses occurring in vegetable crop production. Plant viruses constitute the major causal factor for the diseases. Tomato plants, belonging to the Solanaceae family, and cucumber, melon, and watermelon plants, belonging to the Cucurbitaceae family, have shown the most severe disease symptoms. These symptoms are primarily attributed to infections by viruses belonging to the *Tobamovirus* genus, in the *Virgaviridae* family. The prevalent route of tobamovirus infection is via mechanical plant manipulations [1]. The tobamoviruses are highly stable and kept infectious in soil containing buried virus-contaminated plants [2], on various agricultural facility tool surfaces, in seeds [3], and upon adhering to beneficial pollinator body parts [4, 5]. Two tobamovirus species that had a conspicuous effect on vegetable crop production in various countries and caused severe disease symptoms in host plants are the *Tomato brown rugose fruit virus* (ToBRFV) that infected solanaceous plants [6, 7] and *Cucumber green mottle mosaic virus* (CGMMV) that infected cucurbitaceous plants [8]. An important strategy to reduce viral infection of cultivated crops is to practice hygiene during planting and to divide the planting procedures between workers. The use of appropriate chemicals for disinfection of trellising ropes, planting trays in nurseries, and the various agricultural tools, before planting, is highly recommended [9]. Importantly, the applications of highly sensitive methods to disclose virus-infected seeds [6, 10] increase the probability to sow virus-free seeds. The various maneuvers currently available for tobamoviral disease management and future strategies to alleviate tobamoviral infections are discussed below.

## 2. Tobamovirus worldwide spread

Viruses belonging to the *Tobamovirus* genus are positive-sense single-stranded RNA viruses that infect a wide range of plant species. *Tobacco mosaic virus* (TMV), first described by Mayer in 1886 [11], is the prototype of this genus, in the *Virgaviridae* family. Tobamoviruses infect vegetable crops mostly solanaceous and cucurbitaceous plants, ornamental plants, weeds, and medicinal plants. In the recent years, the spread of tobamoviruses that infect two major cultivated vegetable crops, the solanaceous and cucurbitaceous plants, has increased. The *Tomato mottle mosaic virus* (ToMMV) that infected tomato plants (*Solanum lycopersicum*) had spread in America and Spain [12, 13]. In the Middle East, ToBRFV had broken the highly durable resistance-conferring allele *Tm*-$2^2$ [6] that was introgressed into *Lycopersicon esculentum* from *L. peruvianum* [14]. Phylogenetic tree analysis showed that ToBRFV and ToMMV were clustered in separate clades [6]. ToBRFV infection of tomato plants has recently occurred in Mexico [15], Germany [16], and the USA [17]. A worldwide infection of the cucurbitaceous plants has occurred due to the spread of the tobamovirus CGMMV, first reported by Ainsworth in 1935 [8, 18]. Excluding few reports on CGMMV-resistant plants, commercial cultivars resistant to CGMMV are scarce [19, 20].

## 3. Genome organization

The genome organization of the tobamoviruses ToBRFV and CGMMV resembles in general that of TMV [21, 22]. The virus single-stranded RNA genome encodes four known proteins: short (126 or 129 kDa) and long (183 or 186 kDa) replicase-associated proteins. The long component is the outcome of a translational read-through of a termination codon of the short component. In addition, a movement protein (MP) of ~30 kDa and a coat protein (CP) of ~17 kDa are translated from sub-genomic RNA. A putative fifth 54 kDa protein resides between the two replicase-associated proteins [23]. Recently, in Solanaceae-infecting tobamoviruses, a sixth protein of 4–5 kDa has been identified, which is encoded by a region in the genome overlapping the open reading frames (ORFs) of the MP and the CP [24–26].

## 4. Particle pathogenicity and systemic disease spread

ToBRFV infection of solanaceous plants induced pathogenic systemic symptoms of narrowing leaves and yellow and brown spotted fruits. CGMMV infection of cucurbitaceous plants resulted in systemic mottle mosaic leaves and fruits as well as yellowing fruit flesh combined with necrotic peduncles (**Figure 1**). Increased severity of the symptoms could occur due to a variety of mixed infections. For example, the solanaceous tomato plants infected by both ToBRFV and the abundant tospovirus *Tomato spotted wilt virus* (TSWV) showed severe fruit necrosis (**Figure 1d**), and the cucurbitaceous cucumber plants infected by both CGMMV and the *Pythium* species *P. spinosum* showed plant wilting and collapse [27] (**Figure 1j**).

The virulence factors that caused the severe symptoms occurring upon tobamovirus infection have not been established yet excluding the virulence factor of TMV upon infection of *Nicotiana benthamiana* that was identified as the orf6-expressed protein, which occurs in Solanaceae-infecting tobamoviruses [24]. Similarly, the mechanism of *Tm*-$2^2$ resistance breaking by ToBRFV has not been discovered yet. The viral MP is the avirulence factor recognized by the plant resistance-conferring protein *Tm*-$2^2$ [28]. Mutational analysis of the MP revealed that a change of two amino acids could overcome the resistance conferred by the *Tm*-$2^2$ allele [29]. However, the MP modifications that have occurred during the evolvement of ToBRFV are still unknown, although in bioinformatics approach several potential mutations were identified in the MP of ToBRFV. In the Cucurbitaceae-infecting CGMMV, a single amino acid substitution at the replicase site resulted in symptom attenuation [30], conferring a role for the replicase in viral virulence mechanism.

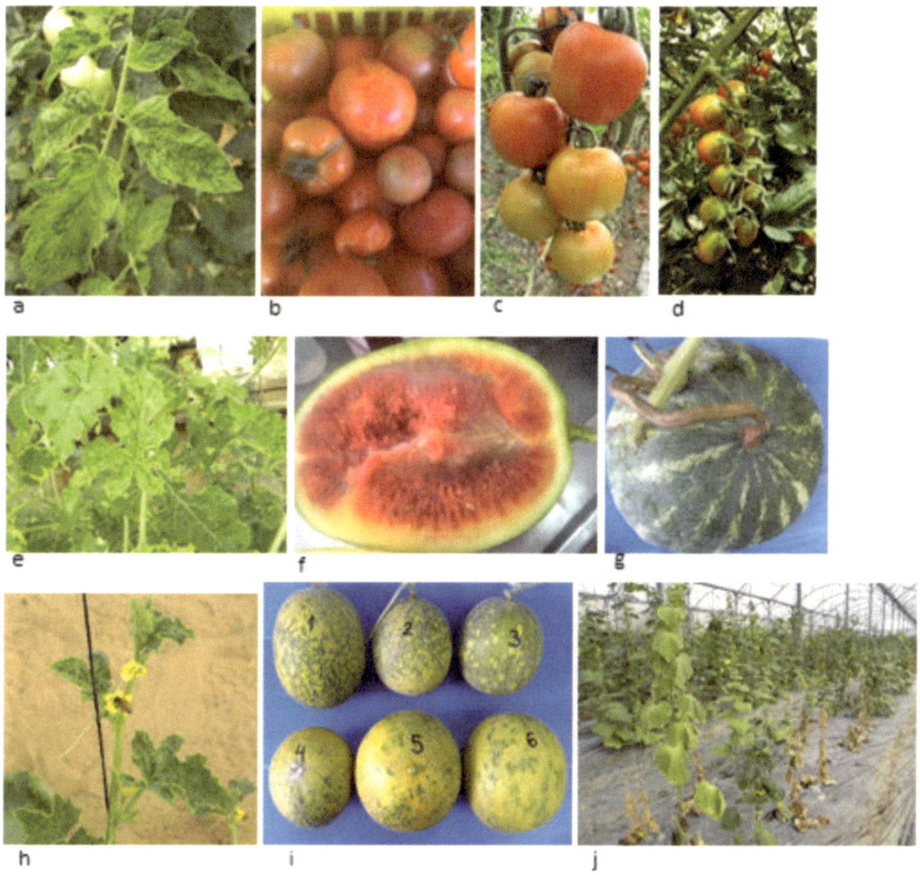


**Figure 1.**
*Tomato brown rugose fruit virus (ToBRFV) and Cucumber green mottle mosaic virus (CGMMV) infected vegetables. (a–d) ToBRFV-infected plants; (e–j) CGMMV-infected plants. (a) Narrowing tomato leaves with mosaic pattern. (b, c) Yellow and brown spotted tomato fruits. (d) Brown spotted and necrotic tomato fruits infected by both ToBRFV and Tomato spotted wilt virus. (e) Mottle mosaic pattern on watermelon leaves. (f) Yellowing and necrotic watermelons. (g) Necrotic peduncle. (h) Mosaic pattern on melon leaves. (i) Various manifestations of mottle mosaic melons. (j) Collapse of cucumber plants infected by both CGMMV and Pythium spinosum.*

The tobamovirus CP molecules constitute the capsid of the virion, which is ~300 nm long and 18 nm wide. For viral RNA encapsidation, *ca*. 2000 CP subunits form a right-handed helix in which each subunit binds three nucleotides. There are electrostatic interactions between charged amino acid residues that contribute to CP subunit interactions and particle stability, which is strengthened by hydrophobic contacts in the capsid [31] and carboxylate interactions between subunits [32]. Tobamovirus particles can survive 90°C heating and years of storage [31, 33].

Tobamovirus encapsidation is necessary for long-distance movement of the virus in the plant but is dispensable for cell-to-cell movement [34, 35]. Since viruses are localized in the symplast, it is necessary to maneuver cell-to-cell movement. Viral MP binds RNA and increases the plasmodesmata size exclusion limit [36]. The virus could then be transmitted via the widened cytoplasmic continuity that was formed between cells [37]. In addition to the MP effect on viral cell-to-cell movement, a role for the short replicase-associated protein in cell-to-cell viral movement was also observed, although the mechanism of the replicase effect is still unclear [38].

Tobamovirus CP is required for long-distance viral dissemination [34, 39]. It is required for viral movement across the boundary between vascular parenchyma and companion cells [40]. It is not quite clear, however, whether the CP is necessary for interactions with host factors [39]. In the phloem, virus particles follow photo-assimilate transportation [41]. However, mechanisms of entry and egress from the phloem differ [42, 43]. For example, egress from the phloem involves the activity of the host plant pectin methylesterase [44].

Viral genome replication that occurs in the epidermis and mesophyll cells induces plant resistance programs such as the RNA silencing process [45, 46]. Plant RNA silencing is triggered by viral double-stranded RNA precursors, which are processed by RNase III Dicer-like protein to small interfering RNA duplexes (siRNA), 21–24 nucleotide long [47, 48]. The siRNAs are stabilized by HUA ENHANCER1 (HEN1), which catalyzes methylation at the 3′ end, generating 2′-*O*-methylated siRNAs [49]. The methylation prevents uridylation and degradation of the siRNA duplexes [49, 50]. Single-stranded siRNAs direct ARGONAUTE (AGO) protein residing in RNA-induced silencing complex (RISC) to silence posttranscriptionally complementary RNA by endonucleolytic activity [51]. Importantly, small RNA duplexes that are formed by the plant silencing mechanism function also as silencing signals that spread via the plasmodesmata between cells and systemically through the phloem [52, 53]. Establishing silencing process systemically can lead to degradation of newly infecting viruses prior to viral replication [54]. Viruses counteract the plant silencing process by the expression of silencing suppressors [55, 56]. The tobamovirus short protein associated with the replicase, such as the 126 kDa protein of TMV [57] or ToMV [58] interferes with the methylation of the siRNA duplexes catalyzed by HEN1 and thereby induces degradation of the siRNAs [54]. Viral RNA silencing suppressors are therefore positive factors in viral long-distance movement [39]. However, the contribution of the replicase-associated protein to viral entry into the phloem is not clear yet but could not be attributed to suppression of RNA silencing [33].

## 5. Modes of infection

### 5.1 Primary infections

#### *5.1.1 Seeds*

Tobamoviruses are seed-borne viruses, although the average of reported seed to seedling transmission ratios was only 4.1% [3]. Low viral transmission ratios in grow-out experiments are commonly indicative of uninfected embryos. Seed coat contamination could occur due to physical attachment between the seeds and the fruit flesh. However, there were also reports on ToMV infecting the endosperm of tomato plant seeds [1]. The tobamovirus passage through the maternal seed coat to the endosperm, which originates from both maternal and paternal sources, is enigmatic in the face of the uninfected embryos [3]. The consequence of endosperm infection is problematic, in particular, for considerations of the appropriate seed disinfection procedures. CGMMV-infected cucurbitaceous seeds are the most challenging for disinfection practices. Seeds from symptomatic CGMMV-infected cucurbit plants showed tobamoviral infection of both the seed coat and the perisperm-endosperm (PE) envelope underlying the seed coat [59, 60], which is characteristic to cucurbits [61, 62]. Importantly, the PE envelope is comprised of endospermic cells on top of which noncellular lipid and callose layers were formed [61, 62]. A similar question is raised therefore regarding CGMMV occurrence in the PE envelope in the face of the uninfected embryos [59, 60]. Tobamoviral dispersal emerging from infected seeds could occur via physical manipulations of the seeds upon sowing, seed to seedling transmission, and seed coat contamination of the soil.

#### *5.1.2 Soil*

Tobamovirus soil contamination primarily occurs due to buried plant debris originated from tobamovirus-infected crops [63]. Using a serological method for ToMV detection, a high primary infection ratio, of up to 80%, apparently occurred in the tomato plants grown in the contaminated soil [63]. Under field conditions as well, ToMV was detected in soil containing tomato debris of crops originated from a previous year planting [2]. ToMV was also recovered from forest soil in which the mineral fraction had more virus than the organic fraction [64]. Clay in the soil adsorbs a high fraction of tobamovirus particles [65], which could be visualized by scanning electron microscopy. Similarly, CGMMV inoculum buried in the ground for overwintering contaminated the soil [66]. Soil contamination was apparent by CGMMV detection in the soil supernatant, by inoculating uninfected cucurbit plants with the soil supernatant and by planting uninfected cucurbit plants in the contaminated soil [66]. Various soil types mediate CGMMV dispersal in various efficiencies, which could be attributed to root damage in the case of rock containing soil.

#### *5.1.3 Beneficial pollinators*

Bumblebees (*Bombus terrestris*) are essential beneficial pollinators of tomato crop cultivation. Bumblebee hives that were placed in ToBRFV-infected tomato-growing areas were ToBRFV contaminated [5]. The virus was detected in the hive components: the comb, the enveloping cotton, and the nectar. ToBRFV in the hives was infectious as studied by inoculating the laboratory test plant *Nicotiana tabacum* cv. Samsun with virus purified from the hive comb. ToBRFV adhered to the bumblebee body parts, primarily the abdomen, suggesting that ToBRFV could be transmitted by buzz pollination. Importantly, bumblebee hives from ToBRFV-infected tomato greenhouses placed in a new greenhouse of uninfected tomato plants constituted carriers of a primary infectious inoculum. ToBRFV infection ratios of the newly infected tomato plants were 12–60%. The ToBRFV infection ratios were positively correlated with bumblebee activity [5].

### 5.2 Secondary disease spread

Tobamovirus disease spread is abiotic. Mechanical manipulations during crop cultivation and the commonly associated plant injury constitute a major route for tobamovirus disease spread. Low concentrations of tobamovirus contamination could establish the disease spread in a growing area due to mechanical manipulations [1]. For effective tobamovirus disease transmission, leaf or root injury seems imperative. Although the most common way of tobamovirus disease spread is via physical attachment, root-to-root viral transmission ratios in tobamovirus-contaminated soil are low [67]. Similarly, seeds sown in tobamovirus-contaminated soil showed low infection ratios when compared to seedling planting, which could involve plant injury [68]. However, high concentrations of the contaminating tobamoviruses and repeated exposure to the infectious source reduce the impact of injury as a necessary determinant in tobamovirus disease spread [63, 65].

### *5.2.1 Irrigation water*

Humidity preserves tobamovirus particle viability in soil. Infectious tobamovirus particles of TMV and ToMV were found in environmental waters such as ponds and streams. The occurrence of the tobamoviruses was visualized by electron microscopy, and the infectivity of the tobamovirus particles was examined in a biological assay on laboratory test plants [69]. A quantitative and sensitive approach to detect the tobamoviruses in environmental waters was also applied using sensitive reverse-transcription real-time PCR analysis [70]. Apparently, there were environmental water samples that tested positive for ToMV without the usual sample concentration step. Dispersal of the Cucurbitaceae-infecting tobamovirus CGMMV via irrigation water was tested, for example, in laboratory facilities in the Volcani Center, Israel. In the middle of a planting tray of cucumber (*Cucumis sativus*) plants, one plant was sap-inoculated with the virus and was then separated from adjacent plants by an open plastic vessel to prevent any mechanical transmission of the virus via any other way than that of the irrigation dripping system that was applied. The results inspected a month later showed that CGMMV infection ratios ranged between 36 and 91%, while the control plants were CGMMV free (Dombrovsky and Darzi, unpublished data). CGMMV transmission efficiency via dripping and flooding irrigation systems was examined in a glasshouse experiment. The distances of CGMMV infection of watermelon (*Citrullus lanatus* Thunb.) plants by dripping and flooding irrigation systems were 1.9 and 2.3 m, respectively [71]. CGMMV was also detected in a river close to a farm of CGMMV-infected muskmelon (*Cucumis melo*) and watermelon plants [72].

### *5.2.2 Plant manipulations*

Contaminated hands, pruning shears, knives, trellising ropes, and grafting procedures are the most common means for effective tobamovirus transmission. Attempts to quantitate the contribution of mechanical contact to tobamovirus disease spread revealed that a high number of repeated contacts between TMV-infected tobacco leaves and uninfected plants were positively correlated with increased tobamovirus transmission efficiency [63]. Interestingly, there was no correlation between the TMV quantity in the source leaves and the efficiency of viral transmission. Several characteristics of the source of infection could also affect transmission efficiency, such as leaf age and the viral source, whether it was the outcome of systemic spread or it was the primary inoculated material. However, the effects of these parameters on TMV disease spread were not conclusive [73]. Quantitating the disease transmission ratios of the Cucurbitaceae-infecting CGMMV in cucumber plants was conducted, for example, by touching the plants with CGMMV-contaminated hands. CGMMV contamination analyzed serologically 3 weeks post the infection procedure spread down the row, sequentially, and the infection ratio was 86% [68]. The contribution of agro-technical work of pruning and trellising to CGMMV disease spread was monitored in an experiment conducted in commercial cucumber greenhouses [68]. In the greenhouses, 5–11 scattered CGMMV-infected plants, which constituted 0.4–0.5% of the plants, were identified, and a survey was conducted on the effects of the intensive agro-technical activities on CGMMV disease spread. The percent increase in infected plants due to agro-technical practice for 40 days, in the various greenhouses, was in the range of 11–32% [68].

#### *5.2.3 Beneficial pollinators*

Beneficial pollinators do not only constitute a primary source of tobamovirus disease spread, as was observed in ToBRFV spread analysis [5], but could also promote secondary viral spread between tobamovirus-infected and uninfected plants. Hives containing bumblebees (*Bombus terrestris* L.) placed in a greenhouse of TMV-infected tomato plants (*Lycopersicon esculentum* L. cv. Momotaro) spread the TMV infection to adjacent uninfected tomato plants planted in the greenhouse. TMV viral particles attached to the bumblebee body parts were visualized by electron microscopy and tested positive for TMV in a serological assay. TMV viral particles isolated from the hive components were infectious, as analyzed in a biological assay using *Nicotiana glutinosa* seedlings for inoculation [74]. Regarding the Cucurbitaceae-infecting tobamovirus CGMMV, the honeybee *Apis mellifera* promoted disease spread between infected melon seedlings, which constituted a primary viral source, and adjacent uninfected plants [4]. Efficient secondary viral transmission between the plants occurred when the uninfected plants were placed on the path of the honeybee foraging track, between the beehive and the CGMMV-infected plants.

#### *5.2.4 Weeds*

Volunteer plants such as weeds could have an important role as tobamovirus reservoirs that may constitute a source of infection. Apparently, weed species could constitute asymptomatic reservoirs of the Cucurbitaceae-infecting tobamovirus CGMMV [75, 76]. Among the weed species susceptible to CGMMV infection that did not show any conspicuous symptom development and their susceptibility to CGMMV infection which was confirmed by laboratory mechanical inoculations were *Molucella laevis*, *Amaranthus graecizans*, and the medicinal plant *Withania somnifera* [76]. Overwintering of tobamoviruses in the weed hosts could promote the tobamovirus spread between cultivated crops of consecutive growing seasons.

## 6. Management strategies

### 6.1 Sensitive tobamovirus detection methods

In order to prevent the occurrence and establishment of tobamovirus primary infectious source introduced by virus-infected seeds, the appropriate detection methods should be applied. Viral RNA extraction (using Viral RNA Extraction Kit; Bioneer) from ToBRFV-infected tomato (*S. lycopersicum*) seeds (Luria and Dombrovsky, unpublished data) and CGMMV-infected cucumber (*C. sativus* Derben) and melon (*C. melo* Raanan) seeds were successfully executed [60]. Next-generation sequencing (NGS) platform has been successfully applied for detection of the tobamoviruses ToBRFV [6] and CGMMV [77]. The NGS detection method is highly sensitive when compared to the most commonly used serological assays (enzyme-linked immunosorbent assay, Western blot) and the genome sequence analysis performed after PCR amplification. ToBRFV-infected tomato seeds mixed with uninfected seeds in a ratio of 1:600 were successfully detected by the NGS method (Luria and Dombrovsky, unpublished data). Viral RNA extractions, which are easy to perform and need a small amount of starting material, were successfully applied in the NGS analysis [78]. The use of the new technology based on a single-molecule sequencing such as the Oxford Nanopore sequencing platform was successfully applied for detection of plant viruses and bacteria and the detection of the tobamovirus ToBRFV in infected tomato seeds. The sensitivity ratio for detection of ToBRFV-infected tomato seeds by applying the Oxford Nanopore sequencing platform was 1:200 virus-infected seeds mixed with uninfected seeds [10]. Application of sensitive methods for tobamovirus detection in seeds is most critical and needs to be developed for CGMMV-infected cucurbitaceous seeds, in which the viral particles accumulate in the PE envelope underlying the seed coat [59, 60].

### 6.2 Alleviating soil-associated tobamovirus infectivity

Soil fumigation with pesticides such as methyl bromide, which had an effect on a wide range of plant pathogens, was successfully used in various crop production facilities. However, since the elimination of its use due to its high toxicity and the detrimental effect on the ozone, several other chemicals such as chloropicrin (trichloronitromethane) had been used [79]. Unlike methyl bromide, many newly used chemicals had no effect on weeds or plant debris, and their efficiency in inactivation of tobamoviruses was questioned. A good alternative to those chemicals are products based on strobilurin fungicide, which originally occurred in the mushroom *Strobilurus tenacellus* [80]. Synthetic compounds such as pyraclostrobin (F 500) that protected the tobacco plant *N. tabacum* (cv. Xanthi nc) against TMV infection could be used in soil preplant treatment. Other chemicals that are based on natural products are alkaloids such as phenanthroquinolizidine that can be extracted from several plant families such as the Vitaceae family [81]. Several formulas of the alkaloid exhibited anti-TMV activity [81]. Similarly, quassinoids isolated from *Brucea javanica* showed anti-TMV activity [82]. Recently, the strong antiviral effect of synthesized bioactive tricyclic spirolactones, which are based on natural polycyclic compounds, has been demonstrated on TMV infection of tobacco plants [83]. Interestingly, the antibiotic Ningnanmycin showed anti-TMV activity both by induction of plant resistance against virus and by inhibition of the virus virulence [84].

Soil steaming treatment using low temperatures (50–60°C) for short time periods (several minutes) had been useful for inactivation of most plant pathogens while preserving soil microflora and minerals [85]. However, these steaming conditions could not be applied for disinfection of tobamovirus-contaminated soil [60]. Interestingly, a combination of mild steaming conditions with chemicals such as potassium hydroxide that are exothermal when reacted with water was effectively applied to disinfection of TMV-infected soil. TMV infectivity ratios were reduced to 3.0%. The increase in the persisted heat in the soil and the higher soil pH could have affected TMV stability [86]. Importantly, regarding CGMMV-contaminated soil, application of intermediate medium composed of CGMMV-free compost, which was prepared from cattle feces, into planting pits prior to planting melon (*C. melo*) seedlings, significantly reduced the initiation of primary infectious foci in the growing area. When combining removal of newly identified infected plants at early growth stage, before trellising, with the implementation of intermediate medium, CGMMV infection ratio at 60 days post planting was 0.3% [60]. Recently, growers have implemented growth bags that separate between plants, to grow various vegetable crops in order to reduce tobamovirus disease spread via soil (**Figure 2**).

Grafting vegetable crops on *Tobamovirus*-resistant rootstocks could also separate the cultivated crops from the contaminated soil. In particular, *Solanum gilo* accessions were found resistant to the tobamoviruses TMV, ToMV, and the *Pepper mild mottle virus* (PMMoV). Unfortunately, CGMMV-resistant rootstocks scarcely occur and are difficult to find. Using CGMMV-tolerant rootstocks for grafting cucumber plants in field experiment in Northern Israel resulted in viral infectivity ratios of 0.4–0.8% (2 rows, 250 plants in each row). Concomitant growth of ungrafted cucumber plants had CGMMV infectivity ratios in the range of 16–44% (5 rows, 320 plants in each row) (Dombrovsky and Koren, unpublished data). Importantly, it is preferable to use rootstocks that do not cause any reduction in crop yield. Rotations in crop cultivation could reduce buildup of primary infectious tobamovirus inoculum from contaminated soil [87]. For example, it is possible to plant tomato plants after pepper plant plantings since PMMoV does not infect tomatoes. However, because ToMV infects pepper plants, planting tomato crops should not be followed by pepper plant plantings [87]. Importantly, alternating rice and watermelon cultivation reduced CGMMV infection ratios of the watermelons by tenfold (amounting to 7.3%) when compared to consecutive watermelon cultivation [88].

### 6.3 Hygienic and careful planting procedures

The use of sodium hypochlorite solution on planting facilities and even on seeds was recommended for disinfection of tobamoviruses. However, seeds treated with the hypochlorite solution could show low germination ratios. Trisodium phosphate treatment (TSP) of tobamovirus-infected seeds was also implemented. Importantly, these commonly used disinfection procedures could not be applied for disinfection of tobamovirus-infected cucurbitaceous seeds in which the virus penetrated the seed coat and accumulated in the PE envelope underlying the seed coat [59, 60]. TSP (10%) treatment, combined with heating to 72°C for 72 hours, did not disinfect CGMMV-infected melon (*C. melo* cv. Raanan) seeds. The CGMMV detected in the treated seeds using serological assays and PCR analysis was infectious in a biological assay [60]. However, sodium hypochlorite solution and the new stabilized chlorine product, which has the active ingredient $C_3Cl_3N_3NaO_3$, could be useful for general tobamovirus disinfection of planting facilities [8] such as shears, knives, trellising ropes, planting trays, and irrigation pipes. Careful planting procedures should be implemented, avoiding the infliction of any injury to the plants. Dividing tasks between workers during planting could also reduce secondary tobamovirus

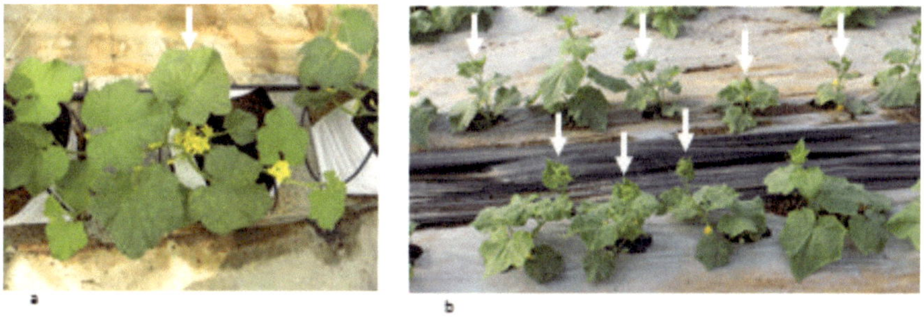


**Figure 2.**
*Limited Cucumber green mottle mosaic virus (CGMMV) infection spread in melon plants grown in growth bags. (a) Melon plants grown in growth bags. (b) CGMMV spread through soil and irrigation water in regular planting of cucumber plants. Arrows mark CGMMV-infected plants.*

infection spread. Weeding the weeds that might be reservoirs of tobamoviruses [76] and supplementing new bumblebee hives for tomato plant cultivation [5] could be important in preventing primary inoculum of tobamovirus infection. Identification and removal of tobamovirus-infected plants in crop cultivation facilities at early stages, before trellising, could reduce secondary tobamovirus disease spread.

### 6.4 Near-future management strategies

In the face of the genetic tobamovirus resistance occurring in tomato plants for many years, such as that of the durable *Tm*-$2^2$ resistance allele [14], a search for ToBRFV-resistant tomato plants could be successful. However, CGMMV-resistant genetic sources for introgression into commercial cucurbitaceous vegetable crop cultivation are scarce [19, 20]. Similarly, sources for CGMMV-resistant rootstocks are limited. Engineering transgenic watermelon rootstocks by transformation of the rootstock *Citrullus lanatus* (Twinser) cv. Gongdae with CGMMV CP gene conferred viral resistance to the plants [89], similar to the phenomenon observed in TMV CP-mediated resistance against TMV [90]. Another approach that could confer viral resistance to susceptible host plants while avoiding the production of transgenic crops is the use of clustered regularly interspaced short palindromic repeats (CRISPR)/Cas9 genome editing technology [91]. This mutagenesis system is targeted by guide RNAs to a desired site in the plant cell genome, where Cas9 endonuclease causes double-stranded DNA breaks. The system exploits host cellular repair mechanisms to confer heritable high fidelity change in the genome. Host endogenous genes, such as the *Arabidopsis thaliana TOM1* and *TOM3* genes, and their homologues in tomato and melon plants, are necessary for tobamovirus replication [92, 93]. The host proteins translated from these genes comprise a complex with the tobamovirus replication protein [94]. These host proteins could be targeted by the CRISPR/Cas9 system. Importantly, RNA silencing of these host genes conferred tobamovirus resistance in *Nicotiana tabacum* [95] and in tomatoes [96]. Interestingly, RNA silencing, which is systemic [52, 53, 97], could be transmitted from rootstocks to scions. Hence, engineering rootstocks alone for tobamovirus resistance by RNA silencing of these host genes could confer resistance to the non-transgenic grafted tomato or melon plants. When using the biocontrol approach, plant defense mechanisms that specifically target the infecting tobamovirus, such as the RNA silencing, could be initiated by infecting the susceptible plants with a stable attenuated virus clone or a mutagenized variant of the virus. For example, several attenuated strains were successfully applied to protect tomato plants against ToMV infection, pepper plants against PMMoV infection [98], and muskmelon and cucumber [99] plants against CGMMV infection. However, mutagenized clones might not always be stable, and symptoms might develop in the susceptible plants. Therefore, in order to implement the cross-protection approach, for example, against ToBRFV that infects tomato plants harboring the *Tm*-$2^2$ resistance allele, it might be beneficial to infect the tomato plants with the stable ToMV that does not show symptoms in the resistant tomato plants. For that purpose, ToMV needs to infect systemically the *Tm*-$2^2$ resistant tomato plants.

## 7. Conclusions

In the recent years, tobamovirus disease spread has been one of the core causes for severe damages observed in various vegetable and ornamental crop productions. Concomitantly, there has been an increase in suggested strategies for tobamovirus disease management. The basic approach of implementing hygienic behavior while planting has been improved by dividing the planting procedures between workers combined with soil disinfection or the use of intermediate tobamovirus-free medium. This new approach reduced tobamovirus infection substantially. Concurrently, new improved soil disinfectants based on naturally occurring products such as the strobilurin fungicide or plant alkaloids have been produced, eliminating possible harmful side effects of the disinfectants on animals and the environment. Improved methods for detection of tobamovirus-infected seeds have been developed as well. In addition, applicable in the near future are methods exploiting new molecular biology techniques, such as genome editing, to develop tobamovirus-resistant plants. Similarly, methods that engage the plant defense system to invoke resistance to tobamoviruses have been developed, such as the use of attenuated viral strains for plant infection or the use of engineered resistant plants as rootstocks.

## Acknowledgements

We thank Amnon Koren, Neta Luria, Elinor Darzi, and Oded Lachman for assistance in data collection.

## Author details

Elisheva Smith and Aviv Dombrovsky*
Institute of Plant Pathology and Weed Research, Agricultural Research Organization, The Volcani Center, Rishon LeZion, Israel

*Address all correspondence to: aviv@agri.gov.il

## References


[1] Broadbent L. The epidemiology of tomato mosaic. XI. Seed transmission of TMV. The Annals of Applied Biology. 1965;(56):177-205

[2] Lanter JM, McGuire JM, Goode MJ. Persistence of tomato mosaic virus in tomato debris and soil under field conditions. Plant Disease. 1982;**66**(7): 552-555

[3] Dombrovsky A, Smith E. Seed transmission of tobamoviruses: Aspects of global disease distribution. In: Advances in Seed Biology. InTech; 2017

[4] Darzi E, Smith E, Shargil D, Lachman O, Ganot L, Dombrovsky A. The honey bee *Apis mellifera* contributes to *Cucumber green mottle mosaic virus* spread via pollination. Plant Pathology. 2018;**67**(1):244-251

[5] Levitzky N, Smith E, Lachman O, Luria N, Mizrahi Y, Bakelman H, et al. The bumblebee *Bombus terrestris* carries a primary inoculum of Tomato brown rugose fruit virus contributing to disease spread in tomatoes. PLoS One. 2019;**14**(1):e0210871

[6] Luria N, Smith E, Reingold V, Bekelman I, Lapidot M, Levin I, et al. A new Israeli tobamovirus isolate infects tomato plants Harboring *Tm*-$2^2$ resistance genes. PLoS One. 2017;**12**(1):e0170429

[7] Salem N, Mansour A, Ciuffo M, Falk B, Turina M. A new tobamovirus infecting tomato crops in Jordan. Archives of Virology. 2016;**161**(2): 503-506

[8] Dombrovsky A, Tran-Nguyen LT, Jones RA. Cucumber green mottle mosaic virus: Rapidly increasing global distribution, etiology, epidemiology, and management. Annual Review of Phytopathology. 2017;**55**(1):231-256

[9] Baker C, Adkins S. Peppers, tomatoes, and tobamoviruses: Division of Plant Industry, Florida Department of Agriculture & Consumer Svcs.; 2000

[10] Chalupowicz L, Dombrovsky A, Gaba V, Luria N, Reuven M, Beerman A, et al. Diagnosis of plant diseases using the nanopore sequencing platform. Plant Pathology. 2018;**68**(2):229-238

[11] Mayer A. Über die Mosaikkrankheit des Tabaks (in German). Die Landwirtschaftliche Versuchs-stationen. 1886;**32**:451-467

[12] Ambros S, Martinez F, Ivars P, Hernandez C, de la Iglesia F, Elena SF. Molecular and biological characterization of an isolate of Tomato mottle mosaic virus (ToMMV) infecting tomato and other experimental hosts in a greenhouse in Valencia, Spain. bioRxiv 063255. 2016; DOI: http://doi.org/10.1101/063255

[13] Webster CG, Rosskopf EN, Lucas L, Mellinger HC, Adkins S. First report of tomato mottle mosaic virus infecting tomato in the United States. Plant Health Progress. 2014;**15**(4):151-152

[14] Lanfermeijer FC, Warmink J, Hille J. The products of the broken *Tm*-2 and the durable *Tm*-$2^2$ resistance genes from tomato differ in four amino acids. Journal of Experimental Botany. 2005;**56**(421):2925-2933

[15] Cambrón-Crisantos JM, Rodríguez-Mendoza J, Valencia-Luna JB, Rangel SA, de Jesús García-Ávila C, López-Buenfil JA. First report of Tomato brown rugose fruit virus (ToBRFV) in Michoacan. Mexican Journal of Phytopathology. 2018;**37**(1):185-192

[16] Menzel W, Knierim D, Winter S, Hamacher J, Heupel M. First report of tomato brown rugose fruit virus infecting tomato in Germany. New Disease Reports. 2019;**39**(1):2044-0588

[17] Ling K-S, Tian T, Gurung S, Salati R, Gilliard A. First report of tomato brown rugose fruit virus infecting greenhouse tomato in the US. Plant Disease. 2019;**103**(6):1439

[18] Ainsworth GC. Mosaic disease of cucumber. The Annals of Applied Biology. 1935;**22**:55-67

[19] Rajamony L, More T, Seshadri V, Varma A. Reaction of muskmelon collections to cucumber green mottle mosaic virus. Journal of Phytopathology. 1990;**129**(3):237-244

[20] Sugiyama M, Ohara T, Sakata Y. Inheritance of resistance to Cucumber green mottle mosaic virus in *Cucumis melo* L.'Chang Bougi'. Journal of the Japanese Society for Horticultural Science. 2007;**76**(4):316-318

[21] Goelet P, Lomonossoff GP, Butler PJ, Akam ME, Gait MJ, Karn J. Nucleotide sequence of tobacco mosaic virus RNA. Proceedings of the National Academy of Sciences of the United States of America. 1982;**79**(19):5818-5822

[22] Ugaki M, Tomiyama M, Kakutani T, Hidaka S, Kiguchi T, Nagata R, et al. The complete nucleotide sequence of cucumber green mottle mosaic virus (SH strain) genomic RNA. The Journal of General Virology. 1991;**72**(7):1487-1495

[23] Zaitlin M. Elucidation of the genome organization of tobacco mosaic virus. Philosophical Transactions of the Royal Society of London. Series B: Biological Sciences. 1999;**354**(1383):587-591

[24] Canto T, MacFarlane SA, Palukaitis P. ORF6 of tobacco mosaic virus is a determinant of viral pathogenicity in *Nicotiana benthamiana*. The Journal of General Virology. 2004;**85**(10):3123-3133

[25] Cooper B. Proof by synthesis of tobacco mosaic virus. Genome Biology. 2014;**15**(5):R67

[26] Morozov SY, Denisenko O, Zelenina D, Fedorkin O, Solovyev A, Maiss E, et al. A novel open reading frame in tobacco mosaic virus genome coding for a putative small, positively charged protein. Biochimie. 1993;**75**(8):659-665

[27] Philosoph AM, Dombrovsky A, Elad Y, Jaiswal AK, Koren A, Lachman O, et al. Combined infection with Cucumber green mottle mosaic virus and *Pythium* species causes extensive collapse in cucumber plants. Plant Disease. 2017;**102**(4):753-759

[28] Chen T, Liu D, Niu X, Wang J, Qian L, Han L, et al. Antiviral resistance protein *Tm*-$2^2$ functions on the plasma membrane. Plant Physiology. 2017;**173**(4):2399-2410

[29] Weber H, Schultze S, Pfitzner A. Two amino acid substitutions in the tomato mosaic virus 30-kilodalton movement protein confer the ability to overcome the *Tm*-2 (2) resistance gene in the tomato. Journal of Virology. 1993;**67**(11):6432-6438

[30] Liu L, Peng B, Zhang Z, Wu Y, Miras M, Aranda MA, et al. Exploring different mutations at a single amino acid position of Cucumber green mottle mosaic virus replicase to attain stable symptom attenuation. Phytopathology. 2017;**107**(9):1080-1086

[31] Gibbs A. Tobamovirus classification. In: Van Regenmortel M.H.V. Fraenkel-Conrat H. editors. The Plant Viruses. The Viruses. Springer: Boston, MA; 1986. p. 167-180

[32] Caspar D. Assembly and stability of the tobacco mosaic virus particle. Advances in Protein Chemistry. 1964;**18**:37-121

[33] Solovyev A, Makarov V. Helical capsids of plant viruses: Architecture with structural lability. The Journal of General Virology. 2016;**97**(8):1739-1754

[34] Saito T, Yamanaka K, Okada Y. Long-distance movement and viral assembly of tobacco mosaic virus mutants. Virology. 1990;**176**(2):329-336

[35] Hilf ME, Dawson WO. The tobamovirus capsid protein functions as a host-specific determinant of long-distance movement. Virology. 1993;**193**(1):106-114

[36] Carrington JC, Kasschau KD, Mahajan SK, Schaad MC. Cell-to-cell and long-distance transport of viruses in plants. The Plant Cell. 1996;**8**(10):1669

[37] Maule AJ, Benitez-Alfonso Y, Faulkner C. Plasmodesmata–membrane tunnels with attitude. Current Opinion in Plant Biology. 2011;**14**(6):683-690

[38] Hirashima K, Watanabe Y. Tobamovirus replicase coding region is involved in cell-to-cell movement. Journal of Virology. 2001;**75**(18):8831-8836

[39] Hipper C, Brault V, Ziegler-Graff V, Revers F. Viral and cellular factors involved in phloem transport of plant viruses. Frontiers in Plant Science. 2013;**4**:154

[40] Ding B, Kwon MO, Warnberg L. Evidence that actin filaments are involved in controlling the permeability of plasmodesmata in tobacco mesophyll. The Plant Journal. 1996;**10**(1):157-164

[41] Maule AJ, Palukaitis P. Virus movement in infected plants. Critical Reviews in Plant Sciences. 1991;**9**(6):457-473

[42] Roberts AG, Cruz SS, Roberts IM, Prior DA, Turgeon R, Oparka KJ. Phloem unloading in sink leaves of *Nicotiana benthamiana*: Comparison of a fluorescent solute with a fluorescent virus. The Plant Cell. 1997;**9**(8):1381-1396

[43] Cheng NH, Su CL, Carter SA, Nelson RS. Vascular invasion routes and systemic accumulation patterns of tobacco mosaic virus in *Nicotiana benthamiana*. The Plant Journal. 2000;**23**(3):349-362

[44] Chen MH, Citovsky V. Systemic movement of a tobamovirus requires host cell pectin methylesterase. The Plant Journal. 2003;**35**(3):386-392

[45] Ding S-W, Voinnet O. Antiviral immunity directed by small RNAs. Cell. 2007;**130**(3):413-426

[46] Conti G, Rodriguez MC, Venturuzzi AL, Asurmendi S. Modulation of host plant immunity by tobamovirus proteins. Annals of Botany. 2017;**119**(5):737-747

[47] Bartel DP. MicroRNAs: Target recognition and regulatory functions. Cell. 2009;**136**(2):215-233

[48] Gasciolli V, Mallory AC, Bartel DP, Vaucheret H. Partially redundant functions of *Arabidopsis* DICER-like enzymes and a role for DCL4 in producing trans-acting siRNAs. Current Biology. 2005;**15**(16):1494-1500

[49] Ren G, Chen X, Yu B. Small RNAs meet their targets: When methylation defends miRNAs from uridylation. RNA Biology. 2014;**11**(9):1099-1104

[50] De Almeida C, Scheer H, Zuber H, Gagliardi D. RNA uridylation: A key posttranscriptional modification shaping the coding and noncoding transcriptome. Wiley Interdisciplinary Reviews: RNA. 2018;**9**(1):e1440

[51] Baumberger N, Baulcombe D. Arabidopsis ARGONAUTE1 is an RNA slicer that selectively recruits microRNAs and short interfering RNAs.

Proceedings of the National Academy of Sciences. 2005;**102**(33):11928-11933

[52] Kalantidis K, Schumacher HT, Alexiadis T, Helm JM. RNA silencing movement in plants. Biology of the Cell. 2008;**100**(1):13-26

[53] Dunoyer P, Schott G, Himber C, Meyer D, Takeda A, Carrington JC, et al. Small RNA duplexes function as mobile silencing signals between plant cells. Science. 2010;**328**(5980):912-916

[54] Vogler H, Akbergenov R, Shivaprasad PV, Dang V, Fasler M, Kwon M-O, et al. Modification of small RNAs associated with suppression of RNA silencing by tobamovirus replicase protein. Journal of Virology. 2007;**81**(19):10379-10388

[55] Silhavy D, Burgyán J. Effects and side-effects of viral RNA silencing suppressors on short RNAs. Trends in Plant Science. 2004;**9**(2):76-83

[56] Voinnet O. Induction and suppression of RNA silencing: Insights from viral infections. Nature Reviews Genetics. 2005;**6**(3):206-220

[57] Ding XS, Liu J, Cheng N-H, Folimonov A, Hou Y-M, Bao Y, et al. The tobacco mosaic virus 126-kDa protein associated with virus replication and movement suppresses RNA silencing. Molecular Plant-Microbe Interactions. 2004;**17**(6):583-592

[58] Kubota K, Tsuda S, Tamai A, Meshi T. Tomato mosaic virus replication protein suppresses virus-targeted posttranscriptional gene silencing. Journal of Virology. 2003;**77**(20):11016-11026

[59] Shargil D, Zemach H, Belausov E, Lachman O, Luria N, Molad O, et al. Insights into the maternal pathway for cucumber green mottle mosaic virus infection of cucurbit seeds. Protoplasma. 2019;**256**(4):1109-1118

[60] Reingold V, Lachman O, Blaosov E, Dombrovsky A. Seed disinfection treatments do not sufficiently eliminate the infectivity of *Cucumber green mottle mosaic virus* (CGMMV) on cucurbit seeds. Plant Pathology. 2015;**64**(2):245-255

[61] Yim K-O, Bradford KJ. Callose deposition is responsible for apoplastic semipermeability of the endosperm envelope of muskmelon seeds. Plant Physiology. 1998;**118**(1):83-90

[62] Ramakrishna P, Amritphale D. The perisperm-endosperm envelope in Cucumis: Structure, proton diffusion and cell wall hydrolysing activity. Annals of Botany. 2005;**96**(5):769-778

[63] Pares RD, Gunn LV, Keskula EN. The role of infective plant debris, and its concentration in soil, in the ecology of tomato mosaic tobamovirus—A non-vectored plant virus. Journal of Phytopathology-Phytopathologische Zeitschrift. 1996;**144**(3):147-150

[64] Fillhart RC, Bachand GD, Castello JD. Detection of infectious tobamoviruses in forest soils. Applied and Environmental Microbiology. 1998;**64**(4):1430-1435

[65] Dornai D, Mingelgrin U, Frenkel H, Bar-Joseph M. Direct quantification of unadsorbed viruses in suspensions of adsorbing colloids with the enzyme-linked-immunosorbent-assay. Applied and Environmental Microbiology. 1993;**59**(9):3123-3125

[66] Li JX, Liu SS, Gu QS. Transmission efficiency of Cucumber green mottle mosaic virus via seeds, soil, pruning and irrigation water. Journal of Phytopathology. 2016;**164**(5):300-309

[67] Koh S, Li H, Sivasithamparam K, Admiraal R, Jones M, Wylie S. Low root-to-root transmission of a tobamovirus, yellow tailflower mild mottle virus, and

resilience of its virions. Plant Pathology. 2018;**67**(3):651-659

[68] Reingold V, Lachman O, Belausov E, Koren A, Mor N, Dombrovsky A. Epidemiological study of *Cucumber green mottle mosaic virus* in greenhouses enables reduction of disease damage in cucurbit production. The Annals of Applied Biology. 2016;**168**(1):29-40

[69] Jeżewska M, Zarzyńska-Nowak A, Trzmiel K. Detection of infectious tobamoviruses in irrigation and drainage canals in Greater Poland. Journal of Plant Protection Research. 2018;**58**(2):202-205

[70] Boben J, Kramberger P, Petrovič N, Cankar K, Peterka M, Štrancar A, et al. Detection and quantification of Tomato mosaic virus in irrigation waters. European Journal of Plant Pathology. 2007;**118**(1):59-71

[71] Li JX, Liu SS, Gu QS. Transmission efficiency of *Cucumber green mottle mosaic virus* via seeds, soil, pruning and irrigation water. Journal of Phytopathology. 2015;**5**(5):300-309

[72] Vani S, Varma A. Properties of cucumber green mottle mosaic virus isolated from water of river Jamuna. Indian Phytopathology. 1993;**46**(2):118-122

[73] Sacristán S, Díaz M, Fraile A, García-Arenal F. Contact transmission of tobacco mosaic virus: A quantitative analysis of parameters relevant for virus evolution. Journal of Virology. 2011;**85**(10):4974-4981

[74] Okada K, Kusakari S, Kawaratani M, Negoro J, Ohk ST, Osak T. Tobacco mosaic virus is transmissible from tomato to tomato by pollinating bumblebees. Journal of General Plant Pathology. 2000;**66**:71-74

[75] Boubourakas I, Hatziloukas E, Antignus Y, Katis N. Etiology of leaf chlorosis and deterioration of the fruit interior of watermelon plants. Journal of Phytopathology. 2004;**152**(10):580-588

[76] Shargil D, Smith E, Lachman O, Reingold V, Darzi E, Tam Y, et al. New weed hosts for *Cucumber green mottle mosaic virus* in wild Mediterranean vegetation. European Journal of Plant Pathology. 2016;**148**(2):473-480

[77] Kehoe MA, Jones RA, Coutts BA. First complete genome sequence of Cucumber green mottle mosaic virus isolated from Australia. Genome Announcements. 2017;**5**(12):e00036-e00017

[78] Luria N, Smith E, Sela N, Lachman O, Koren A, Dombrovsky A. Insights into a watermelon virome contribute to monitoring distribution of whitefly-borne viruses. Phytobiomes. 2019;**3**(1):2471-2906

[79] Duniway J. Status of chemical alternatives to methyl bromide for pre-plant fumigation of soil. Phytopathology. 2002;**92**(12):1337-1343

[80] Sauter H, Steglich W, Anke T. Strobilurins: Evolution of a new class of active substances. Angewandte Chemie, International Edition. 1999;**38**(10):1328-1349

[81] Wang Z, Feng A, Cui M, Liu Y, Wang L, Wang Q. First discovery and stucture-activity relationship study of phenanthroquinolizidines as novel antiviral agents against tobacco mosaic virus (TMV). PLoS One. 2012;**7**(12):e52933

[82] Shen JG, Zhang ZK, Wu ZJ, Ouyang MA, Xie LH, Lin QY. Antiphytoviral activity of bruceine-D from *Brucea javanica* seeds. Pest Management Science: Formerly Pesticide Science. 2008;**64**(2):191-196

[83] Zhu YJ, Wu QF, Fan ZJ, Huo JQ, Zhang JL, Zhao B, et al. Synthesis,

bioactivity and mode of action of 5A5B6C tricyclic spirolactones as novel antiviral lead compounds. Pest Management Science. 2019;**75**(1):292-301

[84] Han Y, Luo Y, Qin S, Xi L, Wan B, Du L. Induction of systemic resistance against tobacco mosaic virus by Ningnanmycin in tobacco. Pesticide Biochemistry and Physiology. 2014;**111**:14-18

[85] van Loenen MC, Turbett Y, Mullins CE, Feilden NE, Wilson MJ, Leifert C, et al. Low temperature–short duration steaming of soil kills soil-borne pathogens, nematode pests and weeds. European Journal of Plant Pathology. 2003;**109**(9):993-1002

[86] Luvisi A, Panattoni A, Materazzi A. Heat treatments for sustainable control of soil viruses. Agronomy for Sustainable Development. 2015;**35**(2):657-666

[87] Albrechtsen SE. Testing methods for seed-transmitted viruses: Principles and protocols. CABI. 2006

[88] Park J-W, Jang T-H, Song S-H, Choi H-S, Ko S-J. Studies on the soil transmission of CGMMV and its control with crop rotation. The Korean Journal of Pesticide Science. 2010;**14**(4):473-477

[89] Park SM, Lee JS, Jegal S, Jeon BY, Jung M, Park YS, et al. Transgenic watermelon rootstock resistant to CGMMV (*Cucumber green mottle mosaic virus*) infection. Plant Cell Reports. 2005;**24**(6):350-356

[90] Bendahmane M, Fitchen JH, Zhang G, Beachy RN. Studies of coat protein-mediated resistance to tobacco mosaic tobamovirus: Correlation between assembly of mutant coat proteins and resistance. Journal of Virology. 1997;**71**(10):7942-7950

[91] Zaidi SS-e-A, Tashkandi M, Mansoor S, Mahfouz MM. Engineering plant immunity: Using CRISPR/Cas9 to generate virus resistance. Frontiers in Plant Science. 2016;**7**

[92] Yamanaka T, Ohta T, Takahashi M, Meshi T, Schmidt R, Dean C, et al. TOM1, an Arabidopsis gene required for efficient multiplication of a tobamovirus, encodes a putative transmembrane protein. Proceedings of the National Academy of Sciences. 2000;**97**(18):10107-10112

[93] Ishikawa M, Okada Y. Replication of tobamovirus RNA. Proceedings of the Japan Academy, Series B. 2004;**80**(5):215-224

[94] Ishibashi K, Ishikawa M. The resistance protein *Tm*-1 inhibits formation of a tomato mosaic virus replication protein-host membrane protein complex. Journal of Virology. 2013;**87**(14):7933-7939

[95] Asano M, Satoh R, Mochizuki A, Tsuda S, Yamanaka T, Nishiguchi M, et al. Tobamovirus-resistant tobacco generated by RNA interference directed against host genes. FEBS Letters. 2005;**579**(20):4479-4484

[96] Ali ME, Ishii Y, Taniguchi J-i, Waliullah S, Kobayashi K, Yaeno T, et al. Conferring virus resistance in tomato by independent RNA silencing of three tomato homologs of Arabidopsis TOM1. Archives of Virology. 2018;**163**(5):1357-1362

[97] Dunoyer P, Brosnan CA, Schott G, Wang Y, Jay F, Alioua A, et al. Retracted: An endogenous, systemic RNAi pathway in plants. The EMBO Journal. 2010;**29**(10):1699-1712

[98] Ichiki T, Nagaoka E, Hagiwara K, Uchikawa K, Tsuda S, Omura T. Integration of mutations responsible for the attenuated phenotype of pepper mild mottle virus strains

results in a symptomless cross-protecting strain. Archives of Virology. 2005;**150**(10):2009-2020

[99] Slavokhotova AA, Istomina EA, Andreeva EN, Korostyleva TV, Pukhalskij VA, Shijan AN, et al. An attenuated strain of *Cucumber green mottle mosaic virus* as a biological control agent against pathogenic viral strains. American Journal of Plant Sciences. 2016;**7**(05):724-732

Chapter 4

# Plant Metabolites in Plant Defense Against Pathogens

*Xóchitl S. Ramírez-Gómez, Sandra N. Jiménez-García, Vicente Beltrán Campos and Ma. Lourdes García Campos*

## Abstract

Medicinal plants are widely used worldwide to treat various diseases. Its widespread use is due in part to the cultural acceptance of traditional medicine in different regions of the world, as well as its effectiveness in treating various diseases. Many of its active substances or secondary metabolites are formed to a response of various situations that generate stress in their habitat, such as sudden changes in environmental temperature, humidity, rain, drought, and infections by phytopathogens (fungi, bacteria, viruses, nematodes, protozoa). The production of these secondary metabolites is a mechanism of defense of plants. In this context, the objective of this chapter is to study the secondary metabolites of medicinal plants that could have a promising application in the control of different phytopathogens in crops of agricultural and economic interest.

**Keywords:** medicinal plants, phytopathogens, secondary metabolites, pesticides, biotic and abiotic elicitors

## 1. Introduction

Phytopathogens generally attack plants during their growth, causing alterations in their cellular metabolism and/or interfering with the absorption of nutrients [1]. The crops of cereals, vegetables, and fruits are affected by these organisms during harvest and postharvest [2]. However, one of the main control measures to eradicate phytopathogens is the use of pesticides. Although they are effective, easy to access, and easy to use, they have several disadvantages, generate resistance, and are considered toxic substances, not only for bacteria, fungi, viruses, protozoa, and nematodes but also for the humans, animals, and the environment [3, 4]. In this context, the pesticides can induce acute and chronic toxicity, to persist in the environment and pollute soil and water. So, they are easily incorporated into the food chain, bioaccumulation, and biomagnification [5]. Regarding their toxicity mechanisms, it has been described that they can act as endocrine disruptors and as reactive species that generate oxidative stress in the cell [6–9].

On the other hand, the study of medicinal plants as possible natural sources of obtaining active compound (secondary metabolites) against phytopathogens has gained increasing interest in recent years, due to several aspects, mainly that they are obtained from a natural source through the production or synthesis of secondary metabolites considered as nontoxic such as phenols, flavonoids, terpenes, alkaloids, etc. [10–13]. Another advantage is that phytopathogens still do not develop resistance to the antifungal, antimicrobial, and nematicide effect of the phytochemical compounds produced by some medicinal plants. When carrying out an exhaustive search in the literature, it was found that the potential use of the secondary metabolites obtained from medicinal plant extracts is fungicide [14–16]. Most of the research in this area focuses on evaluating the effects of these active compounds on fungi such as *Fusarium*, maybe because it is one of the main phytopathogens that cause economic losses mainly in cereal crops and health problems by their aflatoxins [17, 18]. This chapter shows an overview of the recent research on this topic, emphasizing the effect of biotic and abiotic elicitors on the secondary metabolite production, as well as a brief description of the scientific name of the plant, metabolites with antifungal and antibacterial effect, and their limitations and perspectives of its use in the biological control of phytopathogens.

## 2. Pesticides in the control of phytopathogens

In the market, there are a variety of pesticides that are used alone or in combination to eradicate, control, or prevent pests [4]. Pesticides can be classified according to the chemical group to which they belong, to their selectivity toward a certain phytopathogen, its mechanism of action, and its use or application. However, the most widely used for their effectiveness and a broad spectrum of activity against various pests and diseases in plants are insecticides, herbicides, and fungicides [4, 19].

Pesticides used in agriculture mainly contaminate the soil by direct application and water by leaching, and it is very easy for them to be present either in trace quantities or high in food and to enter the food chain, which facilitates its accumulation and biomagnification [5, 20]. In general pesticides are considered dangerous substances for living beings since they can produce acute or chronic toxicity; however the magnitude of the poisoning depends on several aspects to be considered such as the physicochemical characteristics of the pesticide, the concentration, the exposure time, the route of entry to organisms, their toxicodynamics and toxicokinetics (absorption, distribution, half-life, metabolism, and elimination), as well as the use of mixtures of different pesticides, the components of their formulation, and the general state of health of the individual [21, 22]. All these aspects influence that pesticides represent a risk or danger for those who use them in the fields of cultivation, as well as for those who consume foods that contain substances in trace quantities in prolonged consumption.

Regarding its toxicity, it has been described that pesticides act as endocrine disruptors and generators of free radicals and enzymatic inhibitors [8, 9]. Unfortunately, the cellular targets to which most of these pesticides are directed coincide with cellular targets that are also present in man, such as the case of the mechanisms of action of organophosphorus insecticides, which inhibit the activity of acetylcholinesterase enzyme present in different insects; unfortunately man and other mammals also have acetylcholinesterase, so their toxicity is not selective toward the pests that they wish to control, but they also affect man, and depending on the magnitude of the poisoning, they can cause death [19–22]. However, until today an ideal pesticide does not exist, and the correct use of herbicides, fungicides, insecticides, etc. has many benefits to control plagues and increase the yield of the crops [19].

## 3. Secondary metabolites of medicinal plants as biological control of phytopathogens

There are several methods of biological control against phytopathogens. The use of extracts of medicinal plants to eradicate diseases in crops caused mainly by viruses, bacteria, and fungi is one of them [23]. The above makes sense if we analyze the fact that plants have mechanisms to protect themselves from both biotic and abiotic stress agents. That is, if the phytopathogens (biotic agents) are attacking the plants, why not think what the plant does to defend itself?

In this context, it is interesting to analyze the secondary metabolism of plants know which phytochemical substances are produced and what biological activity they present.

### 3.1 The bioactive potential of secondary metabolites derived from the medicinal plant

Plants are formed by a primary metabolism that is responsible for the physiological processes and development of the plant, such as lipids, carbohydrates, and proteins [23]. The secondary metabolism is not essential in the basic processes of plants. However, these bioactive compounds play an important role in the defense of plants, and these secondary metabolites can be classified as phenolic compounds, carotenoids, terpenes, alkaloids, and sulfur compounds, among others, as shown in **Table 1** [24].

Phenolic compounds are aromatic substances formed during the passage of the shikimic acid pathway or mainly the mevalonic pathway. These can be divided into insoluble compounds such as condensed tannins, lignins, and hydroxamic acids bound to the cell walls, and soluble compounds are phenolic acids, flavonoids, and kinases [25]. Carotenoids are lipophilic molecules and are found in plants giving orange tones. The importance of these compounds is the intervention they have in photosynthesis, and they also protect the photosynthetic apparatus from excess

| Classification | Types | Example |
|---|---|---|
| **Terpenes** | Monoterpene | Geraniol |
| | Sesquiterpenes | Humulene |
| | Diterpenes | Cafestol |
| | Sesterpenes | Geranylfarsol |
| | Triterpenes | Squalene |
| | Sesquarterpenes | Ferrugicadiol |
| | Tetraterpenes | Lycopenes |
| | Polyterpenes | Gutta-percha |
| **Phenolics** | Coumarin | Hydroxycoumarins |
| | Furano-coumarins | Psoralin |
| | Lignin | Resveratrol |
| | Flavonoids | Quercitin |
| | Isoflavonoids | Genistein |
| | Tanins | Tanins acid |
| **N Containing Compounds** | Alkaloids | Cocaine |
| | Cyanogenic glucosides | Dhurrin |
| | Non-Protein amino acids | Canavanin |
| **S Containing compounds** | Glutathione | |
| | Glucosinolate | β-D-Glucopyrinose |
| | Thionins | |
| | Defensins | |
| | Allinin | |

**Table 1.**
*Types of plant secondary metabolites.*

energy [25]. The carotenoid contents in plants are affected by various factors, such as plant development, stress conditions, postharvest conditions, or cooking treatments, but the interest of these compounds has been increasing due to their potential antioxidant activity [26]. Terpenes are lipid-soluble compounds that include one- or more five-carbon isoprene units, which are synthesized by all organisms through two pathways, mevalonate and deoxy-D-xylulose [27]. Terpenoids are classified according to the number of isoprene units they contain; terpenes and terpenoids are basic constituents of many types of plant essential oils [28]. Alkaloids are bioactive compounds that generally contain nitrogen derived from an amino acid of great importance because it has physiological and medicinal properties, for example, caffeine, nicotine, morphine, atropine, and quinine [29].

Now well, all these compounds mentioned above help the plants to develop complex defense systems against different types of stress for the survival or the systematic forces in their metabolism for resistance against pests and diseases. Stress provoked in the plant involves several signaling response pathways for pathogens and insects, and some of these response pathways are induced by the microorganisms themselves. Also, the plants have specific recognition and signaling systems allowing them to detect the pathogens and initiate an effective defense response [30, 31]. The defence system broadest have the plants against pathogens are the phenolic compounds (phenylpropanoids and flavonoids). These substances have different mechanisms of action they can dissociate the ions of the phenolic hydroxyl and forming phenolates, ionic and hydrogen bonds with peptides and proteins causing a high astringency and protein denaturation. In the other hand, they interfere with the pathogen's cell signalling compounds and affect their physiological activities through enzymatic inhibition, DNA alkylation and altering their reproductive system [31]. The compounds with allelopathic effects affect positively or negatively on the ecosystem's structure to remove or eliminate microorganisms from the plants. Some phenolic compounds are allelochemicals that have been shown to have an activity as antibiotics, antifungals, and antipredator [31]. Phenolic acids, such as benzoic, hydroxybenzoic, vanillic, and caffeic, have antimicrobial and antifungal properties produced by the inhibition of enzymes. Caffeic, chlorogenic, sinapic, ferulic, and p-coumaric acids have antioxidant activity by the inhibition of oxidation of lipids and the elimination of reactive oxygen species. These effects are important to the plant defense [32].

### 3.2 Improving production of plant secondary metabolites through biotic and abiotic stresses

Classification of secondary metabolites related to the defense of plants is commonly used in the form of synthesis and accumulation of phytochemicals with interaction effect of the pathogenic plant against plant insect, virus, fungi, and antibacterial compounds. For example, phytoalexins are produced very quickly after infection of a pathogen producing toxicity to an ambiguous environment of fungi or bacteria [33, 34].

Phenylpropanoids and flavonoids have hydroxyl groups that contain phenolic compounds, which dissociate into phenolate ions, and the phenolic hydroxyl groups form ionic bonds and hydrogen bonds with peptides and protons, producing a high astringency and denaturation that thus show an antifungal effect acting together with cellular signaling compounds and physiological activities or acting on the parts of the pathogen, reproductive system, enzymatic inhibition, etc. [35]. The properties of the proteins change with any change in protein conformation, for example, by changing the three-dimensional structure forming covalent bonds with SH, OH or free amino groups there is inactivation or protein function loss. When polyphenols of the plants bind to some proteins of phytopathogens are less toxic for them but can protect the plant of abiotic elicitors [36]. On the other hand, phytoalexins are induced against the attack of microbes and insects activated by β-glucosidase by the release of biocidal aglycones [37]. In the same way act the benzoxazinoids (BX), these phytochemical compounds are produced and released by tissue damage and hydrolysis by β-glucosidase and act as insect repellents too [38].

At present, several biotechnological strategies have been used to increase the productivity of secondary metabolites, using different inducers of secondary metabolites such as at the cellular, organic, and plant levels, as well as the most effective methods to improve the synthesis of these secondary metabolites in endemic and medicinal plants [39]. These secondary metabolites accumulate in plants when they are prone to various stress types, inducers, or signal molecules. Thus, there are different modulating factors of secondary metabolites, as well as microbial, physical, or chemical effects such as abiotic or biotic elicitors, inducing the biosynthesis of specific compound that plays an important role in the adaptations of plants to stress conditions, and these phenomena cause a greater synthesis and accumulation of secondary metabolites [40]. In **Table 2** the authors focus on the abiotic elicitors that are substances of biological origin such as proteins and carbohydrates that are initiator compounds or coupling responses at the cellular level activating several enzymes or signaling canals. There are also microorganisms and chemical compounds with elicitor effect that stress the plant and produce the expression of a greater amount of metabolites or new metabolites which cause physiological changes in the plant against pathogens. As shown in **Table 2**, glycoprotein-type proteins produce phytoalexins that have been used to identify ion channels in cell membranes and thus transfer signals by external stimuli, as demonstrated by Alami [41] where the *Plantanus x acerifolia* cultures were applied to an inducer of *Ceratocystis fimbriata* f. sp. These, in turn, induced the synthesis of phytoalexins (hydroxycoumarin, scopoletin, and umbelliferone), and upon isolating the glycoprotein produced the synthesis of coumarin by 80%. On the other hand, oligogalacturonic acids are found in the cell wall of the plant inducing the biosynthesis of phytoalexins, whereas chitin is found in the cell wall of fungi, generating signaling factors in plants such as *Hypericum perforatum* production stress in the plant and increasing the production of phenolic compounds for their defense against pathogens [39, 42]. Rhizobacteria function as modelers of secondary metabolites with pharmacological activity. Rhizobacteria colonize the rhizospheres of the plants and improve the growth of the plant, being localized in the bark or root nodules acting as inducers of the enzymes that participate in the metabolic pathways of bioactive compounds and jasmonic acid biosynthesis; these act as signal transducers [43, 44]. Other signal inducers are the mycorrhizal fungi that help the plant to absorb more water and show defense against other pathogens such as fungi, bacteria, or parasites that affect the roots of the plant. These mycorrhizal fungi produce secondary metabolites such as phenolic compounds and alkaloids, among others [45–48]. Elicitors such as salicylic acid, jasmonic acid, hydrogen peroxide, chitosan, etc. act as plant hormones in the expression of genes interacting as target signaling causing a physiological response in the plant which increases the production of phenolic compounds, vitamin C, carotenoids, or defense stimuli against pathogens; there are also synergistic effects between salicylic acid and jasmonic acid providing resistance against pathogens by the induction of the octadecanoic acid pathway [49–52, 53].

On the other hand, **Table 3** shows some research that has the influence of different abiotic elicitors that are considered substance and that are not of biological origin such as salt, drought, light or heavy metals, and temperature, among others. **Table 3** shows different perspectives of research on medicinal or aromatic plants in hydroponic crops, outdoors, and the application of elicitors in different stages of growth or postharvest. For example, heavy metals such as $Al^{3+}$, $Cr^{3+}$, $Co^{2+}$, $Ni^{2+}$,

| Classification | Elicitor/ Species | Compounds | Plant Species | References |
|---|---|---|---|---|
| Proteins | Glycoprotein | Coumarin | *Plantanus acerifolia* | [41] |
| Carbohydrates | Chitosan | Phytoalexin | *Nicotiana tabacum*<br>*Eschscholzia californica* | [54] |
| | Ologogalacturonic acid | Saponin | *Panax ginseng* | [55] |
| | Ologogalacturonic acid | Trans-resveratrol<br>Viniferins | *Vitis vinifera* | [56] |
| | Chitin<br>Pectin | Hipericin<br>Pseudohypericin | *Hipericum perforatum* | [39] |
| | Chitin | Phenilpropanoid<br>Naphtodianthrone | *Hipericum perforatum* | [42] |
| | Chitosan | Curcumin | *Curcuma longa* L. | [40] |
| | Chitosan | Withaferin | *Wiyhania somnifera* | [57] |
| Plant growth promoting rhizobacteria (PGPR) | *Pseudomonas putida*<br>*Pseudomonas fluorescens* | Cis-Thujone Camphor<br>1,8-cineole | *Salvia officinalis* | [58] |
| | *Pseudomonas fluorescens*<br>*Bacillus subtilis*<br>*Azospirillum brasilense*<br>*Bacillus solanum* | γ- terpinene Trans-sabinene hydrate<br>Cis- sabinene hydrate<br>Thymol | *Origanum majoricum* | [59] |
| | *Glomus aggregatum*<br>*Bacillus coagulans*<br>*Trichoderma harzianum* | Phenols<br>Tannins<br>Flavonoids<br>Saponins<br>Alkaloids | *Solanum viarum* | [43] |
| | *Bacillus polymyxa*<br>*Pseudomonas putida*<br>*Azotobacter chroococcum*<br>*Glomus intraradices* | Stevioside | *Stevia rebaudiana* | [42] |
| | *Bacillus subtilis* | Phenolic compounds (gallic, cinnamic, ferulic acid) | *Ocimum basilicum* | [60] |
| | *Pseudomonas flurescens*<br>*Azopirillum brasilense* | Monoterpenes<br>Phenolic compounds | *Tagetes minuta* | [61] |
| Fungus | *Fusarium oxysporum*<br>*Botrytis cinerea* | Phenylpropanoid<br>Naphtodianthrone | *Hypericum perforatum* | [42] |
| | *Phytopthora megaspema*<br>*Rhizopus arrhizus* | Alkaloids (tropane) | *Datura stramonium* | [45] |
| | *Aspergillus niger* | Rosmarinic acid | *Ocimum basilium* | [46] |
| | *Rhizostonia solani* | Sesquiterpenes | *Hyoscyamus muticus* | [47] |
| Phytohormones | Abscisic acid<br>Gibberellin | Phenolic acids<br>Tanshinones | *Salvia miltiorrhiza* | [48, 62] |
| | Ethylene | Anthocyanin | *Fragaria ananassa* | [63] |
| | Gibberellic acid | Caffeic acid derivatives | *Echinacea pupurea* | [64] |
| Elicitors | Salicylic acid | Stilbene<br>Tanshinones<br>Monoterpene<br>Gymnemic acid | *Vitis vinifera*<br>*Salvia miltiorrhiza*<br>*Houttuynia cordata*<br>*Gymnema sylvestre* | [49-52] |
| | Methyl salicilate | Withaferin A | *Withania somnifera* | [57] |
| | Methyl Jasmonate | Anthocynin<br>Stilbene<br>Trans-resveratrol<br>Rosmarinic acid<br>Saponin<br>Soyasaponin | *Vitis vinifera*<br>*Mentha piperita*<br>*Glycyrrhiza globa* | [56, 53, 54] |
| | Jasmonic acid | Plumgagin | *Plumbago indica*<br>*Plumbago rosea* | [53] |

**Table 2.**
*Effect of biotic elicitor on the production of various secondary metabolites in plants [54–64].*

| Classification | Elicitor/ Species | Compounds | Plant Species | References |
|---|---|---|---|---|
| Heavy metals | $Al^{3+}$, $Cr^{3+}$, $Co^{2+}$, $Ni^{2+}$, $Cu^{2+}$, $Zn^{2+}$, $Cd^{2+}$ | Sesquiterpenoid<br>Lubimin<br>3-hydroxylubimin | *Datura stramonium* | [70, 71] |
| | $Ag^{+}$ | Atropine | *Salvia castanea*<br>*Datura metel* | [72] |
| | $Cd^{2+}$, $Co^{2+}$, $Ag^{+}$ | Resveratrol | *Vitis vinifera* | [73] |
| | $Ca^{2+}$, $Mg^{2+}$, $Mn^{2+}$, $n^{2+}$, $Cu^{2+}$, $Fe^{2+}$, $Co^{2+}$ | Betalain | *Beta vulgaris* | [74] |
| Temperature | High temperature | Hypericin<br>Hyperforin<br><br>Ginsenoside | *Hypericum perforatum*<br><br><br>*Panax quinqufolius* | [65, 75] |
| | Low temperature | Melatonin<br>Anthocyanin | *Rhodiola cremulata*<br>*Melastoma malabathricum* | [66, 78] |
| Light | UV-B light | Vinblastine<br>Vincristine | *Catharanthus roseus* | [66] |
| | UV-C irradiation | Flavonoid<br>Stilbene | *Catharanthus roseus* | [78] |
| | Light radiation | Anthocyanins | *Melastoma malabathric* | [77] |
| Salinity | Salinity | Sorbitol<br>Jasmonic acid<br>Flavonoids<br>Anthocyanin<br>GABA<br>Phenylpropeno | *Lycopersicum esculentum*<br>*Hordeum vulgare*<br>*Brivillea ilicifolia*<br>*G. Arenaria*<br>*Sesamum indicum* | [67-79] |
| Drought | Drought stress | Rosmarinic<br>Ursolic<br>Oleanolic acid | *Prunella vulagaris* | [80] |
| | Water Stress | Salvianolic acid | *Salvia miltiorrhiza* | [68] |
| | Drought | Steviol glycosides | *Stevia rebaudiana* | [69] |
| | Water<br>Osmotic imbalance | Hypericin | *Hypericum perforatum* | [81] |

**Table 3.**
*Effect of abiotic elicitor on the production of various secondary metabolites in plants [70–81].*

$Cu^{2+}$, $Zn^{2+}$, and $Cd^{2+}$, among others, are considered high toxicity compounds depending on the concentrations applied in the sprinkler system or because they are used as biocontrol since they alter the production of metabolites in plants. Similarly, Zobayed [65] demonstrated that the temperature in high concentrations in *Panax quinqufolius* improves the senescence of the leaves and produces a greater quantity of bioactive compounds in the root of the plant. So the investigations using high or low temperatures demonstrate the production of secondary metabolites, but the temperatures that have been investigated the most are the low producing physiological changes in the plant, increasing the lignification by the production of suberin in the cell wall and the metabolites such as sorbitol, raffinose, proline, melatonin, anthocyanins, etc. However, light by means of ultraviolet radiations generates the production of essential oils and phenolic compounds and decreases the production of toxic compounds in some plants [66]. On the other hand, salinity and drought produce death leading to cellular dehydration or osmotic stress and in certain concentrations can reduce the growth or development of plants but alter many physiological and metabolic processes that stimulate the production of polyphenolic compounds, anthocyanins, terpenes, and alkaloids, among others. Salinity can be produced in plants by ionic or osmotic means and drought by environmental or intentional changes due to water deficit which are always accompanied by temperature or solar radiation [67–69]. Then we can say that the biotic and abiotic factors are modular secondary metabolites influencing the metabolic level and the production of secondary metabolites. Therefore, the current research focuses on the use of elicitors, for the regulation of metabolic pathways, and target signaling in genes that influence the overproduction of secondary metabolites using various applications but taking care of the production performance of fruits, vegetables, or different plants.

Recent studies focused on evaluating the secondary metabolites of medicinal plants that are active against phytopathogens show that the potential use that these compounds can have in the future is for the control of phytopathogenic fungi, mainly against different species of *Fusarium* [14–16]. In this regard, the most active compounds have been found mainly in the essential oil obtained from the aerial parts of various medicinal plants, which suggests that the bioactive compounds are liposoluble; this may explain why they are active mainly against fungi, because the cell wall of these specimens are composed mainly of ergosterol, the active liposoluble compounds present in the essential oil to easily cross the cell wall of the fungus and in the interior act on their cell target, or they can alter the permeability of the wall of the fungus [82]. It can cause rupture and lysis of the fungal cell; however, it is necessary to study the toxicodynamics of these substances in order for them to know how to act in the fungi cell. On the other hand, the antifungal activity has been evaluated in *vitro*, by the agar diffusion and microdilution method; in general terms the range of the evaluated IC50 varies in a range that goes from 0.0035 to 8 mg/ml of the extract. It is important to mention that one of the main limitations of these studies is that this activity has only been evaluated at the laboratory level [83–85]. **Table 4** shows different types of extracts made with medicinal plants, and their biological activity reported *in vitro* tests at the laboratory level.

Finally, in the realization of a retrospective of the secondary metabolite modulating factors in our workgroup, Garcia-Mier [95] demonstrated that the use of mixtures of elicitors such as jasmonic acid, hydrogen peroxide, and chitosan in different concentrations applied in various stages of plant development of the sweet bell red pepper and in different stages of ripening of the fruit has a positive effect on the increase of polyphenolic and carotenoid compounds, where the results showed that the maturation stage of 95% produces a greater quantity of bioactive compounds. On the other hand, Vargas-Hernández [96] demonstrated that the foliar application of hydrogen peroxide in *Capsicum chinense* Jacq. has an effect on the antimicrobial activity, where the different concentrations of hydrogen peroxide potentiated the production of secondary metabolites such as flavonoids, capsaicin, and dihydrocapsaicin, where these metabolites had an effect on microorganisms such as *Staphylococcus aureus*, *Escherichia coli*, *Streptococcus mutant*, *Salmonella thompson*, *Listeria monocytogenes*, *Streptococcus faecalis*, and *Candida albicans*, and the results showed that the application of hydrogen peroxide increases the inhibitory effect against pathogenic microorganisms, showing greater activity against *S. aureus*, *S. Thompson*, and *C. albicans* in the jaguar variety, while the variety Chichen-Itza was more potent against *E. faecalis* and *E. coli*. Also, Zunun-Pérez [97] evaluated the effect of modulating factors of secondary metabolites by spray application that is performed in *Capsicum annuum* L. in weekly applications and 1 day before collection with elicitors such as hydrogen peroxide, salicylic acid, and oligosaccharide of xyloglucan on capsiate concentration and the expression of genes such as phenylalanine ammonia-lyase, aminotransferase, capsaicin synthase, and β-keto acyl synthase where the results showed that hydrogen peroxide in weekly applications significantly increases capsiate concentrations and gene expression and the yields of the production of the plant are not affected by the application of these elicitors.

| Medicinal Plant | Type of Extract | Phytochemistry Compounds | Biological Activity Aginst | Reference |
|---|---|---|---|---|
| *Acacia farnesiana* | Hydroalcoholic extract | Tannins<br>Flavonoids<br>Saponins<br>Alkaloids<br>Triterpenes<br>Quinones | *Pyricularia grisea*<br>*Phythophthora parasitica* var. *nicotianae* | [86] |
| *Artemisia herba alba* | Aqueous extract | Tannins<br>Flavonoids<br>Saponins<br>Steroids<br>Alkaloids | *Fusarium graminearum*<br>*Fusarium sporotrichioides* | [87] |
| *Asphodelus tenuifolius* | Aqueous extract | Tannins<br>Flavonoids<br>Steroids<br>Alkaloids | *Fusarium graminearum*<br>*Fusarium sporotrichioides* | [87] |
| *Bauhinia galpinii* | Methanol:Dichloromethane extract | Phenols<br>Flavonoids | *Aspergillus parasiticus*<br>*Aspergillius flavus* | [88] |
| *Breonadia salicina* | Hexane and Methanol extracts | No data | *Penicillium janthinellum*<br>*Trichoderma harzianum*<br>*Fusarium oxysporum* | [89] |
| *Bucida buceras* | Hexane, Dichloromethane, Acetone and Methanol extracts | No data | *Penicillium janthinellum*<br>*Penicillium expansum*<br>*Trichoderma harzianum*<br>*Fusarium oxysporum* | [89] |
| *Carpobrotus eludis* | Methanol:Dichloromethane extract | Phenols<br>Flavonoids | *Aspergillus parasiticus* | [88] |
| *Cotula cinerea* | Aqueous extract | Tannins<br>Flavonoids<br>Saponins<br>Alkaloids | *Fusarium graminearum*<br>*Fusarium sporotrichioides* | [87] |
| *Euphorbia guyoniana* | Aqueous extract | Tannins<br>Flavonoids<br>Saponins<br>Steroids<br>Alkaloids<br>Anthocyanins | *Fusarium graminearum*<br>*Fusarium sporotrichioides* | [87] |
| *Harpephyllum caffrum* | Acetone and Methanol extracts<br><br>Methanol:Dichloromethane extract | No data<br><br>Phenols<br>Flavonoids | *Penicillium janthinellu*,<br>*Trichoderma harzianum*<br>*Fusarium oxysporum*<br><br>*Aspergillus parasiticus*<br>*Aspergillus ochraceous* | [88, 89] |
| *Maesa lanceolata* | Methanol:Dichloromethane extract | Phenols<br>Flavonoids | *Aspergillus parasiticus* | [88] |
| *Milletia grandis* (E. Mey) | Aqueous, Methanol:Dichloro methane extracts | Phenols<br>Flavonoids | *Aspergillus ochraceous*<br>*Fusarium graminearum*<br>*Furasium oxysporum* | [88] |
| *Morinda citrifolia* L. | Essential oil | Methyl octanoate,<br>Octanoic acid,<br>Ethyl octanoate,<br>Isopentyl hexanoate,<br>3- Methyl-2-butenyl hexanoate,<br>3-Methylbutyl octanoate,<br>Methylbutyl-2-enyl octanoate | *Exserohilum turcicum* | [90] |
| *Olinia ventosa* | Hexane, Dichloromethane, Acetone and Methanol extracts | No data | *Trichoderma harzianum* | [89] |
| *Parthenium hysterophorus* | Hydroalcoholic extract | Tannins<br>Flavonoids<br>Saponins<br>Amino acids<br>Triterpenes<br>Phenols | *Pyricularia grisea*<br>*Phytophthora parasitica* var. *nicotianae*.<br>*Phythophthora parasitica*<br>*Fusarium oxysporium*<br>*Stemphylium solani* Weber | [86] |
| *Pluchea carlinensi* | Hydroalcoholic extract | Phenols<br>Tannins<br>Flavonoids<br>Saponins<br>Steroids<br>Alkaloids<br>Quinone | *Pyricularia grisea*<br>*Phytophthora parasitica* var. *nicotianae*.<br>*Phythophthora parasitica*<br>*Fusarium oxysporium*<br>*Stemphylium solani* Weber | [86] |

| | | | | |
|---|---|---|---|---|
| *Ricinus communis* | Methanol:Dichloromethane extract | Phenols Flavonoids | *Aspergillus parasiticus* *Fusarium verticillioides* | [88] |
| *Salvia africana- lutea* L. | Methanol:Dichloromethane extract | Propanoic acid, Dodecane Phosphoric acid, Glycerol, Succinic acid, Malic acid Pentadecane, Rythronic acid, Xylitol, Ribitol, 2-keto-1-gluconic acid, 1,3-dibromobicyclon, D-fructose, Fructose oxime, D-glucose, D- | *Fusarium verticillioides* *Fusarium proliferatum* | [91] |
| | | mannose, D-galactose, Sedoheptulose, o-methyloxime, Galactonic acid, Hexadecanoic acid Myo-inositol, Mannitol Caffeic acid, Octadecanoic acid, Alpha-D-glucopyranoside, Octacosane | | |
| *Solanum panduriforme* | Methanol:Dichlomethane extract | Phenols Flavonoids | *Aspergillius parasiticus* *Aspergillius ochraceous* *Fusarium graminearum* *Fusarium oxysporum* | [88] |
| *Solidago canadensis L.* | Essential oil | Germacrene D, limonene, α-pinene, β-elemene, and bornyl acetate. Camphene, α-caryophyllene, sesquisabinene bicyclosesquiphellandrene, β-cadinene, β-caryophyllene, β-pinene, β-sabinene Hydrocarbon monoterpenes, Oxygenated monoterpenes, Sesquiterpene hydrocarbons | *Monilinia fructicola* *Botrytis cinerea* *Aspergillus niger* *Penicillium expansum* *Bacillus megaterium* *Clavibacter michiganensis* *Xanthomonas campestris* *Pseudomonas fluorescens* *Pseudomonas syringae* pv. *phaseolicola* | [92] |
| *Thymus capitatus* | Essential oil | Thymol Carvacrol | *Aspergillus niger* *Aspergillus oryzae* *Penicillium digitatum* *Fusarium solani* | [93] |
| *Vangueria infausta* | Dichloromethane and Acetone extracts | No data | *Aspergillius parasiticus* *Trichoderma harzianum* | [89] |
| *Viola odorata L.* | Methanol:Water extract | Cyclotides: cyO2, cyO3, cyO13, and cyO19 | *Fusarium oxysporum* *Fusarium graminearum* *Fusarium culmorum* *Mycosphaerella fragariae* *Botrytis cinerea* *Pseudomonas. syringae* pv. *syringae* *Pectobacterium atrosepticum* *Dickeya dadantii* | [94] |
| *Waburgia salutaris* | Methanol:Dichlomethane extract | Phenols Flavonoids | *Aspergillius parasiticus* *Aspergillius ochraceous* *Fusarium verticillioides* *Fusarium oxysporum* | [88] |
| *Xylotheca kraussiana* | Dichloromethane and Acetone extracts | No data | *Trichoderma harzianum* *Fusarium oxysporum* | [89] |
| *Ziziphus mucronata* | Methanol:Dichlomethane extract | Phenols Flavonoids | *Fusarium graminearum* | [88] |

**Table 4.**
*Secondary metabolites of medicinal plants with biological activity against phytopathogens [86–94].*

## 4. Conclusions

The phytochemicals that produce medicinal plants derived from their secondary metabolism represent a safe and effective alternative to control various phytopathogens that affect various crops of agricultural products of economic and nutritional interest. There are different challenges in the use of biopesticides obtained from medicinal plants, such as evaluating the costs of obtaining these compounds on a large scale or exploring the possibility of them being obtained through chemical synthesis to increase yield and reduce costs. On the other hand, the various studies that exist on the effectiveness of these compounds are only at the laboratory level, which is why it is still necessary to explore and evaluate their effectiveness at the greenhouse and field levels.

## Acknowledgements

The authors would like to acknowledge the University of Guanajuato for the grant of this publication.

## Conflict of interest

The authors declare no conflict of interest.

## Author details

Xóchitl S. Ramírez-Gómez[1*], Sandra N. Jiménez-García[2], Vicente Beltrán Campos[1] and Ma. Lourdes García Campos[1]

1 Department of Clinical Nursing, Division of Health Sciences and Engineering, University of Guanajuato, Celaya, Guanajuato, Mexico

2 Department of Nursing and Obstetrics, Division of Health Sciences and Engineering, University of Guanajuato, Celaya, Guanajuato, Mexico

*Address all correspondence to: xosofira2002@yahoo.com.mx

## References


[1] Jones JDG, Dangl JL. The plant immune system. Nature. 2006;**444**: 323-329. DOI: 10.1038/nature05286

[2] FHIA. Post-Harvest Deterioration of Fresh Fruits and Vegetables by Fungi and Bacteria [Internet]. 2007. Available from: http://www.fhia.org.hn/dowloads/fhia_informa/fhiainfdic2007.pdf [Accessed: 04 January 2019]

[3] Gene SM, Hoekstra PF, Hannam C, White M, Truman C, Hanson ML, et al. The role of vegetated buffers in agriculture and their regulation across Canada and the United States. Journal of Environmental Management. 2019;**243**: 12-21. DOI: 10.1016/j.jenvman.2019.05.003

[4] Sun C, Chen L, Zhai L, Liu H, Jiang Y, Wang K, et al. National assessment of spatiotemporal loss in agricultural pesticides and related potential exposure risks to water quality in China. Science of the Total Environment. 2019;**677**:98-107. DOI: 10.1016/j.scitotenv.2019.04.34

[5] Katagi T. Bioconcentration, bioaccumulation, and metabolism of pesticides in aquatic organisms. Reviews of Environmental Contamination and Toxicology. 2010;**204**:1-132. DOI: 10.1007/978-1-4419-1440-8_1

[6] Pelkonen O, Bennekou SH, Crivellente F, Terron A, Hernandez AF. Integration of epidemiological findings with mechanistic evidence in regulatory pesticide risk assessment: EFSA experiences. Archives of Toxicology. 2019:1-10. DOI: 10.1007/s00204-019-02467-w

[7] Panseri S, Chiesa L, Ghisleni G, Marano G, Boracchi P, Ranghieri V, et al. Persistent organic pollutants in fish: Biomonitoring and cocktail effect with implications for food safety. Food Additives & Contaminants. Part A, Chemistry, Analysis, Control, Exposure & Risk Assessment. 2019;**36**:601-611. DOI: 10.1080/19440049.2019.1579926

[8] Hao Y, Zhang H, Zhang P, Yu S, Ma D, Li L, et al. Chlorothalonil inhibits mouse ovarian development through endocrine disruption. Toxicology Letters. 2019;**303**:38-47. DOI: 10.1016/j.toxlet.2018.12.011

[9] Abolhassani M, Asadikaram G, Paydar P, Fallah H, Aghaee-Afshar M, Moazed V, et al. Organochlorine and organophosphorus pesticides may induce colorectal cancer; a case-control study. Ecotoxicology and Environmental Safety. 2019;**178**: 168-177. DOI: 10.1016/j.ecoenv.2019.04.030

[10] Żaczek M, Weber-Dąbrowska B, Górski A. Phages in the global fruit and vegetable industry. Journal of Applied Microbiology. 2015;**118**:537-556. DOI: 10.1111/jam.12700

[11] Pino-Otín MR, Ballestero D, Navarro E, González-Coloma A, Val J, Mainar AM. Ecotoxicity of a novel biopesticide from *Artemisia absinthium* on non-target aquatic organisms. Chemosphere. 2019;**216**:131-146. DOI: 10.1016/j.chemosphere.2018.09.071

[12] Pino-Otín MR, Val J, Ballestero D, Navarro E, Sánchez E, González-Coloma A, et al. Ecotoxicity of a new biopesticide produced by *Lavandula luisieri* on non-target soil organisms from different trophic levels. Science of the Total Environment. 2019;**671**: 83-93. DOI: 10.1016/j.scitotenv.2019.03.293

[13] Yamada T, Hamada M, Floreancig P, Nakabachi A. Diaphorin, a polyketide synthesized by an intracellular symbiont of the Asian citrus psyllid, is potentially harmful for biological control agents. PLoS One. 2019;**14**:e0216319. DOI: 10.1371/journal.pone.0216319

[14] Mafakheri H, Mirghazanfari SM. Antifungal activity of the essential oils of some medicinal plants against human and plant fungal pathogens. Cellular and Molecular Biology. 2018;**64**:13-19

[15] Isaac GS, Abu-Tahon MA. *In vitro* antifugal activity of medicinal plant extract against *Fusarium oxysporum* F. sp. *lycopersici* race 3 the causal agent of tomato wilt. Acta Biologica Hungarica. 2014;**65**:107-118. DOI: 10.1556/ABiol.65.2014.1.10

[16] Askarne L, Talibi I, Boubaker H, Boudyach EH, Msanda F, Saadi B, et al. Use of Moroccan medicinal plant extracts as botanical fungicide against citrus blue mould. Letters in Applied Microbiology. 2013;**56**:37-43. DOI: 10.1111/lam.12012

[17] Mohamed EZ. Impact of mycotoxins on humans and animals. Journal of Saudi Chemical Society. 2011;**15**: 129-144. DOI: 10.1016/j.jscs.2010.06.006

[18] Molina A, Chavarría G, Alfaro-Cascante M, Leiva A, Granados-Chinchilla F. Mycotoxins at the start of the food chain in Costa Rica: Analysis of six Fusarium toxins and ochratoxin a between 2013 and 2017 in animal feed and aflatoxin M1 in dairy products. Toxins. 2019;**11**:E312. DOI: 10.3390/toxins11060312

[19] Thiour-Mauprivez C, Martin-Laurent F, Calvayrac C, Barthelmebs L. Effects of herbicide on non-target microorganisms: Towards a new class of biomarkers? Science of the Total Environment. 2019;**684**:314-325. DOI: 10.1016/j.scitotenv.2019.05.230

[20] Tahir HM, Basheer T, Ali S, Yaqoob R, Naseem S, Khan SY. Effect of pesticides on biological control potential of *Neoscona theisi* (Araneae: Araneidae). Journal of Insect Science. 2019;**19**:pii:17. DOI: 10.1093/jisesa/iez024

[21] Brunton LL, Chabner BA, Knollman B. Goodman & Gilman's the Pharmacological Basis of Therapeutics. 12th ed. Vol. 17-39. United States: McGraw-Hill; 2012. pp. 123-143

[22] Katzung BG, Masters SB, Trevor AJ. Basic & Clinical Pharmacology. 12th ed. United States: McGraw-Hill; 2013. pp. 37-68

[23] Jimenez-Garcia SN, Guevara-Gonzalez RG, Miranda-Lopez R, Feregrino-Perez AA, Torres-Pacheco I, Vazquez-Cruz MA. Functional properties and quality characteristics of bioactive compounds in berries: Biochemistry, biotechnology, and genomics. Food Research International. 2013;**54**:1195-1207. DOI: 10.1016/j.foodres.2012.11.004

[24] Jimenez-Garcia SN, Vazquez-Cruz MA, Guevara-Gonzalez RG, Torres-Pacheco I, Cruz-Hernandez A, Feregrino-Perez AA. Current approaches for enhanced expression of secondary metabolites as bioactive compounds in plants for agronomic and human health purposes—A review. Polish Journal of Food and Nutrition Sciences. 2013;**63**:67-78. DOI: 10.2478/v10222-012-0072-6

[25] Khalid M, Rahman S-u, Bilal M. Role of flavonoids in plant interactions with the environment and against human pathogens—A review. Journal of Integrative Agriculture. 2019;**18**:211-230. DOI: 10.1016/s2095-3119(19)62555-4

[26] Zhao C, Liu Y, Lai S, Cao H, Guan Y, San Cheang W, et al. Effects of domestic cooking process on the chemical and biological properties of dietary phytochemicals. Trends in Food Science and Technology. 2019;**01**:55-66. DOI: 10.1016/j.tifs.2019.01.004

[27] Sahebi M, Hanafi MM, van Wijnen AJ, Akmar ASN, Azizi P, Idris AS, et al. Profiling secondary metabolites of plant defence mechanisms and oil palm in

response to *Ganoderma boninense* attack. International Biodeterioration and Biodegradation. 2017;**122**:151-164. DOI: 10.1016/j.ibiod.2017.04.016

[28] Valduga AT, Gonçalves IL, Magri E, Delalibera FJR. Chemistry, pharmacology and new trends in traditional functional and medicinal beverages. Food Research International. 2019;**120**:478-503. DOI: 10.1016/j.foodres.2018.10.091

[29] Chakraborty P. Herbal genomics as tools for dissecting new metabolic pathways of unexplored medicinal plants and drug discovery. Biochime Open. 2018;**6**:9-16. DOI: 10.1016/j.biopen.2017.12.003

[30] Jamwal K, Bhattacharya S, Puri S. Plant growth regulator mediated consequences of secondary metabolites in medicinal plants. Journal of Applied Research on Medicinal and Aromatic Plants. 2018;**9**:26-38. DOI: 10.1016/j.jarmap.2017.12.003

[31] Frérot B, Leppik E, Groot AT, Unbehend M, Holopainen JK. Chemical signatures in plant-insect interactions. In: Sauvion N, Thiéry D, Calatayud PA, editors. Insect-Plant Interact a Crop Prot Perspect. 1st ed. London, United Kingdom: Academic Press; 2017. pp. 139-177. Available from: http://www.sciencedirect.com/science/article/pii/S0065229616300982

[32] McCutcheon SC, Jørgensen SE. Phytoremediation. In: Jørgensen SE, Fath BD, editors. Encyclopedia of Ecology. 1st ed. Oxford: Academic Press; 2008. pp. 2751-2766. Available from: http://www.sciencedirect.com/science/article/pii/B9780080454054000690

[33] Hounsome N, Hounsome B, Tomos D, Edwards-Jones G. Plant metabolites and nutritional quality of vegetables. Journal of Food Science. 2008;**73**:48-65. DOI: 10.1111/j.1750-3841.2008.00716.x

[34] VanEtten HD, Sandrock RW, Wasmann CC, Soby SD, McCluskey K, Wang P. Detoxification of phytoanticipins and phytoalexins by phytopathogenic fungi. Canadian Journal of Botany. 1995;**73**:518-525. DOI: 10.1139/b95-291

[35] Morrissey J, Lou GM. Iron uptake and transport in plants: The good, the bad, and the ionome. Chemical Reviews. 2009;**109**:4553-4567. DOI: 10.1021/cr900112r

[36] Zaynab M, Fatima M, Abbas S, Sharif Y, Umair M, Zafar MH, et al. Role of secondary metabolites in plant defense against pathogens. Microbial Pathogenesis. 2018;**124**:198-202. DOI: 10.1016/j.micpath.2018.08.034

[37] Seppänen SK, Syrjälä L, Von Weissenberg K, Teeri TH, Paajanen L, Pappinen A. Antifungal activity of stilbenes in *in vitro* bioassays and in transgenic *Populus* expressing a gene encoding pinosylvin synthase. Plant Cell Reports. 2004;**22**:584-593. DOI: 10.1007/s00299-003-0728-0

[38] Del Cueto J, Møller BL, Dicenta F, Sánchez-Pérez R. β-Glucosidase activity in almond seeds. Plant Physiology and Biochemistry. 2018;**126**:163-172. DOI: 10.1016/j.plaphy.2017.12.028

[39] Gadzovska Simic S, Tusevski O, Maury S, Delaunay A, Joseph C, Hagège D. Effects of polysaccharide elicitors on secondary metabolite production and antioxidant response in *Hypericum perforatum* L. shoot cultures. Scientific World Journal. 2014;**2014**:609649. DOI: 10.1155/2014/609649

[40] Sathiyabama M, Bernstein N, Anusuya S. Chitosan elicitation for increased curcumin production and stimulation of defence response in turmeric (*Curcuma longa* L.). Industrial Crops and Products. 2016;**89**:87-94. DOI: 10.1016/j.indcrop.2016.05.007

[41] Alami I, Mari S, Clérivet A. A glycoprotein from *Ceratocystis fimbriata*

f. sp. *platani* triggers phytoalexin synthesis in *Platanus × acerifolia* cell-suspension cultures. Phytochemistry. 1998;**48**:771-776. DOI: 10.1016/S0031-9422(97)00892-3

[42] Gadzovska Simic S, Tusevski O, Maury S, Delaunay A, Lainé E, Joseph C, et al. Polysaccharide elicitors enhance phenylpropanoid and naphtodianthrone production in cell suspension cultures of *Hypericum perforatum*. Plant Cell, Tissue and Organ Culture. 2015;**122**: 649-663. DOI: 10.1007/s11240-015-0798-z

[43] Hemashenpagam N, Selvaraj T. Effect of arbuscular mycorrhizal (AM) fungus and plant growth promoting rhizomicroorganisms (PGPR's) on medicinal plant *Solanum viarum* seedlings. Journal of Environmental Biology. 2011;**32**:579-583

[44] Vafadar F, Amooaghaie R, Otroshy M. Effects of plant-growth-promoting rhizobacteria and arbuscular mycorrhizal fungus on plant growth, stevioside, NPK, and chlorophyll content of *Stevia rebaudiana*. Journal of Plant Interactions. 2013;**9**:128-136. DOI: 10.1080/17429145.2013.779035

[45] Kurosaki F, Yamashita A, Arisawa M. Involvement of GTP-binding protein in the induction of phytoalexin biosynthesis in cultured carrot cells. Plant Science. 2001;**161**:273-278. DOI: 10.1016/S0168-9452(01)00407-1

[46] Bais HP, Walker TS, Schweizer HP, Vivanco JM. Root specific elicitation and antimicrobial activity of rosmarinic acid in hairy root cultures of *Ocimum basilicum*. Plant Physiology and Biochemistry. 2002;**40**:983-995. DOI: 10.1016/S0981-9428(02)01460-2

[47] Singh G, Gavrieli J, Oakey JS, Curtis WR. Interaction of methyl jasmonate, wounding and fungal elicitation during sesquiterpene induction in *Hyoscyamus muticus* in root cultures. Plant Cell Reports. 1998;**17**:391-395. DOI: 10.1007/s002990050412

[48] Yang D, Ma P, Liang X, Wei Z, Liang Z, Liu Y, et al. PEG and ABA trigger methyl jasmonate accumulation to induce the MEP pathway and increase tanshinone production in *Salvia miltiorrhiza* hairy roots. Physiologia Plantarum. 2012;**146**:173-183. DOI: 10.1111/j.1399-3054.2012.01603.x

[49] Xu A, Zhan JC, Huang WD. Effects of ultraviolet C, methyl jasmonate and salicylic acid, alone or in combination, on stilbene biosynthesis in cell suspension cultures of *Vitis vinifera* L. cv. Cabernet Sauvignon. Plant Cell, Tissue and Organ Culture. 2015; **122**:197-211. DOI: 10.1007/s11240-015-0761-z

[50] Hao X, Shi M, Cui L, Xu C, Zhang Y, Kai G. Effects of methyl jasmonate and salicylic acid on tanshinone production and biosynthetic gene expression in transgenic *Salvia miltiorrhiza* hairy roots. Biotechnology and Applied Biochemistry. 2015;**62**:24-31. DOI: 10.1002/bab.1236

[51] Xu YW, Lv SS, Zaho D, Chen JW, Yang WT, Wu W. Effects of salicylic acid on monoterpene production and antioxidant systems in *Houttuynia cordata*. African Journal of Biotechnology. 2012;**11**:1364-1372. DOI: 10.5897/AJB11.1524

[52] Chodisetti B, Rao K, Gandi S, Giri A. Gymnemic acid enhancement in the suspension cultures of *Gymnema sylvestre* by using the signaling molecules—Methyl jasmonate and salicylic acid. *In Vitro* Cellular & Developmental Biology—Plant. 2015;**51**:88-92. DOI: 10.1007/s11627-014-9655-8

[53] Krzyzanowska J, Czubacka A, Pecio L, Przybys M, Doroszewska T, Stochmal A, et al. The effects of jasmonic acid and methyl jasmonate on rosmarinic acid production in *Mentha piperita* cell

suspension cultures. Plant Cell, Tissue and Organ Culture. 2012;**108**:73-81. DOI: 10.1007/s11240-011-0014-8

[54] Hayashi H, Huang P, Inoue K. Up-regulation of soyasaponin biosynthesis by methyl jasmonate in cultured cells of *Glycyrrhiza glabra*. Plant & Cell Physiology. 2003;**44**:404-411. DOI: 10.1093/pcp/pcg054

[55] Hu X, Neill S, Cai W, Tang Z. Hydrogen peroxide and jasmonic acid mediate oligogalacturonic acid-induced saponin accumulation in suspension-cultured cells of *Panax ginseng*. Physiologia Plantarum. 2003;**118**: 414-421. DOI: 10.1034/j.1399-3054.2003.00124.x

[56] Taurino M, Ingrosso I, D'amico L, De Domenico S, Nicoletti I, Corradini D, et al. Jasmonates elicit different sets of stilbenes in *Vitis vinifera* cv. Negramaro cell cultures. Springerplus. 2015;**4**:49. DOI: 10.1186/s40064-015-0831-z

[57] Gorelick J, Rosenberg R, Smotrich A, Hanuš L, Bernstein N. Hypoglycemic activity of withanolides and elicitated *Withania somnifera*. Phytochemistry. 2015;**116**:283-289. DOI: 10.1016/j.phytochem.2015.02.029

[58] Ghorbanpour M, Hatami M, Kariman K, Dahaji PA. Phytochemical variations and enhanced efficiency of antioxidant and antimicrobial ingredients in *Salvia officinalis* as inoculated with different rhizobacteria. Chemistry & Biodiversity. 2016;**13**: 319-330. DOI: 10.1002/cbdv.201500082

[59] Banchio E, Bogino PC, Santoro M, Torres L, Zygadlo J, Giordano W. Systemic induction of monoterpene biosynthesis in *Origanum majoricum* by soil bacteria. Journal of Agricultural and Food Chemistry. 2010;**58**:650-654. DOI: 10.1021/jf9030629

[60] Banchio E, Xie X, Zhang H, Paré PW. Soil bacteria elevate essential oil accumulation and emissions in sweet basil. Journal of Agricultural and Food Chemistry. 2009;**57**:653-657. DOI: 10.1021/jf8020305

[61] del Rosario Cappellari L, Santoro MV, Nievas F, Giordano W, Banchio E. Increase of secondary metabolite content in marigold by inoculation with plant growth-promoting rhizobacteria. Applied Soil Ecology. 2013;**70**:16-22. DOI: 10.1016/j.apsoil.2013.04.001

[62] Liang Z, Ma Y, Xu T, Cui B, Liu Y, Guo Z, et al. Effects of abscisic acid, gibberellin, ethylene and their interactions on production of phenolic acids in *Salvia miltiorrhiza* bunge hairy roots. PLoS One. 2013;**8**:e72806. DOI: 10.1371/journal.pone.0072806

[63] McSteen P, Zhao Y. Plant hormones and signaling: Common themes and new developments. Developmental Cell. 2008;**14**:467-473. DOI: 10.1016/j.devcel.2008.03.013

[64] Abbasi BH, Stiles AR, Saxena PK, Liu CZ. Gibberellic acid increases secondary metabolite production in *Echinacea purpurea* hairy roots. Applied Biochemistry and Biotechnology. 2012; **168**:2057-2066. DOI: 10.1007/s12010-012-9917-z

[65] Zobayed SMA, Afreen F, Kozai T. Temperature stress can alter the photosynthetic efficiency and secondary metabolite concentrations in St. John's wort. Plant Physiology and Biochemistry. 2005;**43**:977-984. DOI: 10.1016/j.plaphy.2005.07.013

[66] Binder BYK, Peebles CAM, Shanks JV, San K-Y. The effects of UV-B stress on the production of terpenoid indole alkaloids in *Catharanthus roseus* hairy roots. Biotechnology Progress. 2009;**25**: 861-865. DOI: 10.1002/btpr.97

[67] Tari I, Kiss G, Deér AK, Csiszár J, Erdei L, Gallé A, et al. Salicylic acid increased aldose reductase activity and

sorbitol accumulation in tomato plants under salt stress. Biologia Plantarum. 2010;**54**:677-683. DOI: 10.1007/s10535-010-0120-1

[68] Liu H, Wang X, Wang D, Zou Z, Liang Z. Effect of drought stress on growth and accumulation of active constituents in *Salvia miltiorrhiza* bunge. Industrial Crops and Products. 2011;**33**:84-88. DOI: 10.1016/j.indcrop.2010.09.006

[69] Gupta P, Sharma S, Saxena S. Biomass yield and steviol glycoside production in callus and suspension culture of *Stevia rebaudiana* treated with proline and polyethylene glycol. Applied Biochemistry and Biotechnology. 2015;**176**:863-874. DOI: 10.1007/s12010-015-1616-0

[70] Threlfall DR, Whitehead IM. The use of biotic and abiotic elicitors to induce the formation of secondary plant products in cell suspension cultures of solanaceous plants. Biochemical Society Transactions. 1988;**16**:71-75. DOI: 10.1042/bst0160071

[71] Furze JM, Rhodes MJ, Parr AJ, Robins RJ, Withehead IM, Threlfall DR. Abiotic factors elicit sesquiterpenoid phytoalexin production but not alkaloid production in transformed root cultures of *Datura stramonium*. Plant Cell Reports Germany. 1991;**10**:111-114. DOI: 10.1007/BF00232039

[72] Shakeran Z, Keyhanfar M, Asghari G, Ghanadian M. Improvement of atropine production by different biotic and abiotic elicitors in hairy root cultures of *Datura metel*. Turkish Journal of Biology. 2015;**39**:111-118. DOI: 10.3906/biy-1405-25

[73] Cai Z, Kastell A, Speiser C, Smetanska I. Enhanced resveratrol production in *Vitis vinifera* cell suspension cultures by heavy metals without loss of cell viability. Applied Biochemistry and Biotechnology. 2013;**171**:330-340. DOI: 10.1007/s12010-013-0354-4

[74] Savitha BC, Thimmaraju R, Bhagyalakshmi N, Ravishankar GA. Different biotic and abiotic elicitors influence betalain production in hairy root cultures of *Beta vulgaris* in shake-flask and bioreactor. Process Biochemistry. 2006;**41**:50-60. DOI: 10.1016/j.procbio.2005.03.071

[75] Jochum GM, Mudge KW, Thomas RB. Elevated temperatures increase leaf senescence and root secondary metabolite concentrations in the understory herb *Panax quinquefolius* (Araliaceae). American Journal of Botany. 2007;**94**:819-826. DOI: 10.3732/ajb.94.5.819

[76] Zhao Y, Qi L-W, Wang W-M, Saxena PK, Liu C-Z. Melatonin improves the survival of cryopreserved callus of *Rhodiola crenulata*. Journal of Pineal Research. 2011;**50**:83-88. DOI: 10.1111/j.1600-079X.2010.00817.x

[77] Chan LK, Koay SS, Boey PL, Bhatt A. Effects of abiotic stress on biomass and anthocyanin. Biological Research. 2010;**43**:127-135. DOI: /S0716-97602010000100014

[78] Liu W, Liu C, Yang C, Wang L, Li S. Effect of grape genotype and tissue type on callus growth and production of resveratrols and their piceids after UV-C irradiation. Food Chemistry. 2010;**122**:475-481. DOI: 10.1016/j.foodchem.2010.03.055

[79] Bor M, Seckin B, Ozgur R, YIlmaz O, Ozdemir F, Turkan I. Comparative effects of drought, salt, heavy metal and heat stresses on gamma-aminobutyric acid levels of sesame (*Sesamum indicum* L.). Acta Physiologiae Plantarum. 2009;**31**:655-659. DOI: 10.1007/s11738-008-0255-2

[80] Chen Y, Guo Q, Liu L, Liao L, Zhu Z. Influence of fertilization and drought

stress on the growth and production of secondary metabolites in *Prunella vulgaris* L. The Journal of Medicinal Plants Research. 2011;**5**:1749-1755

[81] Pavlík M, Vacek J, Klejdus B, Kubáň V. Hypericin and hyperforin production in St. John's wort *in vitro* culture: Influence of saccharose, polyethylene glycol, methyl jasmonate, and agrobacterium tumefaciens. Journal of Agricultural and Food Chemistry. 2007; **55**:6147-6153. DOI: 10.1021/jf070245w

[82] Butassi E, Svetaz LA, Zhou S, Wolfender JL, Cortés JCG, Ribas JC, et al. The antifungal activity and mechanisms of action of quantified extracts from berries, leaves and roots of *Phytolacca tetramera*. Phytomedicine. 2019;**16**:152884. DOI: 10.1016/j.phymed.2019.152884

[83] Talibi I, Askarne L, Boubaker H, Boudyach EH, Msanda F, Saadi B, et al. Antifungal activity of Moroccan medicinal plants against citrus sour rot agent *Geotrichum candidum*. Letters in Applied Microbiology. 2012;**55**:155-161. DOI: 10.1111/j.1472-765X.2012.03273.x

[84] Anaruma ND, Schmidt FL, Duarte MC, Figueira GM, Delarmelina C, Benato LA, et al. Control of *Colletotrichum gloeosporioides* (penz.) Sacc. In yellow passion fruit using *Cymbopogon citratus* essential oil. Brazilian Journal of Microbiology. 2010; **41**:66-73. DOI: 10.1590/S1517-83822010000100012

[85] Zhao W, Xu LL, Zhang X, Gong XW, Zhu DL, Xu XH, et al. Three new phenanthrenes with antimicrobial activities from the aerial parts of *Juncus effusus*. Fitoterapia. 2018;**130**:247-250. DOI: 10.1016/j.fitote.2018.09.007

[86] Rodríguez AT, Morales D, Ramírez MA. Efecto de extractos vegetales sobre el crecimiento *in vitro* de hongos fitopatógenos. Cultivos Tropicales. 2000;**21**:79-82

[87] Salhi N, Saghir SAM, Terzi V, Brahmi I, Ghedairi N, Bissati S. Antifungal activity of aqueous extracts of some dominant Algerian medicinal plants. BioMed Research International. 2017;**2017**:7526291. DOI: 10.1155/2017/7526291

[88] Mongalo NI, Dikhoba PM, Soyingbe SO, Makhafola TJ. Antifungal, anti-oxidant activity and cytotoxicity of south African medicinal plants against mycotoxigenic fungi. Heliyon. 2018;**4**: e00973. DOI: 10.1016/j.heliyon.2018.e00973

[89] Mahlo SM, Chauke HR, McGaw L, Eloff J. Antioxidant and antifungal activity of selected medicinal plant extracts against phytopathogenic fungi. African Journal of Traditional, Complementary, and Alternative Medicines. 2016;**13**:216-222. DOI: 10.21010/ajtcam.v13i4.28

[90] Costa E, Silva J, de Sousa Carlos Mourão D, de Oliveira Lima FS, de Almeida Sarmento R, Sunti Dalcin M, et al. The efficiency of noni (*Morinda citrifolia* L.) essential oil on the control of leaf spot caused by *Exserohilum turcicum* in maize culture. Medicines. 2017;**4**:60. DOI: 10.3390/medicines4030060

[91] Nkomo MM, Katerere D, Vismer H, Cruz TT, Stephane S, Balayssac SS, et al. Fusarium inhibition by wild populations of the medicinal plant *Salvia africana*-lutea L. linked to metabolomic profiling. BMC Complementary and Alternative Medicine. 2014;**14**(99):2-9. DOI: 10.1186/1472-6882-14-99

[92] Elshafie HS, Grul'ová D, Baranová B, Caputo L, De Martino L, Sedlák V, et al. Antimicrobial activity and chemical composition of essential oil extracted from *Solidago canadensis* L. growing wild in Slovakia. Molecules. 2019;**24**:1206. DOI: 10.3390/molecules24071206

[93] Tabti L, Amine Dib ME, Gaouar N, Samira B, Tabti B. Antioxidant and antifungal activity of extracts of the aerial parts of *Thymus capitatus* (L.) Hoffmanns against four phytopathogenic fungi of *Citrus sinensis*. Jundishapur Journal of Natural Pharmaceutical Products. 2014;**9**:49-54. DOI: 10.17795/jjnpp-13972

[94] Slazak B, Kapusta M, Strömstedt AA, Słomka A, Krychowiak M, Shariatgorji M, et al. How does the sweet violet *Viola odorata* L. fight pathogens and pests-cyclotides as a comprehensive plant host defense system. Frontiers in Plant Science. 2018;**9**:1296. DOI: 10.3389/fpls.2018.01296

[95] Garcia-Mier L, Jimenez-Garcia SN, Guevara-González RG, Feregrino-Perez AA, Contreras-Medina LM, Torres-Pacheco I. Elicitor mixtures significantly increase bioactive compounds, antioxidant activity, and quality parameters in sweet bell pepper. Journal of Chemistry. 2015;**2015**:8. DOI: 10.1155/2015/269296. Article ID: 269296

[96] Vargas-Hernández M, Torres-Pacheco I, Gautier F, Álvarez-Mayorga B, Cruz-Hernández A, García-Mier L, et al. Influence of hydrogen peroxide foliar applications on *in vitro* antimicrobial activity in *Capsicum chinense* Jacq. Plant Biosystems. 2017; **151**:269-275. DOI: 10.1080/11263504.2016.1168494

[97] Zunun-Pérez AY, Guevara-Figueroa T, Jimenez-Garcia SN, Feregrino-Pérez AA, Gautier F, Guevara-González RG. Effect of foliar application of salicylic acid, hydrogen peroxide and a xyloglucan oligosaccharide on capsiate content and gene expression associated with capsinoids synthesis in *Capsicum annuum* L. Journal of Biosciences. 2017; **42**:245-250. DOI: 10.1007/s12038-017-9682-9

Chapter 5

# Sisal Bole Rot: An Important but Neglected Disease

*Valter Cruz-Magalhães, Jackeline Pereira Andrade, Yasmim Freitas Figueiredo, Phellippe Arthur Santos Marbach and Jorge Teodoro de Souza*

## Abstract

Sisal (*Agave sisalana*) is one of the main sources of hard natural fibre and raw materials for the industry, medicine and handicrafts. Sisal yields a coarse and strong fibre that is increasingly being used in composite materials for automobiles, furniture, construction and plastic and paper products. Extracts of sisal contain substances with anti-inflammatory, antimicrobial and anthelmintic activities. Sisal is adapted to warm environments with low rainfall and is an excellent option for cultivation in semiarid conditions, where other crops cannot be grown. The world's largest sisal producers are Brazil, Tanzania, China, Kenya and Madagascar. Sisal is a labour-intensive crop with great socio-economical importance as it is cultivated in poor areas employing familiar labour. Sisal bole rot is the main disease of sisal, responsible for substantial losses in producing countries. The disease is caused by certain species of the genus *Aspergillus*, especially the ones belonging in the section *Nigri*. The main symptoms are yellowing of the aerial parts and the red-coloured rot of the bole, which causes the plant to die. In this review we are going to address the taxonomy of the causal agents, disease diagnosis and epidemiology and disease management, with emphasis on biological control.

**Keywords:** *Aspergillus welwitschiae*, *Agave sisalana*, biological control, disease management, semiarid regions

## 1. Introduction

*Agave sisalana* Perr. ex. Engelm is a monocotyledonous, xerophytic, succulent plant that belongs in the *Asparagaceae* family. The genus *Agave* has more than 200 species, and Mexico is their centre of origin and dispersion, where they have high economic importance and several industrial applications [1, 2]. This genus is able to grow in different conditions, as well as to show excellent adaptation to environments with warm climate, high luminosity and prolonged droughts [3, 4]. Tolerance to abiotic stresses is a striking feature of *A. sisalana*, which confers good performances to this species under conditions that limit the development of most plants [4]. This tolerance is related to morphological and physiological characteristics, such as the CAM metabolism (crassulacean acid). This type of metabolism allows for greater efficiency in water use, higher carbon uptake during the night and low nutritional demand when compared to C3 and C4 plants [1, 5–7].

Sisal is a monocarpic plant, and the emission of an inflorescence characterises the end of its vegetative cycle, which can occur between 8 and 30 years. The plant multiplies vegetatively through bulbils produced on the inflorescence pole or by stolons that emerge from the rhizome (subterraneous stem) of adult plants. The use of bulbils is the most common form of propagation, but stolons can also be used. The production of seeds is rare, and induction techniques are necessary when this is the objective [8–10]. Most species of *Agave* are highly endemic and have high levels of genetic variation within populations and low differentiation between populations [11]. This limited diversity hinders the establishment of germplasm banks and the search for genes that confer desirable characteristics to these plants.

*Agave sisalana* is a good producer of hard natural fibres [1]. The fibre extracted from this plant occupies the sixth position of importance and represents 2% of the world production of plant fibres [12]. This product is extracted from the leaves of the plant and is traditionally used in the manufacture of cords and ropes [9]. In addition, it is widely used in various industrial sectors. Amongst several applications, sisal fibre has been increasingly used in the reinforcement of building materials, furniture, panels and automobile upholstery [1, 12, 13]. In addition to the various applications and industrial uses, sisal fibre has advantages over synthetic fibres for having lower density (lighter) and lower production cost and is biodegradable and recyclable. Therefore, the use of sisal fibre fits in the growing world tendency that favours the use of sustainable natural resources with less environmental impact [14, 15].

There has been a growing interest in the use of waste or by-products from *Agave* species in biotechnological processes [16, 17]. After fibre extraction the residue is usually discarded [18]. This residue accounts for 98% of the total biomass of the plant and has potential to be used as raw material for biofuels, especially because it is not directly used as food [6, 12, 19]. In order to exploit the economic value of this material, a joint initiative between the Common Fund for Commodities, the United Nations Industrial Development Organization (UNIDO) and the Tanzanian sisal industry financed the first commercial plant for the production of biogas [12]. In addition to some medicinal properties reported [20, 21], *A. sisalana* also produces compounds that have different biological properties [18] of great interest in the pharmaceutical industry such as hecogenin [12, 21–23]. All of the above features place sisal as a strategic species to be exploited in tropical semiarid regions and in temperate latitudes with drought resulting from global climate change [16, 19, 24].

The main world producers of sisal fibre are Brazil, Tanzania, China, Kenya and Madagascar [25]. Other countries, such as Mexico, South Africa, Mozambique, Angola, Indonesia, Thailand, Haiti and Cuba, also produce but in smaller quantities. According to FAO reports, in 2011 Brazil alone produced more than 111 thousand tons of sisal fibre [12].

In Brazil, the semiarid region of Bahia province (northeastern Brazil) is responsible for more than 95% of the country's sisal production [26]. Other provinces that produce smaller amounts of sisal in Brazil are Paraiba, Rio Grande do Norte and Ceará [27]. It is estimated that more than 150,000 families are directly linked to the producing chain of this crop, totalling more than 700,000 small farmers, and more than half a million direct and indirect jobs are involved in activities related to the maintenance, harvesting, extraction and processing of fibre [28–30]. In this sense, sisal has an important economic and social role of the semiarid region of Brazil.

Sisal management is simple because this plant exhibits tolerance to various abiotic stresses. Even under minimal management conditions, the plant presents good development and consequently good fibre production, with low nutritional requirements [12]. However, although it presents all these adaptive advantages to stress conditions, the main problem is of phytosanitary origin. Sisal bole rot, the main disease of sisal, has caused considerable damage to the crop [31]. This disease causes the death of infected plants, and despite the economic and social importance of sisal, there are few government efforts to control the disease.

In this chapter we introduce the sisal bole rot disease, a neglected disease that represents the main challenge for sisal production in Brazil and other countries of the world. In addition, we discuss some aspects involved in its symptomatology, aetiology, epidemiology and management. The majority of the results that will be shown were obtained in Brazil, where most of the research on sisal bole rot was done.

## 2. Bole rot disease: symptoms and epidemiology

The disease was first reported in production areas of Tanzania and Brazil [31, 32]. In Brazil, since the 1990s, the commercial production of sisal has been

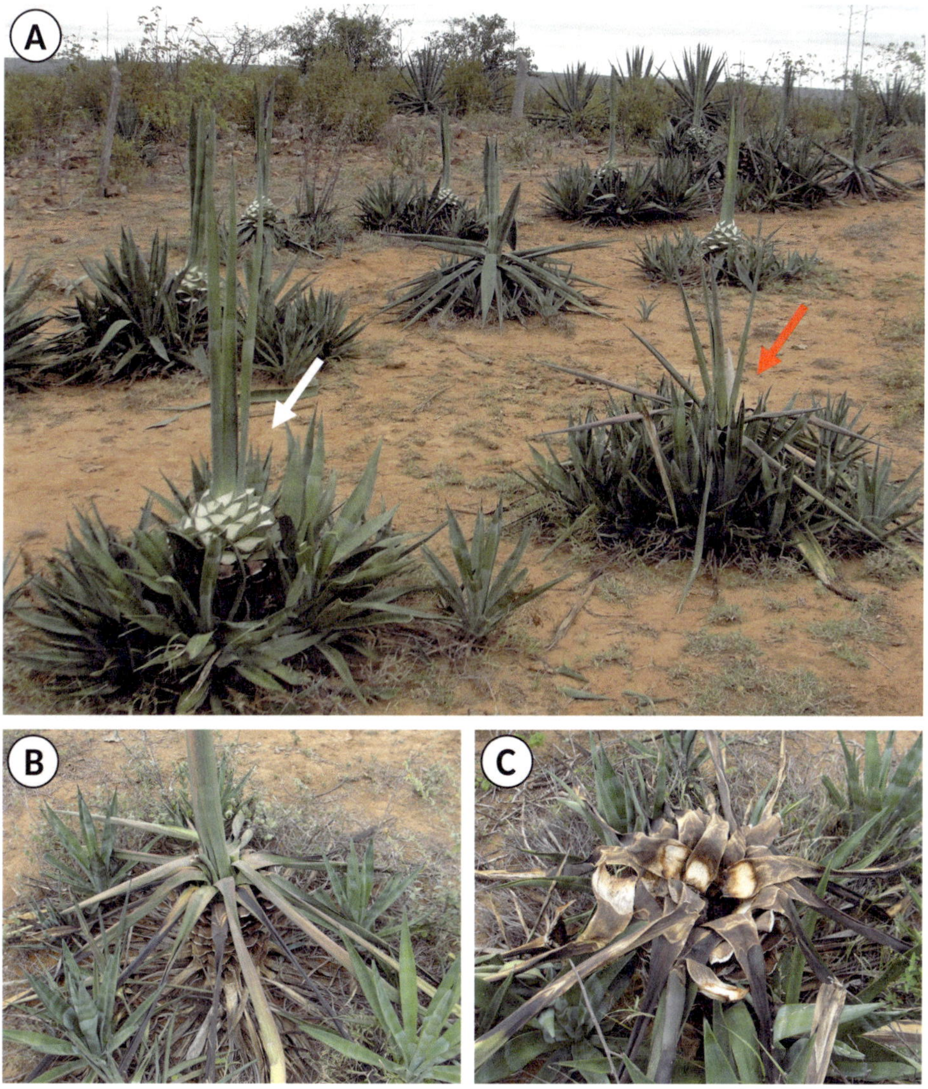


**Figure 1.**
*Adult sisal plants under field conditions. (A) Healthy adult plant (white arrow) after leaf harvest for fibre extraction next to an adult plant showing the external symptoms of sisal bole rot (red arrow). The diseased plant has wilted and yellowish leaves that cannot be used for fibre extraction and therefore was not harvested. (B) and (C) Plants killed by the pathogen.*

declining due to economical crises and the occurrence of this disease [33]. Diseased plants produce leaves that are not suitable for fibre extraction as they lose their turgescence, and although these diseased plants survive for some time, they die with the progress of the disease (**Figure 1**) [35]. Plants at advanced stages of the disease are easily identified by the symptoms, which include wilting and yellowing of the aerial part (**Figure 1A**). The main internal symptom of the disease is rotting of the stem with reddening of the tissues, a response of the plant to fungal colonisation. It is thought that there is no relationship between the phenological stage of the plant and the establishment of the disease, since the fungus is capable of infecting both plantlets (**Figure 2E**) and adult plants (**Figures 1** and **2**).

It was reported that the pathogen depends on mechanical injuries and natural openings, mainly on physiologically stressed plants, to start the infection process [32]. In this sense, it is possible that wounds made by insects or by tools used in crop management, such as harvest of the leaves and cultural practices, are ways of pathogen penetration [32, 35, 36]. The histopathology of diseased plants showed that the pathogen penetrates the tissues of the host from the outside, that is, from the epidermis to the parenchyma and later to the central cylinder of the plant [37].

Abreu [36] studied the spatiotemporal distribution of sisal bole rot in producing areas of Bahia Province, Brazil, and found that the disease was present in all

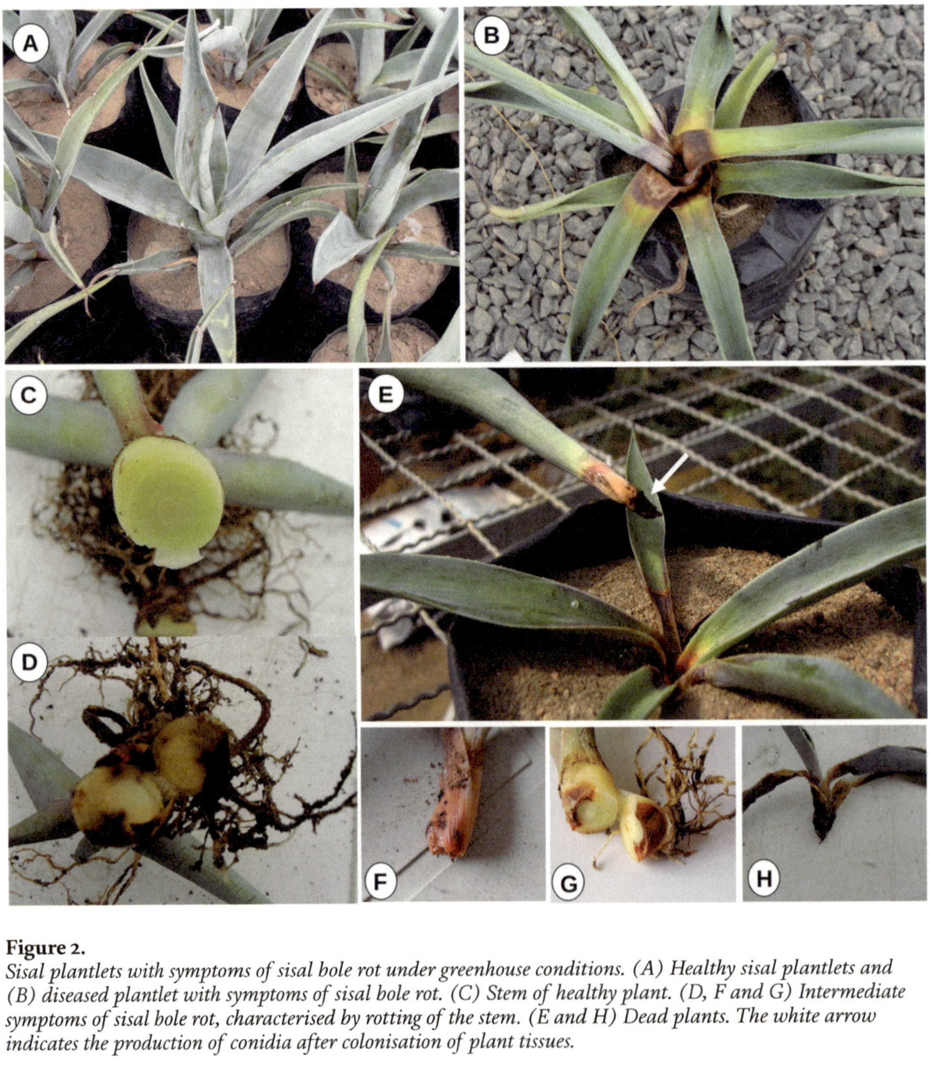


**Figure 2.**
*Sisal plantlets with symptoms of sisal bole rot under greenhouse conditions. (A) Healthy sisal plantlets and (B) diseased plantlet with symptoms of sisal bole rot. (C) Stem of healthy plant. (D, F and G) Intermediate symptoms of sisal bole rot, characterised by rotting of the stem. (E and H) Dead plants. The white arrow indicates the production of conidia after colonisation of plant tissues.*

the studied farms (prevalence of 100%) and, on average, 35% of the plants were infected by the pathogen. This study also showed that the distribution of the disease occurs randomly in the cultivated areas [36]. In the case of sisal bole rot, incidence evaluations are more important than severity, as there are no measures that slow down the progress of the disease.

The lack of more studies on epidemiological aspects of sisal bole rot in different areas where the disease occurs directly impacts the establishment of phytosanitary management practices. More information on these aspects could contribute to the development of strategies to reduce the incidence of the disease. For the moment, what is known is that preventive measures should be employed to avoid the establishment of the pathogen in the area.

## 3. Causal agents

The disease was first observed in areas of sisal production in Tanzania in the 1930s but was only reported in the 1950s [32]. The causal agent was isolated from diseased plant parts and identified as *Aspergillus niger*. In this study, the authors reported fruiting bodies of *A. niger* in exposed plant tissues and also pointed out that the occurrence of the disease was linked to environmental conditions and the nutritional status of the plant [32]. The first report of this disease in Brazil also occurred in the 1950s, when Machado [38] described a rot of the base of sisal

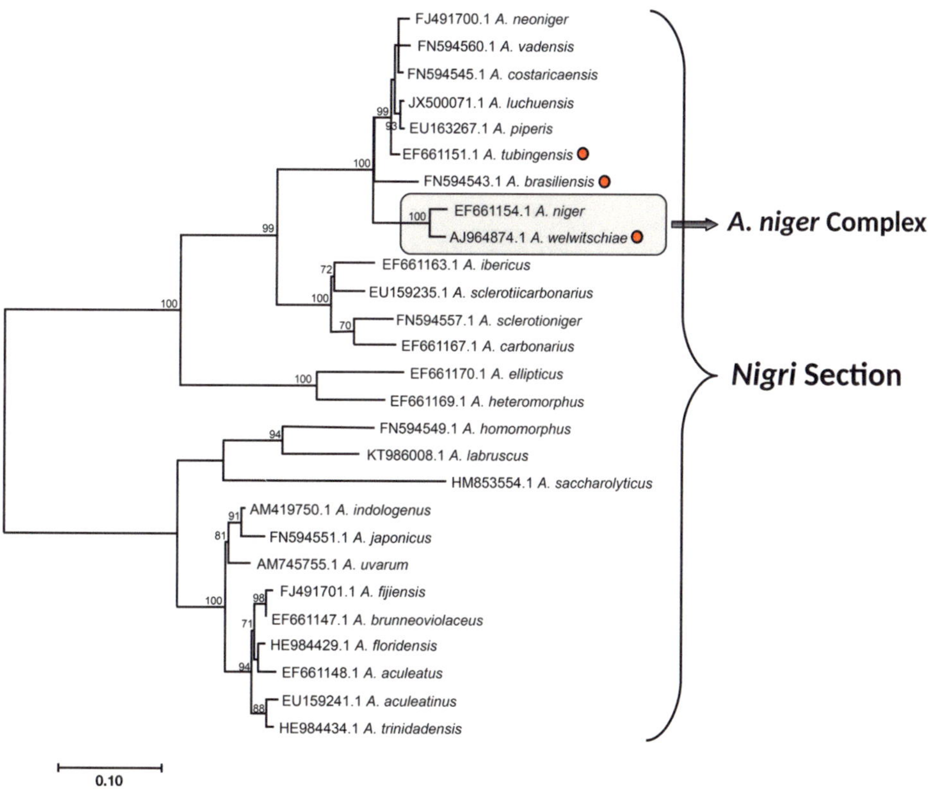


**Figure 3.**
*Phylogenetic tree of the 27 valid species belonging in the Nigri section of Aspergillus. The red circles indicate species shown to cause sisal bole rot in the A. niger complex. The tree was constructed with sequences of the calmodulin gene, with 456 nucleotides aligned using the maximum likelihood (ML) method and the K2 + G + I substitution model. The bootstrap analysis was performed with 1000 resamplings. The scale represents the number of substitutions per site.*

stem in the province of Paraíba, Brazil [39]. In Bahia, the largest sisal-producing province in Brazil, the disease was first noticed in a commercial plantation by researchers from the Agency for Agricultural Development of Bahia (EBDA) and Embrapa Semiárido (Brazilian Agricultural Research Institute) in the municipality of Santaluz [33].

In Tanzania and in Brazil, the disease was initially associated with the species *A. niger*. The aetiology of the disease was determined by Koch's postulates from tissue fragments of diseased sisal plants [40]. Species of the genus *Aspergillus* are filamentous fungi belonging in the phylum *Ascomycota* [41]. *Aspergillus niger* and other closely related species form a cluster of morphologically similar species, collectively known as the section *Nigri* (**Figure 3**). The *Nigri* section is comprised of 27 valid species that contain the *A. niger* complex (**Figure 3**). All these species have as main characteristic the formation of black-coloured conidia, uniseriate or biseriate conidiophores and dark colonies (**Figure 4**) [42]. The taxonomy of the section *Nigri* is very complex because many species of this group are difficult to distinguish morphologically [41]. The morphological criteria were the only ones used to identify these species for a long time, and for this reason, many species were misidentified [43, 44].

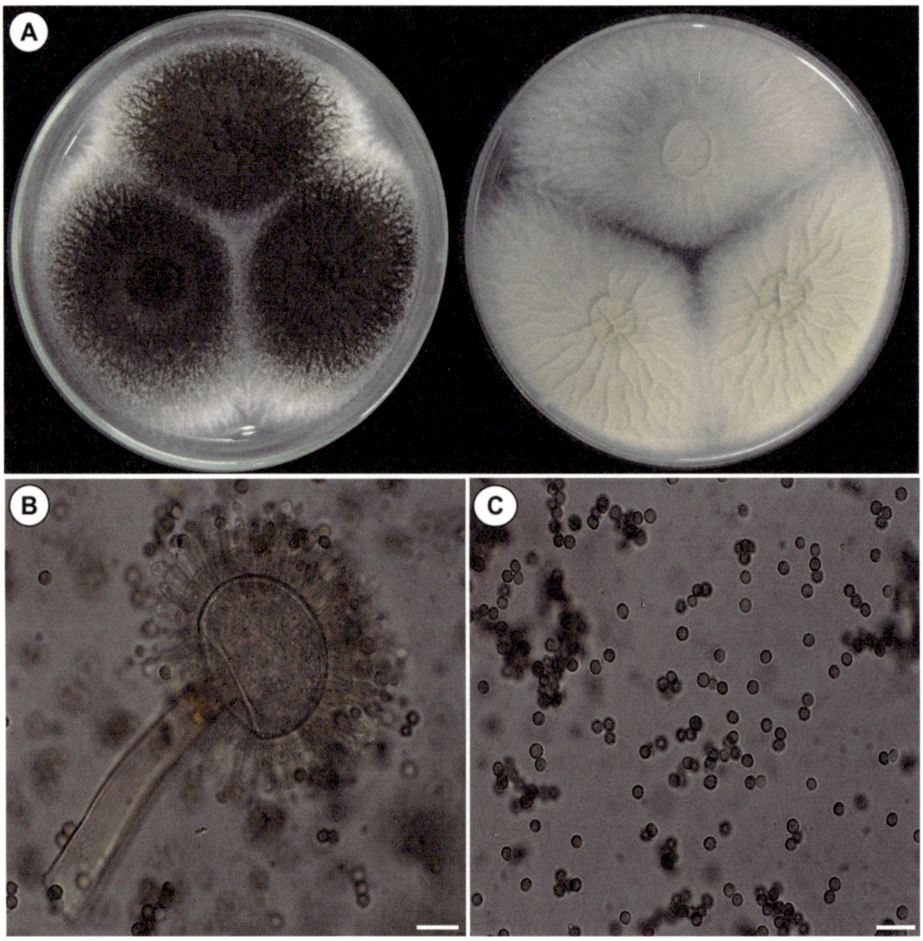


**Figure 4.**
*Macro- and micromorphology of Aspergillus welwitschiae isolated from diseased sisal plants. (A) Obverse and reverse of a plate containing mycelial growth of colony on Blakeslee's malt extract (MEAbl), growing at 25°C for 7 days. (B) Conidiophores of A. welwitschiae and (C) conidia. Scale bars =10 µm.*

The polyphasic taxonomy integrates molecular, physiological, metabolite production and morphological data for the identification and description of new species of the section *Nigri* [45–48]. The regions recommended for the identification and description of species in the genus *Aspergillus* are fragments of the ITS region of the ribosomal DNA, calmodulin (*caM*), beta-tubulin (*benA*) and the beta subunit of the RNA polymerase (*rpb2*). However, caM sequences were proposed as the most informative markers for the section *Nigri* [49]. The gene *benA* is very informative for the uniseriate/aculeatus clade; however, care must be taken not to use the wrong set of primers (Bt2a/Bt2b) that can also amplify *tubC*, a paralog of *benA*, resulting in misidentification. The alternative primer pair ben2f/Bt2b should be used instead [50]. The other methods used in the polyphasic approach include growth on different media and temperatures, production of secondary metabolites and measurement of all fungal structures [44, 45].

The initial studies implicated only *A. niger* as the cause of bole rot disease because the authors only took the morphological features of the pathogen into account [32, 40]. Further studies including sequences of the ITS region of the ribosomal DNA and a fragment of the transcription and elongation factor of the RNA polymerase (tef1-alpha) also identified *A. brasiliensis* and *A. tubingensis* in addition to *A. niger* as agents of the disease [31]. Recently, Duarte et al. [37] identified molecular phylogeny strains of *Aspergillus* sp. of the section *Nigri* obtained from diseased plants using a fragment of the calmodulin gene and proposed that *A. welwitschiae* and not *A. niger* is the causal agent of sisal bole rot disease. However, these authors did not include *A. niger* in their study, and therefore, further investigations are still needed to evaluate the ability of other species in the section *Nigri* to cause the disease, including *A. niger*.

## 4. Disease management

There are no effective control methods available for bole rot disease [51]. Mechanical lesions are used by the pathogen as penetration sites, and this has direct implications for crop management since leaf harvest causes wounds in the plant [32, 36]. Additionally, the pathogen may be spread through the use of tools contaminated in diseased plants.

Most farmers use plantlets from stolons to establish new plantations, and infected plant material contributes to the spread of the disease to new areas. Therefore, the establishment of new areas using healthy plant material is thought to be one of the most effective ways to prevent the introduction of the pathogen. Removal and destruction of diseased plants from the plantations, balanced fertilisation to prevent stresses and disinfestation of the tools used in diseased plants are other measures recommended to decrease the incidence and avoid the spread of the disease to new areas [52].

Another method investigated to manage the disease is the use of antagonistic microorganisms [53, 34]. Chemical control was never investigated probably because the causal agents are soilborne fungi and farmers have little financial resources. Biological control is an environmentally friendly and viable method to control plant pathogens [54, 45]. Antagonistic bacteria were shown to have potential to control the bole rot disease [53, 34]. Several strains of an undescribed species of *Burkholderia* and strains of *Bacillus* decreased the incidence and severity of the disease under field conditions (**Figures 5** and **6**) [53, 34]. Therefore, it is possible to establish programmes aimed at the development of biological products to manage the disease in the field.

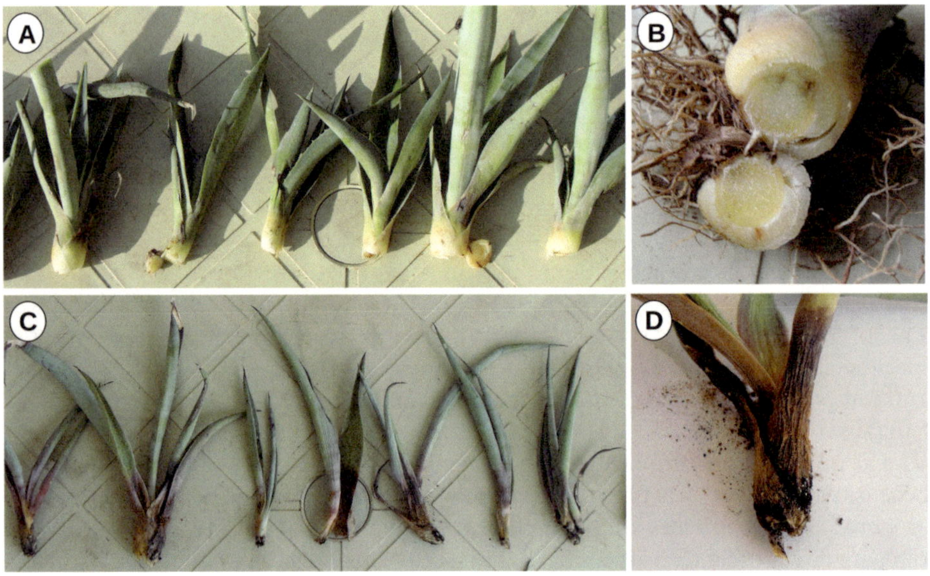


**Figure 5.**
*Management of sisal bole rot disease with antagonistic bacteria. (A) and (B) Plantlets treated with Burkholderia sp. and inoculated with the pathogen A. welwitschiae in the field. (C) and (D) Sisal plants inoculated with A. welwitschiae only under field conditions (positive control).*

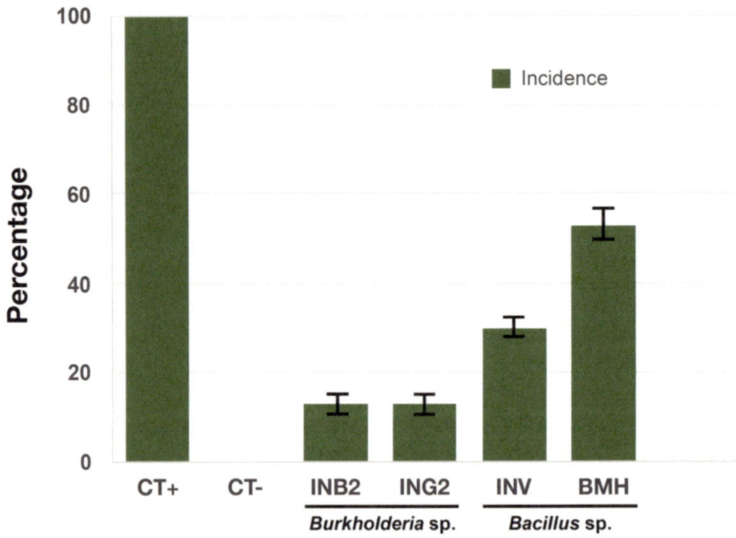


**Figure 6.**
*Incidence of sisal bole rot disease by the application of Burkholderia and Bacillus strains under field conditions. The means represent 25 replicates per treatment. The negative control was treated with water only (CT-) and positive control with A. welwitschiae (CT+). Error bars represent the standard error of the means.*

## 5. Outlook

Little is known about the mechanisms used by the pathogen to infect the plant, although *Aspergillus* shows a typical necrotrophic behaviour [37]. More information on the pathogenicity mechanisms could be obtained by the use of omics tools, such as RNAseq, to identify genes expressed by the pathogen during infection. Other microorganisms can influence the establishment and progress of the disease, and in this sense it will be interesting to study the comparative microbiome of diseased and healthy plants. This information may be used to engineer the microbiome to keep the plants healthy, as it has been attempted for other agricultural crops [55].

Sisal bole rot cannot be controlled by any single method, and therefore, the integration of control measures must be adopted. Resistant cultivars are not available for this crop, and unfortunately there are no breeding programmes focusing on sisal bole rot [9]. Breeding programmes are limited by the low genetic diversity of natural populations out of Mexico.

Preventive measures are thought to be the most effective ways to control bole rot, and these include (i) the use of healthy planting material, (ii) balanced fertilisation to avoid nutritional stresses and (iii) maintaining adequate soil humidity levels to avoid physiological imbalances [52]. When these measures are not able to contain the pathogen, removal of diseased plants is recommended to decrease the source of inoculum of the pathogen [52]. One challenge in this regard is the development strategies to identify diseased plants before the dispersal of pathogen propagules.

Sisal residues are commonly used to fertilise plants in the field [52], but only the fermented residue is suitable for this purpose as fresh residues stimulate the spread of the pathogen [56]. Information such as these could be disseminated to farmers to contribute to the management of the disease. Sisal farmers in many parts of the world do not have access to information on the technical aspects of sisal, depend on familiar labour and have little financial resources to invest in the crop. The information generated so far on the management of the disease through the use of antagonistic bacteria are promising, but it is still necessary to develop it into products that can be used by the farmers. New studies aiming at formulating and distributing biological products should be encouraged to contribute to the sustainability of this crop in the long run. The general lack of research on bole rot classifies it as a neglected disease that deserves more attention from research institutes and the government.

## Acknowledgements

The authors thank the Brazilian agencies CNPq and CAPES for the financial support.

## Author details

Valter Cruz-Magalhães[1], Jackeline Pereira Andrade[2], Yasmim Freitas Figueiredo[1], Phellippe Arthur Santos Marbach[3] and Jorge Teodoro de Souza[1*]

1 Federal University of Lavras, Lavras, MG, Brazil

2 Universidade Estadual de Feira de Santana, Feira de Santana, BA, Brazil

3 Reconcavo da Bahia Federal University, BA, Brazil

*Address all correspondence to: jorge.souza@dfp.ufla.br

## References

[1] Nava-Cruz NY, Medina-Morales MA, Martinez JL, Rodriguez R, Aguilar CN. Agave biotechnology: An overview. Critical Reviews in Biotechnology. 2015, 2015;**35**:546-559. DOI: 10.3109/07388551.2014.923813

[2] Trejo-Torres JC, Gann GD, Christenhusz MJ. The Yucatan Peninsula is the place of origin of sisal (*Agave sisalana*, *Asparagaceae*): Historical accounts, phytogeography and current populations. Botanical Sciences. 2018;**96**:366-379. DOI: 10.17129/botsci.1928

[3] Pinos-Rodríguez JM, Zamudio M, González SS, Mendoza GD, Bárcena R, Ortega ME, et al. Effects of maturity and ensiling of *Agave salmiana* on nutritional quality for lambs. Animal Feed Science and Technology. 2009;**152**:298-306. DOI: 10.1016/j.anifeedsci.2009.05.002

[4] Sarwar MB, Ahmad Z, Rashid B, Hassan S, Gregersen PL, Leyva MDLO, et al. De novo assembly of *Agave sisalana* transcriptome in response to drought stress provides insight into the tolerance mechanisms. Scientific Reports. 2019;**9**:1-14. DOI: 10.1038/s41598-018-35891-6

[5] Kant P. Could Agave be the species of choice for climate change mitigation? In: Working Paper IGREC-11. New Delhi: Institute of Green Economy, IGREC; 2010

[6] Escamilla-Treviño LL. Potential of plants from the genus *Agave* as bioenergy crops. Bio Energy Research. 2012;**5**:1-9. DOI: 10.1007/s12155-011-9159-x

[7] Gross SM, Martin JA, Simpson J, Abraham-Juarez MJ, Wang Z, Visel A. De novo transcriptome assembly of drought tolerant CAM plants, *Agave deserti* and *Agave tequilana*. BMC Genomics. 2013;**14**:563. DOI: 10.1186/1471-2164-14-563

[8] Das T. Micropropagation of *Agave sisalana*. Plant Cell, Tissue and Organ Culture. 1992;**31**:253-255. DOI: 10.1007/BF00036233

[9] Nikam TD. High frequency shoot regeneration in *Agave sisalana*. Plant Cell, Tissue and Organ Culture. 1997;**51**(3):225-228. DOI: 10.1023/A:1005976304198

[10] Nikam TD, Bansude GM, Kumar KA. Somatic embryogenesis in sisal (*Agave sisalana* Perr. ex. Engelm). Plant Cell Reports. 2003;**22**(3):188-194. DOI: 10.1007/s00299-003-0675-9

[11] Eguiarte LE, Aguirre-Planter E, Aguirre X, Colín R, González A, Rocha M, et al. From isozymes to genomics: Population genetics and conservation of Agave in México. The Botanical Review. 2013;**79**(4):483-506. DOI: 10.1007/s12229-013-9123-x

[12] Food and Agriculture Organization (FAO). Future fibres [Internet]. 2019. Available from: http://www.fao.org/economic/futurefibres/fibres/sisal/en/online [Accessed: 01 February 2019]

[13] Bessadok A, Langevin D, Gouanvé F, Chappey C, Roudesli S, Marais S. Study of water sorption on modified *Agave* fibres. Carbohydrate Polymers. 2009;**76**:74-85. DOI: 10.1016/j.carbpol.2008.09.033

[14] Flores-Sahagun TH, Dos Santos LP, Dos Santos J, Mazzaro I, Mikowski A. Characterization of blue *Agave* bagasse fibers of Mexico. Composites Part A: Applied Science and Manufacturing. 2013;**45**:153-161. DOI: 10.1016/j.compositesa.2012.09.001

[15] Martin AR, Martins MA, Mattoso LH, Silva OR. Caracterização química e

estrutural de fibra de sisal da variedade *Agave sisalana*. Polímeros: ciência e tecnologia. 2009;**19**(1):40-46

[16] Yang X, Cushman JC, Borland AM, Edwards EJ, Wullschleger SD, Tuskan GA, et al. A roadmap for research on crassulacean acid metabolism (CAM) to enhance sustainable food and bioenergy production in a hotter, drier world. The New Phytologist. 2015;**207**(3):491-504. DOI: 10.1111/nph.13393

[17] Goldbeck R, Ramos M, Pereira G, Maugeri-Filho F. Cellulase production from a new strain *Acremonium strictum* isolated from the Brazilian biome using different substrates. Bioresource Technology. 2013;**128**:797-803. DOI: 10.1016/j.biortech.2012.10.034

[18] Viel AM, Pereira AR, Neres WE, Dos Santos L, Oliva Neto P, Souza EB, et al. Effect of *Agave sisalana* Perrine extract on the ovarian and uterine tissues and fetal parameters: Comparative interventional study. International Multispeciality Journal of Health. 2017;**3**:129-138

[19] Rodríguez-Garay B. Somatic embryogenesis in *Agave* spp. In: Loyola-Vargas V, Ochoa-Alejo N, editors. Somatic Embryogenesis: Fundamental Aspects and Applications. Cham: Springer; 2016. DOI: 10.1007/978-3-319-33705-0_16

[20] Chen PY, Kuo YC, Chen CH, Kuo YH, Lee CK. Isolation and immunomodulatory effect of homoisoflavones and flavones from *Agave sisalana* Perrine ex Engelm. Molecules. 2009;**14**:1789-1795. DOI: 10.3390/molecules14051789

[21] Debnath M, Mukeshwar P, Sharma R, Thakur GS, Lal P. Biotechnological intervention of *Agave sisalana*: A unique fiber yielding plant with medicinal property. Journal of Medicinal Plant Research. 2010;**4**:177-187

[22] Carneiro F d S, de Oliveira Domingos Queiroz SR, Rodrigues Passos A, Neves do Nascimento M, Souza dos Santos K. Embriogênese somática em *Agave sisalana* Perrine: indução, caracterização anatômica e regeneração. Pesquisa Agropecuária Tropical. 2014;**44**:3

[23] Sidana J, Singh B, Sharma OP. Saponins of *Agave*: Chemistry and bioactivity. Phytochemistry. 2016;**130**:22-46. DOI: 10.1016/j.phytochem.2016.06.010

[24] Rajaud A, de Noblet-Ducoudré N. Tropical semi-arid regions expanding over temperate latitudes under climate change. Climatic ChangeClimatic Change. 2017;**144**(4):703-719. DOI: 10.1007/s10584-017-2052-7

[25] Sharma S, Varshney VK. Chemical analysis of *Agave sisalana* juice for its possible utilization. Acta Chimica and Pharmaceutica Indica. 2012;**2**:60-66

[26] IBGE. Instituto Brasileiro de Geografia e Estatística. Sistema IBGE de Recuperação Automática [Internet]. 2015. Available from: http://www.sidra.ibge.gov.br/ [Accessed: 27 February 2015]

[27] Instituto Brasileiro de Geografia e Estatística (IBGE). Levantamento Sistemático da Produção Agrícola [Internet]. 2011. Available from: http://www.sidra.ibge.gov.br/ [Accessed: 2011-08-01]

[28] Mattoso LHC, Ferreira FC, Curvelo AAS. In: Leão AL, Carvalho FX, Frollini E, editors. Lignocellulose-Plastic Composites. São Paulo, Brazil: USP and UNESP; 1997

[29] Silva ORR, Beltrão NEM. O agronegócio do sisal no Brasil. Campina Grande, Brasil: Embrapa-CNPA; 1999

[30] Silva ORRF, Coutinho WM, Cartaxo WV, Sofiatti V, Filho JLS, Carvalho OS,

Costa LD. Cultivo do Sisal no Nordeste Brasileiro. Ministério da Agricultura, Pecuária e Abastecimento, Circular técnica. 2008; 123

[31] Santos POD, Silva ACMD, Corrêa ÉB, Magalhães VC, Souza JTD. Additional species of *Aspergillus* causing bole rot disease in *Agave sisalana*. Tropical Plant Pathology. 2014;**39**(4):331-334. DOI: 10.1590/ S1982-56762014000400008

[32] Wallace GB, Dieckmahns EC. Bole rot in sisal. East African Agricultural. 1952;**18**:24-29. DOI: 10.1080/03670074.1952.11664819

[33] Lima EF, Moreira JDAN, Batista FAS, Silva ORRF, Farias FJC, Araújo AE. Podridão vermelha do tronco do sisal (*Agave sisalana* Perrine.) causada por *Botryodiplodia theobromae* pat. Revista de Oleaginosas e Fibrosas. 1998, 1998;**2**:109-112

[34] Barbosa LO, Lima JS, Magalhães VC, Gava CAT, Soares ACF, Marbach PAS, et al. Compatibility and combination of selected bacterial antagonists in the biocontrol of sisal bole rot disease. Biological Control. 2018;**63**(4):595-605. DOI: 10.1007/s10526-018-9872-x

[35] SÁ JO. Controle biológico da podridão vermelha do sisal (*Agave sisalana* Perrine) com *Trichoderma* spp. e Actinobactérias [MSc thesis]. Cruz das Almas: Universidade Federal do Recôncavo da Bahia; 2019

[36] Abreu KCLDM. Epidemiologia da podridão Vermelha do Sisal no Estado da Bahia [MSc thesis]. Cruz das Almas: Universidade Federal do Recôncavo da Bahia; 2010

[37] Duarte EAA, Damasceno CL, Oliveira TASD, Barbosa LDO, Martins FM, Silva JRDQ, et al. Putting the mess in order: A*spergillus welwitschiae* (and not *A. niger*) is the etiological agent of sisal bole rot disease in Brazil. Frontiers in Microbiology. 2018;**9**:1-21. DOI: 10.3389/fmicb.2018.01227

[38] Machado AA. Sobre a Ocorrência de uma Nova Moléstia do Agave na Paraíba. Technical report. Relatório de uma viagem realizada no município de Campina Grande; 1951

[39] Medina JC. O sisal. Secretaria da Agricultura do Estado de São Paulo. São Paulo, Brazil; 1954

[40] Coutinho WM, Suassuna ND, Luz CM, Suinaga FA, Silva ORRF. Bole rot of sisal caused by *Aspergillus niger* in Brazil. Fitopatologia Brasileira. 2006;**31**:605-605. DOI: 10.1590 S0100-41582006000600014

[41] Varga J, Frisvad JC, Kocsubé S, Brankovics B, Tóth B, Szigeti G, et al. New and revisited species in *Aspergillus* section *Nigri*. Studies in Mycology. 2011;**69**:1-17. DOI: 10.3114/ sim.2011.69.01

[42] Ismail MA. Incidence and significance of black aspergilli in agricultural commodities: A review, with a key to all species accepted to-date. European Journal of Biological Research. 2017;**7**:207-222. DOI: 10.5281/ zenodo.834504

[43] Pitt JL, Hocking AD. Fungi and Food Spoilage. Cambridge: Chapman & Hall; 1997. DOI: 10.1007/978-0-387-92207-2

[44] Samson RA, Houbraken JAMP, Kuijpers AFA, Frank MJ, Frisvad JC. New ochratoxin A or sclerotium producing species in *Aspergillus* section *Nigri*. Studies in Mycology. 2004;**50**:45-61

[45] Varga J, Kocsubé S, Tóth B, Frisvad JC, Perrone G, Susca A, et al. *Aspergillus brasiliensis* sp. nov., a biseriate black *Aspergillus* species with world-wide distribuition. International Journal of Systematic and Evolutionary

Microbiology. 2007;**57**:1925-1932. DOI: 10.1099/ijs.0.65021-0

[46] Noonim P, Mahakarnchanakul W, Varga J, Frisvad JC, Samson RA. Two novel species of *Aspergillus* section *Nigri* from Thai coffee beans. International Journal of Systematic and Evolutionary Microbiology. 2008;**58**:1727-1734. DOI: 10.1099/ijs.0.65694-0

[47] Oliveri C, Torta L, Catara VA. Polyphasic approach to the identification of ochratoxin A-producing black *Aspergillus* isolates from vineyards in Sicily. International Journal of Food Microbiology. 2008;**127**:147-154. DOI: 10.1016/j.ijfoodmicro.2008.06.021

[48] Perrone G, Varga J, Susca A, Frisvad JC, Stea G, Kocsubé S, et al. *Aspergillus uvarum* sp. nov., an uniseriate black *Aspergillus* species isolated from grapes in Europe. International Journal of Systematic and Evolutionary Microbiology. 2008;**58**:1032-1039. DOI: 10.1099/ijs.0.65463-0

[49] Samson RA, Visagie CM, Houbraken J, Hong SB, Hubka V, Klaassen CHW, et al. Phylogeny, identification and nomenclature of the genus *Aspergillus*. Studies in Mycology. 2014;**78**:141-173. DOI: 10.1016/j.simyco.2014.07.004

[50] Hubka V, Kolarik M. Beta-tubulin paralogue tubC is frequently misidentified as the benA gene in *Aspergillus* section *Nigri* taxonomy: Primer specificity testing and taxonomic consequences. Persoonia. 2012;**29**:1-10. DOI: 10.3767/003158512X658123

[51] Embrapa. Cultivo do sisal [Internet]. 2010. Available from http://sistemasdeproducao.cnptia.embrapa.br/FontesHTML/Sisal/CultivodoSisal/doencas.html [Accessed: 25 May 2010]

[52] Suinaga FA, Silva ORRF, Coutinho WM. Cultivo de sisal na região Semi-árida do Nordeste Brasileiro. Campina Grande, Brazil; 2006. p. 44

[53] Magalhães VC, Barbosa LO, Andrade JP, Soares ACF, de Souza JT, Marbach PAS. *Burkholderia* isolates from a sand dune leaf litter display biocontrol activity against the bole rot disease of *Agave sisalana*. Biological Control. 2017;**112**:41-48. DOI: 10.1016/j.biocontrol.2017.06.005

[54] Baker KF. Evolving concepts of biological control of plant pathogens. Annual Review of Phytopathology. 1987;**25**:67-85

[55] Mueller UG, Sachs JL. Engineering microbiomes to improve plant and animal health. Trends in Microbiology. 2015;**23**:606-617. DOI: 10.1016/j.tim.2015.07.009

[56] do Carmo CO, Tavares PF, da Silva RM, Damasceno CL, Sá JO, Soares ACF. Fatores que afetam a sobrevivência de *Aspergillus niger* e sua relação com a podridão vermelha do caule do sisal. Magistra. 2018;**29**:144-153

Chapter 6

# Impact of Climate Change on Plant Diseases and IPM Strategies

*Sahar Abdou Zayan*

## Abstract

There has been a remarkable scientific output on the topic of how climate change is likely to affect plant diseases. Climate change influences the occurrence, prevalence, and severity of plant diseases. Projected atmospheric and climate change will thus affect the interaction between crops and pathogens in multiple ways. This will also affect disease management with regard to timing, preference, and efficacy of chemical, physical, and biological measures of control and their utilization within integrated pest management (IPM) strategies. Prediction of future requirements in disease management is of great interest for agro-industries, extension services, and practical farmers. A comprehensive analysis of potential climate change effects on disease control is difficult because current knowledge is limited and fragmented and due to the complexity of future risks for plant disease management, particularly if new crops are introduced in an area. Uncertainty in models of plant disease development under climate change calls for a diversity of management strategies, from more participatory approaches to interdisciplinary science. Involvement of stakeholders and scientists from outside plant pathology shows the importance of trade-offs. All these efforts and integrations will produce effective crop protection strategies using novel technologies as appropriate tools to adapt to altered climatic conditions.

**Keywords:** climate, change, plant, pathology, agriculture

## 1. Introduction

Climate change is a major concern for agricultural communities worldwide [1, 2]. The agricultural process consists of three main parts, pathogen, host, and environmental conditions, where the relation between them is the main key for the occurrence of infection from its absence (**Figure 1**), where climate change has great effect on all these factors. Changes in climatic parameters greatly affect crop production and susceptibility to pests as well as insect pest longevity. Climate change affects crop pests and disease susceptibility which in turn affects crop health, and these changes cause deviations in farming practices as to cope with the effects of these changes and to prevent a decline in productivity.

Agriculture is an economic activity which is highly reliant on climate and weather in order to produce the food and fiber necessary to sustain human life. Agriculture is, however, an activity which is extremely vulnerable to climate change.

The effects of climate change on agriculture are characterized by various forms of uncertainty. Firstly, there are uncertainties concerning the rate and magnitude

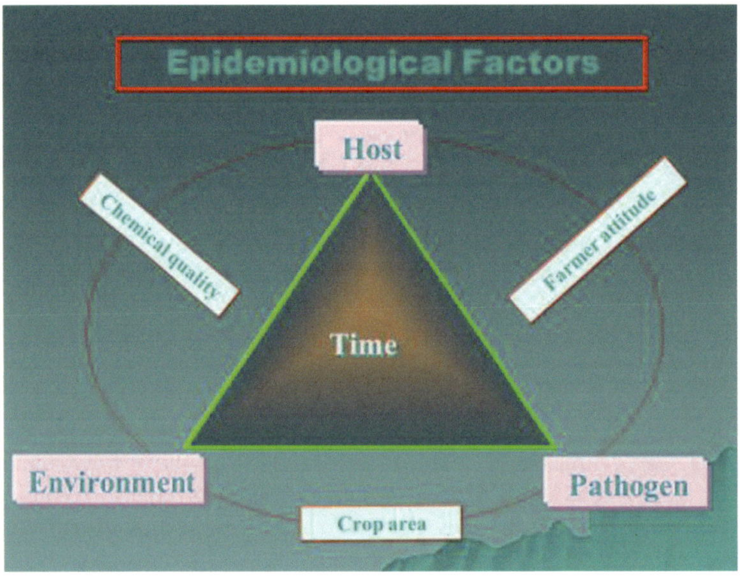


**Figure 1.**
*The relation between the pathogen, host, and environmental conditions which are the main factors required for infections to occur.*

of climate change itself. Secondly, there are uncertainties around the response of agriculture-based outputs, for example, with $CO_2$ fertilization. Thirdly, there are uncertainties as to how society responds or even the aptitude to respond to these expected impacts. Some aspects of climate change research are limited by these uncertainties. Most of these uncertainties cannot be quantified, causing a certain level of ignorance in our understandings of future climate change [3].

It is highly possible that climate change will affect food security at the global, regional, and local levels. Climate change can disturb and reduce food availability as well as lower food quality. For example, increases in temperatures, changes in extreme weather events, changes in precipitation patterns, and reductions in water availability could all result in reduced agricultural productivity. Prevalence of extreme weather conditions can also interrupt food delivery and result in increases in food prices due to low supply after extreme events, which are expected to be more frequent in the future. Moreover, increasing temperatures can contribute to spoilage and contamination.

There are four different future scenarios regarding climate change including A1, A2, B1, and B2. The A1 scenario focuses on rapid increases in global economic development, A2 focuses on rapid regional economic development instead of the global one in A1 scenario, B1 focuses on rapid global environmental development regarding agriculture, and B2 focuses on rapid environmental sustainability on regional and local levels.

## 2. Effect of climate change on plants and plant diseases

A major example for the devastating effects of climate change is floods caused by rising of sea level that can cause the disappearance of low-level lands and major crop losses. Another example is drought, where insufficiencies in water levels in the soil cause plants to lose their biological functions and even become more susceptible to diseases and pests. Climatic conditions contribute to the disease triangle, which involves the presence of a susceptible host, a pathogen, and suitable environmental conditions for infection to occur, and climate change affects environmental conditions whether it be in favor of the host or the pathogen. Examples of these conditions include dew, rain, relative humidity, temperature, aeration (wind), soil moisture, and sunlight intensity.

For any type of crop, the effect exerted by high temperature is highly dependent on the optimal growth and reproduction temperature of the crop. In certain regions, increased temperature may prove beneficial to the types of crops that usually grow there or permit farmers to switch to planting crops that grow in warmer areas. However, that is not always the case; if the higher temperature exceeds a crop's optimum temperature yields will decline, or worse, appearance and infestation of pathogens might occur. Crop yield can be affected by high levels of $CO_2$. A few laboratory experiments showed that high levels of $CO_2$ could positively affect growth. However, certain variables such as varying temperatures, water, ozone, and low nutrient levels may oppose these possible increases in yield. For instance, if the temperature is higher than a crop's optimal temperature requirement, if there are insufficiencies in water and nutrients, increase in yield may be low. Increased levels of $CO_2$ are linked to lower nitrogen and protein content in soybean and alfalfa plants, which results in a great quality reduction. Reduced forage and grain quality can reduce the ability of rangeland and pasture to support livestock which rely on grazing. Although rising $CO_2$ can stimulate plant growth, it also lowers the nutritional value of the majority of food crops. Rising levels of atmospheric carbon dioxide directly affect the concentrations of protein and essential minerals by reducing their content in a variety of plant species, which include rice, soybeans, and wheat. Therefore, the effect of rising $CO_2$ on the crops' nutritional value is considered a possible and indirect threat to human health as well. Moreover, due to the increased use and lowered efficiency of pesticides due to development of pest resistance, human health is additionally threatened by pesticide use as well as their residual toxicity in humans. More extreme temperatures and precipitation might decrease growth in certain crops. As previously mentioned, extreme events such as droughts and floods can decrease yield and damage crops. For instance, increased evening temperatures affected corn yield throughout the US Corn Belt. Additionally, premature budding due to a warmer winter instigated losses equivalent to $220 million of cherries in Michigan in 2010 and 2012.

Moreover, drought has developed into a major problem in regions with increased summer temperatures as this causes dryness in soils. Even though higher irrigation may be possible in certain regions, water supplies may be also lowered in other locations, causing a lower availability of water for irrigation when more is needed. Many weeds, pests, and fungi thrive under warmer temperatures, wetter climates, and increased $CO_2$ levels. Currently, US farmers spend more than $11 billion every year to control weeds, which compete with crops for nutritional resources. The ranges and distribution of weeds and pests are likely to increase with climate change. This could cause new problems for farmers' crops previously unexposed to these species.

Climate change parameters can have effects on both the host and the pathogen, for example, certain degrees of temperature promote pathogen growth, and certain temperatures can cause the host to have higher resistance to pathogenic infections. An example highlighting these events involves wheat and oats, which become more susceptible to rust diseases with increased temperature, while some forage species become more resistant [2]. Moreover, changes in temperature as limited as $CO_2$ changes could cause certain pests to undergo from 1 to 5 additional lifecycles per season, which increases the ability of the pests to overcome plant resistance.

Certain mycotoxins such as fusarium mycotoxins (produced by *Fusarium* spp.) have increased concentrations at harvest due to high humidity and temperature. Humid conditions also increase proliferation of weeds, and weed biomass increases with increasing temperatures.

Certain parameters can have different effects depending on plant physiology, for example, increased $CO_2$ levels can cause a decrease in plant decomposition rates, which results in higher fungal inoculum levels, and these concentrations may induce the production of more fungal spores. On the other hand, high $CO_2$ concentrations may cause physiological changes to plants, causing them to acquire higher resistance to certain pathogens.

Other extreme conditions may include low water levels and soil erosion which causes a decline in soil fertility and hence plant health.

Fungicide activity is also a major determinant factor; climate change may highly affect fungicide efficiency. Highly frequent rainfalls greatly impact the efficiency of contact fungicides, as rain has the ability to sweep and eliminate contact fungicides from the hosts' surface, rendering them ineffective. However, plants with high metabolic rates have increased intake of fungicides and aren't highly affected by this parameter.

In 2008, the International Food Policy Research Institute estimated that due to climate changes, by 2050, 25 million additional children will have malnutrition due to increased consumption of food products with little efforts done to adapt to and deal with these changes. In addition, the yearly costs to deal with the issue by reducing its impacts by 2050 will be $7 billion. It will generally be difficult to deal with international trade of crops due to appearance of unexpected pathogens more frequently (Food and Agriculture Organization of the United Nations, 2008).

## 3. Integrated pest management and mitigating pest management

IPM stands for integrated pest management, according to the Food and Agricultural Organizations (FAO) in the United States, IPM is an ecosystem approach involving crop protection which combines different strategies and practices toward growing healthier crops and minimizing the use of pesticides to protect the environment. It is an analytical method used to analyze the agroecosystem and its different elements in order to optimally manage these elements to control and minimize pests while protecting the environment and the economic health.

That is, the available methods of control (biological, cultural, chemical, and physical) should be considered and rationally applied by the farmers. However, IPM is more than just a tool and collection of control choices. It also comprises precaution techniques (which mainly include monitoring, prevention, early diagnosis, and forecasting) which assist in the control of pest populations as where data is collected, and preventive actions is recommended as explained in **Figure 2**. A significant part in IPM techniques is proper decision-making for any interferences. Every decision made must be justifiable both ecologically and economically. Consequently, control programs which involve systematic application of chemicals which may harm the environment are unacceptable in IPM processes. As an alternative, precedence is given to alternative control techniques as well as preventive methods. IPM has been applied in various countries and areas that differ in their natural, social, and economic circumstances in addition to their levels of agricultural expansion. However, advancement in crop yield and safety may be realized in any existing conditions through the implementation of IPM. The practice of IPM is not a strict and simple form of submission to regulations and rules, but it rather involves taking actions with environmentally friendly approaches through principles and approaches that contribute to the reduction of the use of chemicals and increasing food security to achieve agricultural sustainability. In order to make IPM as effective as possible, it should be modified to local conditions.

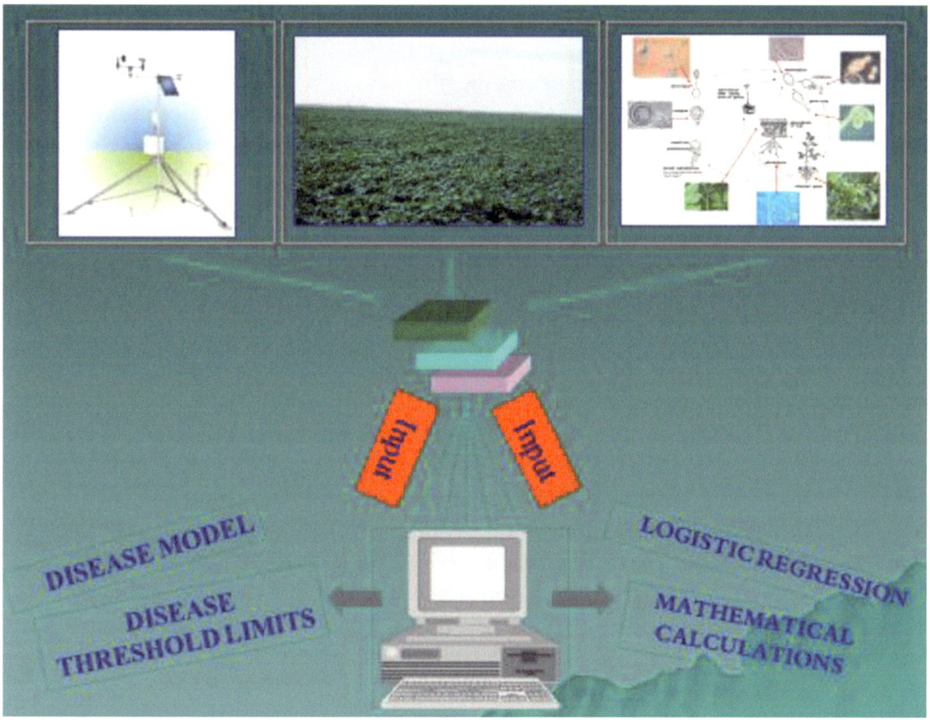


**Figure 2.**
*The correlation between forecasting data input, pathogen studies, and environmental conditions as input and disease modeling to develop preventive measures.*

The process does not involve a single pest management step, but a collection of pest management steps where decisions, evaluations, and control steps have to be made in order to successfully apply the chosen strategy. In IPM practice, farmers who understand the potential of pests when it comes to crop infestation follow a four-step approach. These steps include:

### 3.1 Setting action thresholds

Prior to taking any control decision or action, IPM first sets a threshold, which is a point at which the set of involved variable levels specifies that proper control actions must be made in order to control pest populations. Detection of a pest does not mean a certain control action is required. However, the detection of pests or variables at certain thresholds/levels is the determining factor. Therefore, the level at which pests could develop into threats is extremely important while taking pest management decisions.

### 3.2 Monitoring and identification of pests

A lot of insects, weeds, and other living organisms are not considered pests which require control. Most organisms are not harmful; on the contrary, some of them are useful. IPM programs are to accurately detect and screen for pests, so that proper management decisions can be made in combination with the action deciding thresholds. This process removes the probability that pesticides will be applied when there is no need for their use or that the incorrect type of pesticide will be applied.

### 3.3 Prevention

In order to achieve proper pest control, IPM programs are designed to manage the crop, lawn, or indoor space to prevent the appearance and development of pests. In the case of agricultural crops, this could mean using proper planting methods, for example, rotating between crops, planting resistant plant varieties, and the use of pest-free rootstock. These control techniques can be very useful and efficient in terms of cost and present lower risk to human health and the environment.

### 3.4 Control

Once the previously mentioned variables specify that control actions are needed and that protective approaches are ineffective, IPM programs then assess the appropriate control actions in terms of efficiency and risk. Efficient and low-risk control methods are considered first, including targeted and ecofriendly chemicals, such as pheromones which disrupt pest reproduction, or mechanical control, including trapping and weeding. If data generated by the previously mentioned steps specify that less risky management methods are ineffective, then further pest control attempts should be considered, for example, directed use of pesticides. The use of nontargeted pesticides is a less recommended alternative.

A lot of agricultural growers identify their pests prior to pesticide application. Less risky pesticides such as pheromones are employed by a lower subset of growers. In the end, a lot of these farmers are using IPM techniques. The objective is to make more growers use the proper IPM practices. Mostly, crops produced using IPM techniques are not recognized in the marketplace as organic crops. Growers who use IPM practices have no national certifications in certain countries. Due to the complexity of the IPM pest management techniques, it is not possible to use a single IPM description for all crops and all regions of a country. Many growers of certain crops including strawberries and potatoes are attempting to define what IPM means in their crops case as well as the region of growth. Moreover, certified IPM crops are unavailable in a lot of regions. With definitions, farmers can start to market their crops as IPM-grown, which would give consumers alternative and better options while purchasing their food.

The previously mentioned processes of IPM have been redefined and modified over time, and the IPM pyramid was created to provide an easier understanding of the approach. The IPM pyramid consists of three main processes which include preventive or indirect crop protection, risk assessment or monitoring, and responsive or direct crop protection. The three processes aim to increase the efficiency of each step involving crop breading and maintenance. Preventive crop protection involves the use of certified seeds, cultivars which have high tolerance to pathogens, and enhancement of natural enemies of plant pathogens such as microbiological competitors. Risk assessment and monitoring is the most crucial process in IPM; it involves the use of an early warning forecast system which provides information related to current climate and how it could affect plant health and by using such information and understanding plant physiology and susceptibility to pathogens; one can determine timeframes where plants are most susceptible to pathogens and take countermeasures to prevent or minimize pathogen severity (e.g., through the use of fungicides). Direct crop protection basically involves the countermeasures taken to deal with unfavorable conditions, which include the use of antagonistic microorganisms or application of fungicides.

A simple example for how an integrated system for pest management can be created as illustrated in **Figure 3**; generally in order to create such a system, the main information needed include weather data, crop, and disease information. Through knowing the weather data, which is most commonly obtained from meteorological

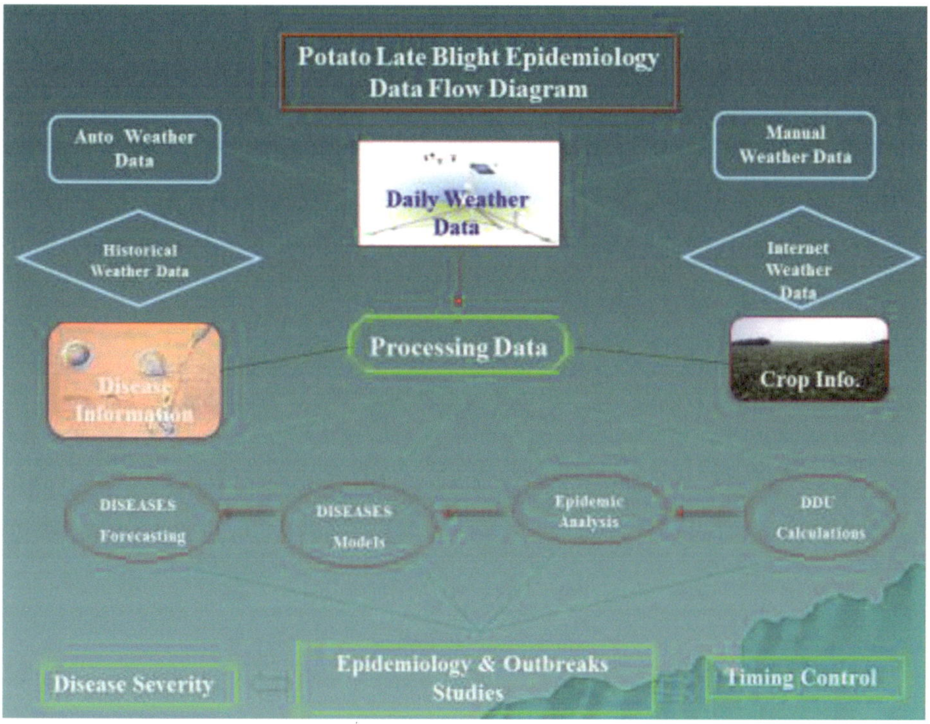


**Figure 3.**
*Example of pathogen epidemiology system in potato late blight and its integrated components.*

stations to obtain micro environment weather data and not that of the macro environment, macro environment data can still be used using certain equations to relate to the micro environment. This would allow the prediction and knowledge of current and upcoming weather conditions, in hand with obtaining information about the crop as in which pests affect the grown crops, optimal growth conditions, and lifetime as well as obtaining specific disease information for diseases which have the capability of affecting said crops. One can create a forecasting tool which helps prevent the spread of certain diseases.

After obtaining information about the disease, in order to create a disease model, its efficiency is determined through several tests. The general scopes of these tests would be the difference between disease spread and crop loss before and after the implementation of the model. Did delaying the use of pesticides until the threshold point for disease spread determined by the model actually cause a positive difference or was the threshold inaccurate? Was there a noticeable increase in crop yield after implementation? Was there any human error in pesticide management and spraying timelines? Several questions can be answered, and through these answers, the efficiency of the model can be determined.

There are several advantages for the use of IPM in mitigating agricultural problems which include:

Slower development of resistance to pesticides: Pesticide resistance can be incurred by the repeated use of pesticides; this would occur if a farmer is using traditional farming methods as pests would develop resistance to the pesticide due to repeated exposure to the pesticides through development of resistance by natural selection; then the resistant genes would be transferred to the offsprings, incurring permanent resistance to a given pesticide. However, this would not occur with reduced and efficient application of pesticides which is a main strategy adopted by IPM systems.

Maintaining a balanced ecosystem: Increased use of pesticides might affect nontarget and beneficial organisms; if these organisms are wiped out, the ecosystem will suffer and in turn results in species loss. IPM eradicates pests while minimizing the damage dealt to nontarget species.

Better cost vs. value: Since pesticides incur the highest cost for a farmer during a growing season. Reducing the use of pesticides proves more cost-efficient on the long run than the price for equipment used to determine thresholds, weather conditions, and application of IPM strategies. This is due to limited and efficient pesticide application.

The disadvantages of using IPM strategies include:

More involvement in the technicalities of the method

All individuals involved have to be educated about the available methods and importance of IPM.

Time and energy consuming

IPM strategies are critical strategies; failure to proceed with certain decisions during the IPM process can prove fatal to the entire process due to the need of different control methods for different pests and the need to monitor the application process.

## 4. Decision support system (DSS)

In order to produce an efficient model, understanding the decision support system is essential. The decision support system is an informatics tool which uses mathematical models such as equations and statistics to help the decision-maker take action. The three main phases of a decision-making system include intelligence, design, and choice; two other subsequent phases include implementation of the decision and monitoring of its effect and outcomes. The decision-making process in IPM is highly complex and dynamic; it requires a high level of organization and constant update of operators; it requires the presence of databases and means to collect data and information as well as tools to handle data. The decision-making process generally provides the capability to identify when difficulties may occur and how to deal with these difficulties depending on data provided.

The main properties of a successful DSS include ease of use, presentation format, system restrictiveness, decisional guidance, feedback, and interaction support:

### 4.1 Ease of use

A DSS system is only beneficial if users perceive a DSS to be easy to use and that using it enhances their performance and productivity. The system should be easy to operate and interact with and requires minimal cognitive efforts; to sum up it should reduce mental effort and time consumed to analyze data and increase comfort of the user.

### 4.2 Presentation format

The way information is presented through the program/system may influence the user's judgment/decision; therefore, the way information is presented through the decision support system should be focused on showing key data in an accurate and favorable format.

### 4.3 System restrictiveness and decisional guidance

These refer to how much a DSS limits the options of the user and to which extent it guides the user toward a certain decision. A good DSS provides a reasonable amount of options within the scope of the topic/field at hand, as well as ample guidance to perform the optimal decision and achieve the most beneficial outcome.

### 4.4 Feedback

The way the system provides messages and the wording of certain commands is important because they promote positive user experience and enhance the decision-making process.

### 4.5 Interaction support

Interaction support means that users are permitted a particular level of interaction with a DSS. The DSS design is the determining factor on the presence as well as the level of interactivity between the user and the system. Users may have control over the system when a certain level of interaction support is present. The received control over the use of a system may have a motivational effect on its use.

The system involves an integration of certain components and interacting factors with a common objective. In the case of pathogen monitoring, a pathogen monitoring system would basically receive input based on environmental factors and properties, and the output is expressed in the form of maps, information, and graphs. The system would then, based on information provided by threshold charts for pathogen favorable growth conditions, give out options that would determine the best possible course of actions in order to prevent disease outbreaks and crop loss.

With this, an integrated model is illustrated. Although the systems are accurate, the main drawbacks include maintenance needs of meteorological stations, the requirement of different systems with different parameters depending on the type of plant, and disease as well as their growth conditions and application of these processes in farms which could be a difficult task due to old farming traditions.

### 4.6 Forecasting and early warning system

Forecasting of pests and diseases appearance in plants is an additional application that demands a consistent and dependable stock of weather data. There are huge losses in yields due to pests and diseases prevalence which could have been controlled in several situations if the appropriate forecasting techniques were available. Consequently, the forecasting and early warning system, within the Plant Pathology Research Institute of the Agricultural Research Center, was established in the same timeframe of system and climate change applications in agriculture.

Prediction of pest, disease prevalence, and progression based on weather data is extremely crucial when planning and implementing control measures.

The idea of forecasting and early warning system has been introduced in 1926; with the appearance of computers and information technology, softwares were developed in order to produce convenient warning systems. Currently, early warning systems are being used to deal with pathogens of certain crops such as faba beans. The main concept involves the use of a mobile telemetry automated weather station system to monitor environmental conditions and softwares to interpret the input; based on the information provided, a decision can be made regarding the protection and maintenance of plant health.

An early warning system is shown in **Figure 4** which is used to predict and prevent the development of chocolate spot in faba beans that has been developed by Dr. Sahar Zayan, Head of the Early Warning Unit, Plant Pathology Research Institute [4].

A set of computer programs have been successfully produced by the unit's work team, and some of them were applied on crop databases in different governorates. These programs have proven to be successful early warning systems, as they predicted the appearance of diseases before infection and before they reached the epidemic level as well as the reduction of the amount of fungicides used for disease resistance.

The first computer simulation model for prediction of late blight in potato was being produced in Egypt by Prof. Dr. Mohsen Abd El Razek Afifi and Dr. Sahar Zayan in the forecasting and early warning unit in the plant pathology research institute, Agricultural Research Center. The model was applied in the fields, and it produced results which assisted in the protection of the potato crops from infection and the reduction of pesticide application periods which was equivalent to 75% in certain regions.

After the construction of the first Egyptian computer model, the creator named it EGY-BLIGHTCAST, and its efficiency was verified in all the computer laboratories (Workstations) as well as the field conditions by the potato producing private sector companies [5]; the model was applied in 1998 and 1999, and it preserved the crop from the risks of epidemic infection; pesticide savings reached 50% in a season and 75% in another, and the productivity increased by a ton and 300 kilograms per acre which was denoted in official reports by the applying company. Afterward the model was developed in 2002 and 2003; it was used in different regions (hotspots of late blight on potato crops) in the main governorates for potato production in Egypt throughout 2004–2008; the methodologies for prediction of late blight were linked and modified based on short-term observation.

Throughout several growing seasons of potato and the analysis of the relation between 24-hour meteorological data which were collected in real-time from the forecasting station (AdconTelemetry A733) and its effect on the possibility of daily infection by diseases triggered by late blight, it is possible for the EGY-BLIGHTCAST (DDIP) model to accurately predict the outbreak of the late blight disease and to drastically reduce the cost of necessary fungicide to control the outbreak when compared to routine spraying programs (schedule based programs)

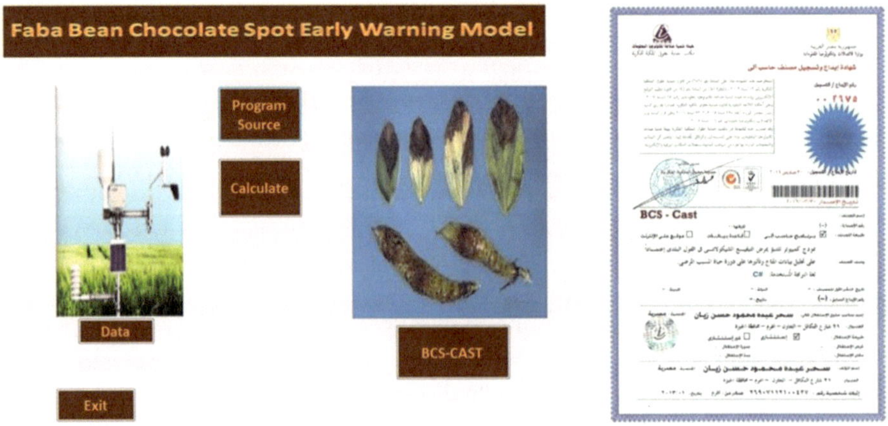


**Figure 4.**
*A certified early warning system for faba bean chocolate spot [4].*

in light of the field conditions. The main roles for the analysis of the model validation system were discussed through a study which was published in the year 2009. Moreover, several computer simulation models were produced on the same basis for a number of important diseases on strategic crops in Egypt, including downy and powdery mildew in grapes—downy mildew in onions and early blight in tomatoes. All of these forecasting models were applied in test fields, and their efficiency in disease prediction was proven as well as the actual savings in application of pesticides used in disease control.

In the year 2015, the system and model production techniques were developed by Dr. Sahar Zayan, and a study was published for a computer model for brown spot on beans which received an Intellectual Property Rights (IPR) license from official authorities in Egypt [6].

With the appearance of climate change phenomena, farmers and decision-makers will need more decision support systems especially plant disease forecasting systems.

## Thanks

I would like to thank my team who helped me in developing this work.

## Author details

Sahar Abdou Zayan
Unit of Forecasting and Early Warning, Plant Pathology Research Institute (ARC), Giza, Egypt

*Address all correspondence to: drsahar.abdo@gmail.com

## References

[1] FAO. Climate Change, Agriculture and Food Security [Internet]. Agriculture Organization. 2008. Available from: http://www.fao.org/faostat/en/#data/RF

[2] Coakley S, Scherm H, Chakraborty S. Climate change and plant disease management. Annual Review of Phytopathology. 1999;**37**(1):399-426

[3] Anita W, Dominic M, Neil A. Climate Change and Agriculture Impacts, Adaptation and Mitigation: Impacts, Adaptation and Mitigation. OECD Publishing; 2010

[4] Zayan S, Morsy M. BCS-CAST: An early warning computerized model for Faba bean chocolate spot in Egypt. In: Proceedings of 5th International Conference on Alternative Methods of Crop Protection; 11-13 March 2015; Lille, France. Lille, France: Association Françoise of Plant Protection (AFPP); 2015

[5] Afifi M, Zayan S. Implementation of Egy-Blight Cast the first computer simulation model for potato late blight in Egypt. In: Proceedings of Agriculture: Africa's "Engine for Growth"-Plant Science & Biotechnology Hold the Key at Roth Amsted Research; Harpenden, UK: Association of Applied Biologists; October 2009. 12-14

[6] Medany M, Zayan S, Fiani D. New communication methodologies in an innovative digital extension system in Egypt. In: The Ciheam Watch Letter no 38 in February 2017 on "Rural Innovation and Digital Revolution in Agriculture". 2017

Section 2

# Host-Pathogen Coevolution

Chapter 7

# Asymptomatic Phytoplasma Reveal a Novel and Troublesome Infection

*Philip Donkersley, Farley W.S. Silva, Murilo S. Alves, Claudine M. Carvalho, Abdullah M. Al-Sadi and Simon L. Elliot*

## Abstract

Asymptomatic infections are by their nature challenging to study and even more difficult to monitor across broad geographical ranges, particularly as methods are reliant on expensive molecular techniques. The plant pathogen that causes Witches' Broom disease of lime (*Candidatus* Phytoplasma aurantifolia) is a major limiting factor in lime production across the Middle East and was recently detected in Brazil, but without the typical symptoms from the Middle East. Here, we discuss the difficulty of monitoring asymptomatic infections and highlight the threat posed by highlight future outbreaks. Asymptomatic infections have important implications for understanding the evolution of pathogens within perennial hosts. We use three model systems of asymptomatic infections: (i) a Phytoplasma and (ii) a bacterial infection of lime (*Citrus aurantifolia*) and (iii) an "out-group" Phytoplasma of Cassava (*Manihot esculenta*) to demonstrate consistency across divergent hosts. We found that although all plants in the study were intentionally infected, assays typically did not confirm this diagnosis. Emergent technologies monitoring gene expression could be used to both study novel biology associated with asymptomatic infections and develop monitoring technologies. We highlight the difficulty of monitoring asymptomatic infections in possible future outbreaks and have important implications for understanding the evolution of pathogens within perennial hosts.

**Keywords:** *Citrus aurantifolia*, acid lime, silent infection, phytoplasma, differentially expressed genes

## 1. Introduction

Vector-borne plant pathogens of perennial crop species provide an opportunity to study the impacts of long-term infections, in terms of epidemiology and vector ecology. Crop diseases directly threaten global food security; an estimated 16% of food production globally is lost despite our efforts to control crop diseases [1]. Perennial crops generally have advantages over annuals in terms of energetic efficiency; for example, constant canopy development increases photosynthesis efficiency [2], which results in 30% increases in carbon turnover than those maintained by annual crops [2]. Pathogens must evolve to infect and reproduce within a single year in annual cropping systems, and thus typically demonstrate more aggressive pathologies [3], which often require multiple hosts, such as potato blight (*Phytophthora infestans*) and wheat rust (*Puccinia graminis*). As the host plant remains in situ after harvest, perennial cropping systems therefore theoretically allow for evolution of slower pathologies, which may be cryptic in nature.

Globally, plant pathogens are spreading faster than ever, due to climate change, increased crop and germplasm trading, failure of border biocontrol and associated spread of vector species. Here, we shall introduce and discuss a complex vector-borne plant pathogens of a perennial tropical cash-crop plant: *Citrus*. *Citrus* is the world's principal fruit crop, with about 60 million megatons grown annually [4]. Limes account for ~5% of global *Citrus* production [4]. Lime is cultivated in tropical, subtropical and temperate regions from 40°N to 40°S [5, 6]. Countries in the Middle East, as well as India, Pakistan, Brazil, Argentina and Mexico grow lime as a key part of their agricultural economies [7, 8].

The production of lime in the Middle East has been markedly impacted by Witches' Broom Disease of Lime (WBDL) [7]. Symptoms of witches' broom disease of lime (WBDL) were first observed in Oman in the 1970s [9]. Infected trees present with "witches' brooms": shoot structures characterized compactness and small, pale green leaves. In the advanced stages of the disease, leaves become dry, brooms become increasingly more prevalent, and fruits become significantly smaller and less marketable. Finally, the tree collapses within 4 or 5 years after infection [10].

Asymptomatic ("silent") infections have recently been detected in lime trees in Brazil [11] and Oman [12]. This silent infection was observed through molecular testing of plant material, yet the host plants themselves show no obvious visible symptoms. These infected trees do however, also collapse within the 5 year post infection period [13], making this asymptomatic variant potentially even more of a threat to global lime production.

Detailed research into this system has been limited, some suggest that the silent infection may be due to ultra-low pathogen titre levels within the host plant [12, 14] or due to different interactions with plant defences [15] or insect vectors [16, 17]. Silent infections are difficult to monitor and pose a significant risk to global food security, given that the limited knowledge we have suggests they may be as destructive as symptomatic [18], but we do not yet know the full extent of their range.

The Phytoplasma "*Candidatus* Phytoplasma aurantifolia" has been identified as the causative agent of WBDL [19]. Phytoplasma are wall-less gram-positive bacteria belonging to the class Mollicutes [20]. They are found in the phloem sieve tubes of plants and in the gut, salivary glands and other organs of Hemipteran insect vectors [21]. Phytoplasma are obligate biotrophic organisms, which lack many essential genes that encode for components of metabolic pathways; and they likely import metabolites such as nucleotides, amino acids, and fatty acids from the host plant [22]. Phytoplasma are the only known organisms that lack ATP-synthase subunits, which are thought to be essential for life [22]. Owing to the inability to culture them *in vitro* and their inaccessibility in host plants [19, 22], the molecular mechanisms that underlie Phytoplasma infections within host plants remain largely unknown [10]. Phytoplasma may be able to overcome plant defences by producing specific proteins: effectors [15]. The effectors (e.g., SAP11 and SAP54) may modulate host plant growth and interactions with the insect vectors [16, 23].

Although studies using proteomics [10, 24] and cDNA-amplified fragment length polymorphism (cDNA-AFLP) [25] have investigated differentially expressed genes (DEGs) in plants infected by "*Ca*. P. aurantifolia," these studies provide only a brief snapshot of gene expression and regulation during infection. Recent developments in high throughput "omics" based approaches now allow a detailed examination of plant pathogen interactions, and these have been applied to symptomatic infections of "*Ca*. P. aurantifolia" in the Middle East [18, 26]. Our study examined DEGs in symptomatic and asymptomatic infections of the Phytoplasma in acid lime trees. Although asymptomatic infections have been linked to fitness benefits in the vectors of this pathogen [17], our knowledge of understanding of gene expression differences in an asymptomatic infection are extremely limited. One way to understand the effects and biology of asymptomatic infections is by developing our knowledge of these differentially expressed genes.

Within this chapter, we shall discuss two studies on asymptomatic infections of crop plants [1]. Reliable detection of asymptomatic plant pathogens is the greatest limitation on controlling and limiting their global spread. We first discuss and test the potential for currently employed molecular tools to misidentify "healthy" plants. We study three asymptomatic infections (a Phytoplasma of lime, a Phytoplasma of cassava and *Citrus* Huanglongbing) and compare the rate of false-negatives detecting the disease [2]. Asymptomatic infections in Brazil represent a novel biology by the Phytoplasma infecting lime trees. This novel pathology needs to be explored to better understand the infection process, and also presents us with an opportunity to design superior detection tools. We compare the gene expression of infected symptomatic and asymptomatic plants using qPCR. These findings provide an important and novel examination of the nature of asymptomatic infections, a poorly understood, emerging area of plant pathology.

## 2. Pathogen detection in the absence of visible symptoms: study system

In order to comprehensively study the most ubiquitous methods used globally for asymptomatic infections of crop plants, we used three model systems: the aforementioned Phytoplasma causing Witches' Broom Disease of Lime (WBDL), a closely related Phytoplasma causing Cassava (*Manihot esculenta* L.) Witches' Broom, and an out group pathogen of lime—"*Candidatus Liberibacter* asiaticus," causative organism of Huanglongbing disease of lime. Data for the first two pathosystems was collected for the present study, whereas data from Huanglongbing came from a previously published study by *Citrus* [27].

### 2.1 Sample locations

Acid lime (*C. aurantifolia* L.) trees were grown on a *Citrus* orchard maintained at Universidade Federal de Viçosa (UFV), Brazil (S20°45′585″; W042°50′908″). The site was chosen as plant material there had previously been found to be infected with "*Ca*. P. aurantifolia," but showing no visible symptoms [17].

Leaf samples of cassava (*M. esculenta*) grown in a glasshouse at UFV and deliberately infected with a cassava witches' broom (Phytoplasma 16SrIII-A) were also taken. For details regarding this pathogen, please see [18]. Although this disease can display typical symptoms of witches' broom (e.g., stunting, leaf chlorosis, deformation, and reduced size), the infections in Brazil do not display symptoms until harvest, when it can cause 100% crop losses [18].

### 2.2 Plant material

*Citrus* leaf samples from Brazil were taken from four 15-year adult trees and 10 1-year saplings; for each adult tree 30 leaves were collected and for saplings 10 samples were collected in a semi-random fashion. Cassava leaf samples were collected from eight 1-year adult plants, 10 leaves were sampled from each cassava plant.

The sampling strategy for both lime Phytoplasma and cassava Phytoplasma aimed to collect a spatially diverse group of samples (orientated on x, y and z axes relative to the trunk), with the position of each leaf sampled noted with respect to its branches from the main trunk. For all sample types locations, leaf midrib samples (the larger vein along the midline of a leaf) were taken. The midribs were immediately frozen in liquid nitrogen after harvesting and then transported to the laboratory, where they were stored at −80°C until total DNA and RNA isolation.

### 2.3 Molecular detection of Phytoplasma

The presence/absence of the Phytoplasma in the leaf samples of both acid lime and cassava was analysed using PCR for Phytoplasma detection. To this end, total DNA was extracted from acid lime leaf samples using the DNeasy Qiagen Plant Mini Prep kit following manufacturer's instructions. Then, total DNA was extracted from the cassava leaf samples following the protocol of [28], with modifications that are detailed in [18].

We then used a nested PCR using universal primers for Phytoplasma detection. Extracted DNA of both *Citrus* and cassava Phytoplasma were amplified using 16S rRNA PCR primers P4 (5′-CAT CAT TTA GTT GGG CAC TT-3′) and 23rev (5′-CGT CCT TCA TCG GCT CTT-3′) in the initial reaction, and the resulting amplicon was diluted (1:10) and used as template DNA for nested PCR amplification using the P3 (5′-GGA TGG ATC ACC TCC TT-3′) and 23rev primers [18, 29, 30].

PCR amplification was carried out using a Loccus Biotechnologia TC9639 Thermal Cycler (LB, São Paulo, Brazil) in 20 μl volumes, such that each reaction contained the following: 2.0 μl (20 pmol) of each primer, 8.0 μl water (DNA-free water; Qiagen, SP, Brazil), 4.0 μl sample extracted DNA and 0.1 μl Invitrogen *Taq* DNA Polymerase (5 U/μl) (ThermoFisher Scientific, Brazil), 1.3 μl MgCl (50 mm) 2.6 μl dNTPs (10 mm), 2.0 μl PCR buffer (200 mm Tris-HCl pH 8.4, 500 mm KCl). For the first round PCR, initial denaturation at 95°C for 3 min, followed by 30 cycles of 95°C for 45 s, 55°C for 45 s and 72°C for 3 min, with a final elongation step at 72°C for 7 min. For the nested reactions, the conditions were 95°C for 3 min, followed by 32 cycles of 95°C for 45 s, 54°C for 45 s and 72°C for 3 min, with a final elongation step at 72°C for 7 min. The resulting amplicon was then visualised on agarose gel electrophoresis using SybrSafe DNA stain to confirm the presence/absence of both Phytoplasma from each leaf sample of each plant host.

Data on the successful amplification of "*Candidatus* C. liberibacter" were obtained from the Coy et al. [27] study. Briefly, this study compares the efficacy of the current method of detection for C. *liberibacter asiaticus* within plant and insect samples is by a presence/absence PCR assay using a 16S rDNA gene target. Specifically they examined these methods for sensitivity to low bacterial titers or suboptimal PCR conditions that can result in false-negatives. This study concluded that the high incidence of false negatives using this system could contributes to the under-reporting of plant pathogen infections. Hence, the data paralleled our present study, and were used for direct comparison of this pathosystem with our own presented here.

## 3. Pathogen detection in the absence of visible symptoms: results and discussion

Detection of "*Ca*. Phytoplasma aurantifolia" by 23S-PCR on asymptomatic acid lime (*C. aurantifolia*) plants showed that all plants sampled in this study were technically infected (**Table 1**), meaning that each plant had at least one sample that positively detected the Phytoplasma. The proportion of samples that failed to detect the pathogen was, on average, in adult trees 38.5% ± 6.62 (n = 3), and in saplings

| Tree | Infected | Detection likelihood (%) |
|---|---|---|
| A | 21/31 | 67.74 |
| B | 24/44 | 54.55 |
| C | 28/45 | 62.22 |
| SA | 5/10 | 50.00 |
| SB | 6/10 | 60.00 |
| SC | 6/10 | 60.00 |
| SD | 6/10 | 60.00 |
| SE | 4/10 | 40.00 |
| SF | 3/10 | 30.00 |
| SG | 3/10 | 30.00 |
| SH | 10/10 | 100.00 |

**Table 1.**
*Results of asymptomatic infections of "Ca. Phytoplasma aurantifolia" detection using 23S-PCR from adult (A–C) and sapling (SA-SH) Citrus acid lime plants.*

46.25% ± 22.6 (n = 10). Within cassava (*Manihot esculenta*), false-negative rate was 48.75% ± 17.3 (n = 8). False-negative molecular tests have also been found in molecular techniques for detecting Huanglongbing infections in *Citrus* plants. Thus particular study found a false-negative rate of 54.9%, using a nested PCR assay [27], and identified that more sensitive molecular tests involving qPCR addressed this issue, albeit not in a manner applicable to growers and germplasm suppliers expecting to provide disease-free planting material [31].

The evidence for false-negative across multiple plant pathosystems has notable implications across the field. One of the base assumptions of plant pathology is the suitability of a biological sample to represent the entire host plant. These false-negatives mean that multiple biological samples per plant may be required to correctly identify the presence of a pathogen. A hypothetical plant with α leaves and a false-negative rate of $\beta$ ± SD, to guarantee a correct identification (under P = 1.00) the minimum sample number (n) must be:

$$n = (\alpha \times \beta) + 1 \tag{1}$$

$$\sum_{k=x}^{\alpha} \binom{\alpha}{k} \beta^k (1 - \beta)^{n-k} \tag{2}$$

Due to the nature of additive probabilities (Eq. (2)), the probability of, for example, 38 continuous false-negatives on a tree of 100 leaves would be P = $4.83^{-22}$. Consequently, a decision support system based on the likelihood of having an infected tree can be developed in order to determine the appropriate number of samples required to avoid a false-negative. For example, for P = 0.05, minimum sample number would be n = 4.19; for P = 0.005, n = 8.94; for P = 0.001, n = 12.25 (**Figure 1a**). For cassava similarly the minimum sample number for the same probabilities would be (in order): n = 3.55, n = 7.20 and n = 9.76 (**Figure 1b**).

Asymptomatic plant pathogens are particularly troublesome within perennial crops as they are not removed at the end of the growing season and act as reservoirs of infectious materials to be dispersed to new hosts by insects (and other vehicles). Persistence of asymptomatic infections in hosts may also cause problems through subtle direct damage or sublethal infections leading to plant-by-plant transmission

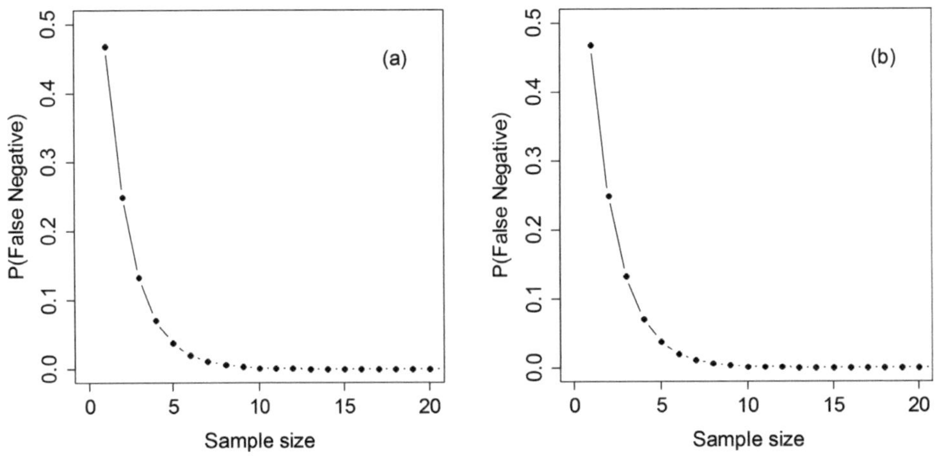


**Figure 1.**
*Probability function for false negatives using PCR-based detection for asymptomatic Phytoplasma infections. The additive probability of sequential false negatives as the sample size increases in (a) Citrus Phytoplasma in adult Citrus trees (false negative rate = 38.5%); (b) cassava Phytoplasma (false negative rate = 48.75%).*

[32]. The use of accurate and timely diagnostic methods is undoubtedly one of the best ways to monitor pathogen ranges in asymptomatic infected plants, and thus avoid dissemination to new hosts and ranges. Generally, traditional methods of identification based on visual symptoms and culturing in laboratories are time-consuming, labour-intensive, costly and have "very low sensitivity and specificity" [33, 34].

Molecular methods are the mainstream alternative to symptomology and laboratory culture. The results of this present (and a previous) study [27] have demonstrated a potential flaw in molecular methods: the frequency of false-negatives. Whereas classical plant pathology can rely on a non-destructive inspection of the entire host plant, culture and molecular methods must only use a small "representative" destructive subsample of the plant. The major limitation to this is the quality of the representation of the host plant within this subsample. We have demonstrated here that a single biological sample from an infected plant may not be representative of the whole plant and therefore multiple samples from within the same host plant can result in different results from molecular testing for pathogens. We found false-negative rates between 38 and 49%, meaning that approximately a minimum of one in three samples would fail to detect a pathogen if taken alone. Although this calls into question the use of single biological samples for identifying pathogens by molecular methods, these methods have to strike a balance between precision and cost [35]. We calculate, based on these false-negative rates, minimum sample numbers (per plant) between 3 and 5 samples, which may make these methods prohibitively expensive for widespread use within agriculture.

By comparison, real-time PCR used to detect and quantify pathogens in symptomless plant tissues is a promising tool to improve our understanding of "silent" infections [36]. Different methods of DNA amplification that rely on conventional and quantitative PCRs have also been developed to detect and identify "*Ca.* Liberibacter" species associated with Huanglongbing (HLB) in *Citrus* [27, 37]. But other simpler methods, such as direct tissue blot immunoassay, have been used to facilitate detection of pathogens in asymptomatic plants of *Citrus* [38]. Molecular tools have been developed for identification of WBDL from field samples [7, 39], but remain prohibitively expensive for widespread implementation by growers. Much research effort and resources have been devoted to development of on-the-spot diagnostics in plant pathology, and have shown success in control and monitoring the spread of some plant diseases (e.g., *Potato Virus Y*), but do not exist for Phytoplasma yet [40]. *In-situ* kits for testing Phytoplasma using immunofluorescence have been developed; but have not been adopted for widespread use yet [34, 41].

## 4. Novel asymptomatic infection biology: study system

Successful identification of asymptomatic infections by the Phytoplasma causing Witches' Broom Disease of Lime (WBDL) provide a unique opportunity to compare the pathology with its' symptomatic counterpart. A recent study by Mardi et al. [26] using a high-throughput genomics approach identified 2805 differentially expressed genes in symptomatically infected *Citrus* plants. This study revealed the key potential molecular pathways through which the Phytoplasma infects and parasitizes its host. Correspondingly, here we studied 25 of these that were differentially expressed by more than 128-fold and 4 further genes identified as significantly differentially expressed in recent infections found in Brazil (Alves et al. unpublished data). These genes allowed us to design a targeted study to understand how the symptomatic and asymptomatic infections differ, and potentially identify some of the "silent" symptoms in this newly emerged pathosystem.

### 4.1 Sample locations

Acid lime (*C. aurantifolia*) trees were grown at the same *Citrus* orchard at UFV mentioned previously. Lime leaves were also collected from cultivated areas in Muscat, Oman (N23°58′591″, E58°40′590″). Omani samples were collected from a farm with symptomatic infected trees (drastic reduction in growth, generalized leaf yellowing and necrosis) and uninfected (healthy tissue).

### 4.2 Plant material

Six *Citrus* plants were sampled each in Brazil and Oman (three symptomatic and three healthy plants), for three biological replicates. Samples from Brazil were confirmed for Phytoplasma by PCR (see Section 2), samples from Oman were confirmed by symptoms (drastic reduction in growth, generalized leaf yellowing and necrosis).

### 4.3 RNA extraction

Total RNA was extracted from the three biological replicates of limes infected with "*Ca*. P aurantifolia" and three healthy acid lime leaves (from both Brazil and Oman) using the RNeasy Plant Mini Kit (Qiagen, SP, Brazil). RNA quantity and quality were determined using a Nano-Drop ND 1000 spectrophotometer (Thermo Scientific, MA, USA). five hundred nanogram of total RNA from each replicate was reverse-transcribed in a 20 μl reaction using 1 μl of Invitrogen SuperScript® III Reverse Transcriptase (Thermo Scientific), 1 μl oligo(dT)$_{18}$ (100 nm), 1 μl dTT (100 mm), 2 μl dNTP (10 mm), 4 μl 5× first-strand buffer (250 mm Tris-HCl (pH 8.3), 375 mm KCl, 15 mm $MgCl_2$) and RNAse free water (Qiagen).

### 4.4 Gene expression

Gene specific primers were designed for 15 genes belonging to key pathways with possible implication in disease progression and resistance identified by Mardi et al. [26] and four by Alves et al. (unpublished). The sequence of primers, amplicon length, optimal primer and enzymatic efficiency for each primer pair is presented in **Table 2**. Mardi genes were amplified only for Brazilian samples,

| Unigene | Forward primer | Reverse primer | Amplicon length (bp) |
|---|---|---|---|
| U352 | TGGCTCTGGATGGCATTG | GTGCTTCTGGGATAGTGA | 133 |
| U2265 | TGCTGCATTGGTTCTGTC | GACTGCAAAGGACTCCAAG | 130 |
| U27316 | ATGCGATACACAACCCAATCT | CGGCCATGAGACCAAAACT | 126 |
| U75775 | GAAGGAGCTGACGTTTTC | CTTCTGCCTCTTCCCTCTC | 160 |
| U26576 | GATTGTCCGCCCAGTAGTG | CACGCGATCAGCCAAACTC | 174 |
| U72184 | CAAAGAGATGGGCAAAGAG | GCCAAATTACAAACCAAACGA | 121 |
| U59125 | TATGGGGATAAGGGGTGT | TGCCACAACTAACCTCCTC | 182 |
| U68165 | CTGCTGAGATTACATGGTT | CTCTTCAGGGAATTGCAC | 147 |
| U68593 | GACTCTCTTTCAATGCCA | TTGAAAGCACAGGTTCCGA | 119 |
| U77887 | CATGCCATCCTCTTCACT | GGGTTGGGTTGAGTATCT | 123 |
| U3869 | CTCCTCCTCCTCCTCCAAAG | GCGAACCCATCACACTACAT | 117 |
| U17275 | AACACCCATTTGCATTCTC | GGTTTGTATGCCTTCGATG | 130 |
| U41653 | GAGAGTAGCAAGACCTCAAG | TATCACCAGCCTCACTTCAC | 114 |
| U17606 | CTCACCGCAGATTTTGAACCAC | ACATCCGTCTTCTCATCCACA | 158 |
| U24969 | GCCTCCGTTTCCAATTCTC | GATACCGAGGATTTCATGGC | 131 |
| WRKY33 | GATGATGAAAATGAACCTGATGCT | CAATTCTTGGCTCCCTCACAGT | 144 |
| WRKY70 | AGACCGGAGAGGATGCTACAAG | CCCATATTTCCTCCATGCAAA | 152 |
| MYBR1 | AATGGATCCAACTTGGTTTTGAA | ATCCAAACTCGCCCTGGTT | 110 |
| JAZ6 | ACAATGATGCAACCCCACTTC | TGCTGCAGCCCTTTCTTTTC | 120 |

**Table 2.**
*Primer sequences for potential infection related differentially expressed genes in Citrus aurantifolia used in qPCR.*

whereas we were able to study the smaller number Alves genes were amplified for both Brazilian and Oman samples.

The selected genes were quantified using the Applied Biosystems StepOne™ Real Time PCR system (Thermo Scientific). qRT-PCR was performed in a 10-µl reaction containing 5 µl of SYBR Green PCR Master Mix, 4 µl of each primer mix (**Table 1**), 50 ng of template cDNA. The thermal cycling conditions consisted of an initial denaturation at 95°C for 5 min, followed by 40 cycles of denaturation at 95°C for 30 s, annealing at 60°C for 30 s, and extension at 72°C for 45 s, and a final extension step at 72°C for 5 min.

The detected expression of selected transcripts was measured using the absolute quantification method. We prepared standard curves for each target gene (0.01–10 ng $\mu l^{-1}$) in order to quantify each genes expression relative to a standard internal control gene. Cycle threshold ($C_T$) value of each gene relative to the internal control gene was used to estimate gene expression in RNA concentration values of ng $\mu l^{-1}$ [42]. Triplicate reactions were used for each sample.

Ubiquitin 1 and Tubulin alpha were used as internal reference genes, with primer sets UBi-IF (5′-TTT CTT CCT CAA CTT CAC TTG TAT CC-3′), UBi-IR (5′-TGG TCA TAG GCT GTT CGA TCA C-3′), α-tub-F (5′-CTG CAA GGG TTC TTG GTG TTC-3′) and α-tub-R (5′-GAT AGG CGT TCC AGT AAC AAC GA-3′), respectively. Standard curves for each gene were examined in the amplification plot and the standard curve plot was prepared in ABI 7500 software v.2.0.6. Reaction efficiency, R square and slope values were calculated by the ABI 7500 software v.2.0.6 program (**Table 3**) and were used to determine the copy number of infection-related RNA in each sample.

| Unigene | Slope | −1/slope | E | E (%) |
|---|---|---|---|---|
| U352 | −4.69701 | 0.212901 | 1.159017 | 115.9 |
| U2265 | −4.99484 | 0.200206 | 1.148863 | 114.9 |
| U27316 | −4.17641 | 0.23944 | 1.180534 | 118.1 |
| U75775 | −1.01071 | 0.989403 | 1.985363 | 198.5 |
| U26576 | −1.69178 | 0.591093 | 1.506388 | 150.6 |
| U72184 | −4.35679 | 0.229527 | 1.17245 | 117.2 |
| U59125 | −4.19476 | 0.238393 | 1.179678 | 117.9 |
| U68165 | −4.67463 | 0.213921 | 1.159836 | 115.9 |
| U68593 | −1.68595 | 0.593137 | 1.508523 | 150.8 |
| U77887 | −1.32334 | 0.755662 | 1.688406 | 168.8 |
| U3869 | −4.3699 | 0.228838 | 1.171891 | 117.2 |
| U17275 | −2.41499 | 0.41408 | 1.332449 | 133.2 |
| U41653 | −4.77939 | 0.209232 | 1.156072 | 115.6 |
| U17606 | −3.94001 | 0.253806 | 1.192349 | 119.2 |
| U24969 | −5.796 | 0.172533 | 1.127035 | 112.7 |
| WRKY33 | — | — | — | 112.8 |
| WRKY70 | — | — | — | 132.5 |
| MYBR1 | — | — | — | 119.1 |
| JAZ6 | — | — | — | 102.7 |

**Table 3.**
*qPCR efficiency values for Phytoplasma related genes in C. aurantifolia.*

### 4.5 Statistical analysis

Analyses of differential gene expression in asymptomatic Phytoplasma infections of acid lime were performed using the *R* statistical software v3.3.2 [43]. Non-metric multidimensional scaling (NMDS) was used to analyse differential gene expression and partition variation between symptomatic/asymptomatic and infected/uninfected groups across all genes [44]. Here, we analysed normalised gene copy number by NMDS using the "*metaMDS*" function [45]. NMDS was performed using the Bray-Curtis dissimilarity index on two ordinal scales for optimal NMDS stress values. Interactions between these and infection type were tested and assigned significance using the "*envfit*" function. Significant differences in DEGs between asymptomatic infected and healthy *Citrus* plants were tested using Student's *t*-tests. Matched gene expression data between Brazil and Oman were further analysed using *post-hoc* Tukey HSD tests to test differential expression based on sample location and symptom type.

## 5. Novel asymptomatic infection biology: results and discussion

Gene expression profiles were determined by qPCR for 15-disease related genes identified previously for infections of "*Ca*. Phytoplasma aurantifolia" in *Citrus aurantifolia* adult trees by Mardi et al. [26]. NMDS showed that a two-dimensional solution was sufficient to achieve low stress values to enable us to interpret disease-related gene expression (stress = 0.049). Infection status (asymptomatic/uninfected) of leaf samples was significantly correlated with the NMDS analysis of gene expression (**Figure 2**, $R^2 = 0.533$, $P < 0.001$), demonstrating clear differences in

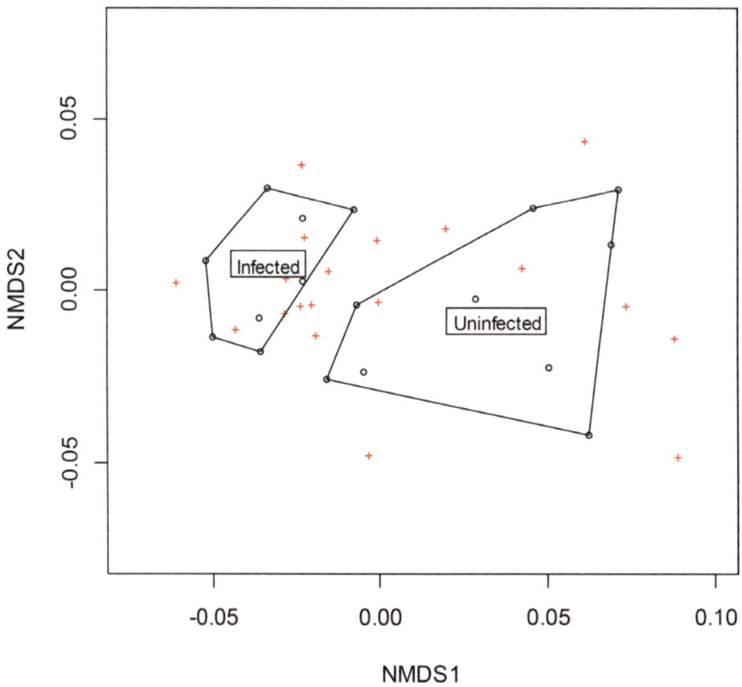


**Figure 2.**
*Surface NMDS ordinations of differential gene expression from samples of "Ca. Phytoplasma aurantifolia" asymptomatic infected and uninfected (healthy) acid lime trees from Brazil denoted by open circles; their position is determined by where they fall on ordinal axes 1 and 2. Red names are species centroids for each Unigene. Polygons indicate clustering of each infection type, which are interpreted as how each gene (and the overall gene expression composition) correlates with the infection properties.*

host plant gene expression in response to infection by this asymptomatic infection. When examining the direction and significance of differential expression of each of these 15-disease related genes, several significant decreases were found (**Table 4**). Expression of four genes related to stress tolerance, cell replication, energy production and protein production (CRT/DRE binding factor; NAC domain-containing protein 71; beta-galactosidase 3; nitrite reductase) were significantly decreased in asymptomatic infected plants. Genes related to immune response (mitogen-activated protein kinase 1; cyclic nucleotide-gated ion channel 1; brassinosteroid insensitive-1-associated receptor kinase) were not significantly differentially expressed however.

| Unigene ID | Transcript | Uninfected expression (ng $\mu l^{-1}$) | Asymptomatic expression (ng $\mu l^{-1}$) | Differential expression | Functional characterisation |
|---|---|---|---|---|---|
| U24969 | Probable LRR receptor-like serine/threonine-protein kinase | 11.22 | 13.67 | NS (p = 0.321) | ABA-signalling |
| U72184 | Zinc finger A20 and AN1 domain-containing stress-associated protein 3 | 8.15 | 7.82 | NS (p = 0.537) | Abiotic stress tolerance |
| U59125 | CRT/DRE binding factor | 12.32 | 7.76 | ↓ (p = 0.050) | Abiotic stress tolerance |
| U27316 | NAC domain-containing protein 71 | 32.74 | 15.30 | ↓ (p = 0.011) | Cell Replication |
| U352 | Beta-galactosidase 3 | 9.74 | 8.47 | ↓ (p < 0.001) | Energy production |
| U68165 | Ent-copalyl diphosphate synthase | 7.54 | 7.38 | NS (p = 0.664) | Growth regulation |
| U77887 | Gibberellin 2-oxidase | 10.24 | 8.20 | NS (p = 0.195) | Growth regulation |
| U41653 | LRR receptor-like serine/threonine-protein kinase GSO1 | 21.27 | 18.40 | NS (p = 0.140) | Growth regulation |
| U26576 | Mitogen-activated protein kinase 1 | 27.04 | 22.42 | NS (p = 0.118) | Immune response |
| U68593 | Cyclic nucleotide-gated ion channel 1 | 17.12 | 16.97 | NS (p = 0.918) | Immune response |
| U17606 | Brassinosteroid insensitive-1-associated receptor kinase | 20.04 | 21.12 | NS (p = 0.453) | Immune response |
| U3869 | Jasmonate ZIM domain-containing protein 6 | 15.42 | 15.73 | NS (p = 0.659) | JA-signalling |
| U17275 | Phytochrome-interacting factor 3 | 6.42 | 6.52 | NS (p = 0.623) | Light response |
| U2265 | Amino acid transporter | 7.85 | 8.38 | NS (p = 0.051) | Protein production |
| U75775 | Nitrite reductase | 17.27 | 12.58 | ↓ (p = 0.001) | Protein production |

*Significant differences were tested by students T test.*

**Table 4.**
*Functional characterisation of DEGs expressed in response to infection by "Ca. P. aurantifolia" and mean differential expression between asymptomatic infected and healthy C. aurantifolia plants.*

The genes MYBR, JAZ6, WRKY37 and WRKY70 were targeted for amplification from samples from both Oman and Brazil (Alves et al. unpublished). MYBR gene expression was not significantly different between Brazil and Oman ($F = 3.725$, $P = 0.067$ **Figure 3a**); *posthoc* tests showed no significant difference between infected/uninfected in Oman ($P = 0.998$) or Brazil ($P = 0.354$). JAZ6 expression was significantly different between Brazil and Oman ($F = 24.016$, $P < 0.001$ **Figure 3b**); *posthoc* tests showed a significant difference between infected/uninfected in Oman ($P = 0.043$), but not Brazil ($P = 0.588$). WRKY70 expression was significantly different between Brazil and Oman ($F = 50.002$, $P < 0.001$ **Figure 3c**); *posthoc* tests showed a significant difference between infected/uninfected both in Oman ($P < 0.001$), and Brazil ($P = 0.004$). WRKY37 expression was significantly different between Brazil and Oman ($F = 9.617$, $P = 0.004$ **Figure 3d**); *posthoc* tests showed a significant difference between infected/uninfected both in Oman ($P < 0.001$), and Brazil ($P < 0.001$).

Disease symptoms are, taken at their most literal, an observable change in host homeostasis in response to the presence of a pathogen. The mechanism underlying symptoms (or lack thereof) within the host plant is broad, but mostly resides in genetic changes (host immune response, genomic mutations, RNA silencing) in either the host or pathogen. The nature of asymptomatic infections is complex and poorly understood. Some may express pathogenesis genes at a lower level and be kept in the host without causing overt symptoms [46].

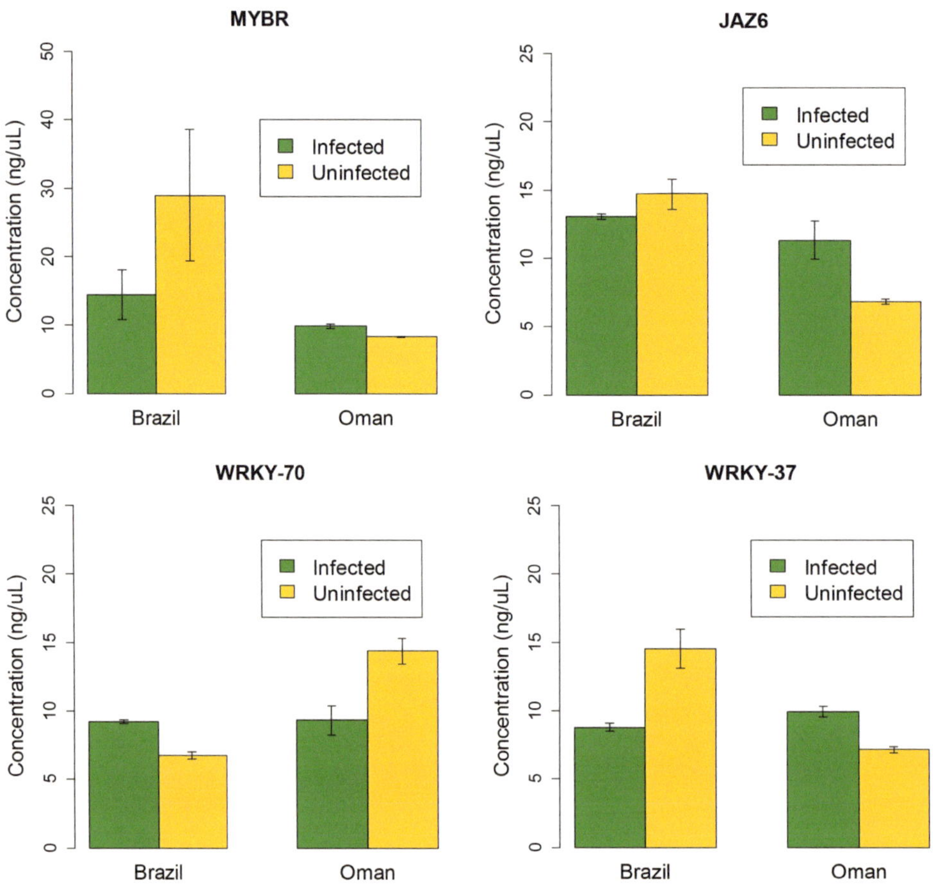


**Figure 3.**
*Differential gene expression of disease-related genes amplified in Brazilian (asymptomatic) and Omani (symptomatic) acid lime trees infected with the Phytoplasma "Ca. Phytoplasma aurantifolia."*

We examined a group of host plant (*C. aurantifolia*) infection related genes identified by [26] in the context of an asymptomatic infection. This previous study established by next generation sequencing of host plant RNA expression (RNAseq) that 2805 genes are differentially expressed in symptomatic infected compared with healthy uninfected plants. Of these, 71 genes were significantly deregulated; of them, 52 were upregulated and 19 down-regulated in response to Phytoplasma infection [26]. Here, using quantitative PCR methods, we studied a subset of these genes that were expressed by more than 128-fold and their differential expression in relation to healthy vs. asymptomatic infected lime plants in Brazil (**Table 4**). We demonstrate that the asymptomatic infection does result in detectable changes in host plant gene expression (**Figure 2**). Specifically, however, no significant change in expression of *Citrus* immune response genes was found here, which would be expected given the asymptomatic nature of the infections (**Table 4**).

Certain genes related to stress tolerance, cell replication and energy production had their expression significantly reduced in infected plants (**Table 4**). The latter may be the best candidate for a "symptom" of these "silent" infections: Phytoplasma are obligate biotrophic organisms and their parasitism may be through host ATP-synthase subunits [22]. When comparing these results with those of [26], the stress tolerance gene also shows a significant reduction in expression in symptomatic infected lime plants. However, cell replication and energy production genes were significantly deregulated in the asymptomatic infections, which was distinct to the symptomatic infection in [26]. This may be one of the first accounts of a significant alteration of gene expression by a host plant infected by an asymptomatic plant pathogen. The demonstrated response by the plant clearly indicates that these are not truly "silent" infections, and perhaps opens up new routes for detecting these pathogens.

Previous research into symptomatic infections of "*Ca*. P. aurantifolia" infecting acid lime has indicated production of several metabolites significantly altered during infection. In Iran, infections are associated with catechin and epicatechin production in leaves [47, 48]. Amino and organic acid concentrations (such as proline, arginine, glutamate, citrate and salicylate) are also significantly increased immediately after inoculation [47]. Studies have shown that "*Ca*. P aurantifolia" also alters the concentration of limonene, ocimene and trans-caryophyllene [7]. Much like the DEGs we have identified in the present study, each of these chemicals could act as measurable indicators to diagnose the infected lime at the early stages of the WBDL progression.

A distinct host plant genomic response to infection by this asymptomatic infection has significant implications for the diseases' insect vectors. Management strategies for insect-vectored pathogens specifically target the vector-plant interactions, relying on monitoring and suppressing these vectors in order to reduce the frequency and severity of disease outbreaks [49]. Many vector-borne plant diseases alter host plant phenotypes in ways that can influence their vectors biology and behaviour [50–52], with significant implications for disease transmission.

Infected plants are often better for their vectors than uninfected in terms of vector growth rates, reproduction and longevity [17, 53]; although the opposite is certainly true in some pathosystems [53] and some vectors actively avoid infected hosts that represent inferior hosts [54]. We have previously demonstrated that an asymptomatic infection results in significant increases in vector life history traits (reproduction and growth rates) than with a symptomatic infection [17]. In future studies, the distinct expression profile detected within the plant host here could be usefully explored in relation to differential gene expression in the insect host, in order to fully understand this vector-host-pathogen complex [16, 23].

We also specifically consider differences between two agricultural loci—the Middle East and South America—by examining a gene set directly related to the plant-pathogen (Phytoplasma) interaction. Four genes (JAZ6, MYBR, WRKY70 and WRKY33) are modulated during Phytoplasma infection in lime trees (**Figure 3**). Interestingly, an inverse expression profile for this gene set could be verified by comparing infected lime trees from Brazil and Oman (**Figure 3**). While JAZ6 and WRKY33 are up-regulated in infected (symptomatic) Omani samples, the same genes present lower gene expression in infected (asymptomatic) Brazilian samples (**Figure 3**). The same inverse relation can be verified for WRKY70, which is down-regulated in infected Omani samples, but presents a significantly higher expression in Brazilian samples (**Figure 3**). Such expression profiles of this gene set represent a signature of symptomatic and asymptomatic Phytoplasma infected plants, which can be used to distinguish earlier Phytoplasma infections. This specific expression profile can be associated to the distinct "*Ca*. P. aurantifolia"-related strains responsible for different infections (symptomatic and asymptomatic) in lime trees. The differential expression of plant transcriptional regulation-related genes reflects the possible action of strain-specific Phytoplasma effectors, as verified for other plant-Phytoplasma interactions [16].

Finally, we should also address the previously reported benefits of asymptomatic infections for their host plants. Asymptomatic infections may result in induced systemic resistance (ISR) [55]: pathogens acquired at low titres elicit a set of systemic plant defences (i.e., oxidative burst, phytoalexins and pathogenesis-related proteins) which prepare hosts to more successfully resist later, more severe infections [56–58]. The use of ISR to induce resistance in plants by application of exogenous (chemical or organic) inducers, has been used in integrated programs of disease management. Pre-inoculation of sour orange (*Citrus aurantium*) seedlings with a hypovirulent isolate of *Phytophthora Citrus* root rot protected them from later infections [59]. Li et al. [60] have also demonstrated the effects chemical inducers on resistance of *Citrus* groves to HLB disease of *Citrus*. Over-expression of an *Arabidopsis* gene (a positive regulator of ISR) in transgenic "Duncan" grapefruit and "Hamlin" sweet orange increased their resistance to *Citrus* canker [61]. Although ISR may be a useful alternative for disease control, it has to be cautiously assessed. In some cases the use of ISR compounds may not provide the expected protection against disease: for example, spraying ISRs onto sweet orange plants did not reduced incidence of *Citrus* canker [59].

## 6. Conclusions

This study has addressed two key questions regarding the nature of asymptomatic infections: [1] that being invisible or "silent" infections (and the consequent reliance on molecular tools for detection) makes them inherently challenging to monitor; and [2] that this organism interacts with its plant host in a distinct manner that we have observed in the present study. The key findings are that asymptomatic infections from three case studies all demonstrate high rates of false-negative discovery; meaning that repeated testing of the same plant can give both negative and positive results and that a single positive result is taken as meaning the plant is infected. We also demonstrate that infection by the Phytoplasma "*Ca*. P aurantifolia" is associated with significantly different genetic expression by its acid lime host, giving a first unique insight into the biology of a "silent" infection.

The Phytoplasma "*Ca*. P aurantifolia" is the aetiological agent of Witches' Broom Disease of Lime (WBDL). Although in the Middle East this disease causes high economic impact on lime production, in Brazil emerging infections are notably symptomless [17]. Asymptomatic infections are not particularly rare in plant pathology. *Colletotrichum* fungi, for example, are symbionts that interact with a range of plants as either symptomatic pathogens or asymptomatic endophytes [62]. Yet we do not understand whether the symbiont can use both strategies or if certain strains display the pathogenic or endophytic strategy. Asymptomatic infections also exists for plant viruses: Pelargonium line pattern virus (PLPV; family Tombusviridae) can be asymptomatic when infecting geranium, which may be due to plant defences such as RNA silencing [63]. In some cases, a resource allocation trade-off mechanism between replication and virulence factor production may explain the emergence of asymptomatic modes of a pathogen, for example, in *Ralstonia solanacearum* populations [64].

As "*Ca.* P. aurantifolia" and other asymptomatic plant pathogens like it spread to novel sites of infection globally [31], and as these infections become more difficult to detect [11], new rapid detection methods will be required in order to effectively detect sources of pathogen and monitor its evolution. This study has presented both the difficulties in monitoring "silent" infections using PCR based methods, but has also identified target genes that behave consistently and distinctly during infection by this Phytoplasma.

## Acknowledgements

This study was financed in part by the Coordenação de Aperfeiçoamento de Pessoal de Nível Superior - Brasil (CAPES) - Finance Code 001.

SLE has been the beneficiary of CNPq productivity grants (grant nos. 309221/2013-7 & 309845/2016-5).

The authors would like to thanks Vale S.A. for financing of the project.

Thanks to SQU for partial support of the work through the grant EG/AGR/CROP/16/01.

## Conflict of interest

The authors declare no conflict of interest.

## Author details

Philip Donkersley[1]*, Farley W.S. Silva[2], Murilo S. Alves[3], Claudine M. Carvalho[3], Abdullah M. Al-Sadi[4] and Simon L. Elliot[2]

1 Lancaster Environment Centre, Lancaster University, Lancaster, United Kingdom

2 Department of Entomology, Universidade Federal de Viçosa, Viçosa, Minas Gerais, Brazil

3 Department of Phytopathology, Universidade Federal de Viçosa, Viçosa, Minas Gerais, Brazil

4 Crop Sciences, Sultan Qaabos University, Oman

*Address all correspondence to: donkersleyp@gmail.com

## References

[1] Oerke E-C, Trapero C, Wilson IW, Stiller WN, Wilson LJ, Wilson C, et al. Crop losses to pests. Ecological Economics. 2016;**7**(3):449-462. DOI: 10.1017/S0021859605005708

[2] Glover JD, Reganold JP, Bell LW, Borevitz J, Brummer EC, Buckler ES, et al. Increased food and ecosystem security via perennial grains. Science. 2010;**328**(5986):1638-1639. DOI: 10.1126/science.1188761

[3] Thrall PH, Biere A, Antonovics J. Plant life-history and disease susceptibility—The occurrence of *Ustilago violacea* on different species within the Caryophyllaceae. Journal of Ecology. 1993;**81**(3):489-498. DOI: 10.2307/2261527

[4] FAO. FAOSTAT: Global Food Production Database. 2018. Available from: http://www.fao.org/statistics/en/

[5] Mukhopadhyay S. *Citrus*: Production, Post Harvest, Disease and Pest Management. Florida: CRC Press; 2010

[6] Samson JA. *Citrus*. In: Tropical Fruits. New York: Longman Scientific and Technical Essex; 1986. pp. 73-138

[7] Al-Yahyai R, Khan I, Al-Said F, Al-Sadi A, Al-Wahaibi A, Deadman M. Status of *Citrus aurantifolia* infected with witches' broom disease of lime in Oman. In: Acta Horticulturae. 2012. pp. 375-382. DOI: 10.17660/ActaHortic.2012.928.50

[8] Donkersley P, Silva FWS, Carvalho CM, Al-Sadi AM, Elliot SL. Biological, environmental and socioeconomic threats to *Citrus* lime production. Journal of Plant Diseases and Protection. 2018;**125**:1-18. DOI: 10.1007/s41348-018-0160-x

[9] Waller JM, Bridge J. Plant diseases and nematodes in the Sultanate of Oman. PANS. 1978;**24**(3):313-326. DOI: 10.1080/09670877809411632

[10] Taheri F, Nematzadeh G, Zamharir MG, Nekouei MK, Naghavi M, Mardi M, et al. Proteomic analysis of the Mexican lime tree response to *candidatus* Phytoplasma aurantifolia infection. Molecular Biosystems. 2011;**7**(11): 3028-3035. DOI: 10.1039/c1mb05268c

[11] Silva FN, Queiroz RB, Souza AN, Al-Sadi AM, Siqueira DL, Elliot SL, et al. First report of a 16SrII-C Phytoplasma associated with asymptomatic acid lime (*Citrus aurantifolia*) in Brazil. Plant Disease. 2014;**98**(11):1577. DOI: 10.1094/pdis-04-14-0431-pdn

[12] Al-Ghaithi AG, Al-Sadi AM, Al-Hammadi MS, Al-Shariqi RM, Al-Yahyai RA, Al-Mahmooli IH, et al. Expression of Phytoplasma-induced witches' broom disease symptoms in acid lime (*Citrus aurantifolia*) trees is affected by climatic conditions. Plant Pathology. 2017;**66**(8):1380-1388. DOI: 10.1111/ppa.12683

[13] Al-Ghaithi AG, Al-Subhi AM, Al-Mahmooli IH, Al-Sadi AM. Genetic analysis of '*Candidatus* Phytoplasma aurantifolia' associated with witches' broom on acid lime trees. Wiles S, editor. PeerJ. 2018;**6**:e4480. DOI: 10.7717/peerj.4480

[14] Al-Sadi AM, Al-Moqbali HS, Al-Yahyai RA, Al-Said FA. AFLP data suggest a potential role for the low genetic diversity of acid lime (*Citrus aurantifolia* Swingle) in Oman in the outbreak of witches' broom disease of lime. Euphytica. 2012;**188**(2):285-297. DOI: 10.1007/s10681-012-0728-7

[15] Bai X, Zhang J, Ewing A, Miller SA, Radek AJ, Shevchenko DV, et al. Living with genome instability: The adaptation of Phytoplasmas to diverse environments of their insect and

plant hosts. Journal of Bacteriology. 2006;**188**(10):3682-3696. DOI: 10.1128/JB.188.10.3682-3696.2006

[16] MacLean AM, Orlovskis Z, Kowitwanich K, Zdziarska AM, Angenent GC, Immink RGH, et al. Phytoplasma effector SAP54 hijacks plant reproduction by degrading MADS-box proteins and promotes insect colonization in a RAD23-dependent manner. PLoS Biology. 2014;**12**(4):e1001835. DOI: 10.1371/journal.pbio.1001835

[17] Queiroz RB, Donkersley P, Silva FN, Al-Mahmmoli IH, Al-Sadi AM, Carvalho CM, et al. Invasive mutualisms between a plant pathogen and insect vectors in the Middle East and Brazil. Royal Society Open Science. 2016;**3**(12):160557. DOI: 10.1098/rsos.160557

[18] de Souza AN, da Silva FN, Bedendo IP, Carvalho CM. A phytoplasma belonging to a 16SrIII-A subgroup and dsRNA virus associated with cassava Frogskin disease in Brazil. Plant Disease. 2014;**98**(6):771-779. DOI: 10.1094/PDIS-04-13-0440-RE

[19] Zreik L, Carle P, Bove JM, Garnier M. Characterization of the Mycoplasma like organism associated with witches'-broom disease of lime and proposition of a *Candidatus* taxon for the organism, *Candidatus* Phytoplasma aurantifolia. International Journal of Systematic Bacteriology. 2009;**45**:449-453. DOI: 10.1099/00207713-45-3-449

[20] Lee I-M, Davis RE, Gundersen-Rindal DE. Phytoplasma: Phytopathogenic mollicutes. Annual Review of Microbiology. 2000;**54**(1):221-255

[21] Hogenhout SA, Oshima K, Ammar ED, Kakizawa S, Kingdom HN, Namba S. Phytoplasmas: Bacteria that manipulate plants and insects. Molecular Plant Pathology. 2008;**9**(4):403-423. DOI: 10.1111/j.1364-3703.2008.00472.x

[22] Oshima K, Kakizawa S, Nishigawa H, Jung HY, Wei W, Suzuki S, et al. Reductive evolution suggested from the complete genome sequence of a plant-pathogenic Phytoplasma. Nature Genetics. 2004;**36**:27-29. DOI: 10.1038/ng1277

[23] Sugio A, Kingdom HN, MacLean AM, Grieve VM, Hogenhout SA. Phytoplasma protein effector SAP11 enhances insect vector reproduction by manipulating plant development and defense hormone biosynthesis. Proceedings of the National Academy of Sciences. 2011;**108**(48):E1254-E1263. DOI: 10.1073/pnas.1105664108

[24] Monavarfeshani A, Mirzaei M, Sarhadi E, Amirkhani A, Khayam Nekouei M, Haynes PA, et al. Shotgun proteomic analysis of the mexican lime tree infected with *Candidatus* Phytoplasma aurantifolia. Journal of Proteome Research. 2013;**12**(2):785-795. DOI: 10.1021/pr300865t

[25] Zamharir MG, Mardi M, Alavi SM, Hasanzadeh N, Nekouei MK, Zamanizadeh HR, et al. Identification of genes differentially expressed during interaction of Mexican lime tree infected with *Candidatus* Phytoplasma aurantifolia. BMC Microbiology. 2011;**11**(1):1-9. DOI: 10.1186/1471-2180-11-1

[26] Mardi M, Karimi Farsad L, Gharechahi J, Salekdeh GH. In-depth transcriptome sequencing of Mexican lime trees infected with *Candidatus* Phytoplasma aurantifolia. PLoS One. 2015;**10**(7):e0130425. DOI: 10.1371/journal.pone.0130425

[27] Coy MR, Hoffmann M, Kingdom Gibbard HN, Kuhns EH, Pelz-Stelinski KS, Stelinski LL. Nested-quantitative PCR approach with improved sensitivity for the detection of low titer levels of

*Candidatus* Liberibacter asiaticus in the Asian *Citrus* psyllid, *Diaphorina citri* Kuwayama. Journal of Microbiological Methods. 2014;**102**:15-22. DOI: 10.1016/j.mimet.2014.04.007

[28] Doyle JJ, Doyle JL. A rapid DNA isolation procedure for small quantities of fresh leaf tissue. Phytochemical Bulletin. 1987;**19**:11-15

[29] Smart CD, Schneider B, Blomquist ÇL, Guerra LJ, Harrison NA, Ahrens U, et al. Phytoplasma-specific PCR primers based on sequences of the 16S-23S rRNA spacer region. Applied and Environmental Microbiology. 1996;**62**(8):2988-2993. DOI: 0099-2240/96/$04.0010

[30] Hodgetts J, Boonham N, Mumford R, Harrison N, Dickinson M. Phytoplasma phylogenetics based on analysis of secA and 23S rRNA gene sequences for improved resolution of candidate species of *Candidatus* Phytoplasma. International Journal of Systematic and Evolutionary Microbiology. 2008;**58**(8):1826-1837. DOI: 10.1099/ijs.0.65668-0

[31] Donkersley P, Blanford JM, Queiroz RB, Silva FWS, Carvalho CM, Al-Sadi AM, et al. Witch's broom disease of lime (*Candidatus* Phytoplasma aurantifolia): Identifying high-risk areas by climatic mapping. Economic Entomology. 2018;**111**(6):2553-2561. DOI: 10.1093/jee/toy248

[32] Stanosz GR, Smith DR, Albers JS. Surveys for asymptomatic persistence of *Sphaeropsis sapinea* on or in stems of red pine seedlings from seven Great Lakes region nurseries. Forest Pathology. 2005;**35**(4):233-244. DOI: 10.1111/j.1439-0329.2005.00407.x

[33] Vu NT, Pardo JM, Alvarez E, Le HH, Wyckhuys K, Nguyen K-L, et al. Establishment of a loop-mediated isothermal amplification (LAMP) assay for the detection of Phytoplasma-associated cassava witches' broom disease. Applied Biological Chemistry. 2016;**59**(2):151-156. DOI: 10.1007/s13765-015-0134-7

[34] Kashyap PL, Kumar S, Srivastava AK. Nanodiagnostics for plant pathogens. Environmental Chemistry Letters. 2017;**15**:7-13. DOI: 10.1007/s10311-016-0580-4

[35] Binns MR, Nyrop JP. Sampling insect populations for the purpose of IPM decision making. Annual Review of Entomology. 2003;**37**:427-453. DOI: 10.1146/annurev.en.37.010192.002235

[36] Luchi N, Capretti P, Pinzani P, Orlando C, Pazzagli M. Real-time PCR detection of *Biscogniauxia mediterranea* in symptomless oak tissue. Letters in Applied Microbiology. 2005;**41**(1):61-68. DOI: 10.1111/j.1472-765X.2005.01701.x

[37] Li W, Hartung JS, Levy L. Evaluation of DNA amplification methods for improved detection of *Candidatus* Liberibacter species associated with *Citrus* Huanglongbing. Plant Disease. 2007;**51**:1-8. DOI: 10.1094/PD-91-0051

[38] Ding F, Duan Y, Paul C, Brlansky RH, Hartung JS. Localization and distribution of *Candidatus* Liberibacter asiaticus in *Citrus* and periwinkle by direct tissue blot immuno assay with an anti-ompa polyclonal antibody. PLoS One. 2015;**10**(5):e0123939. DOI: 10.1371/journal.pone.0123939

[39] Ghosh D, Bhose S, Manimekalai R, Gowda S. Molecular detection of *Candidatus* Phytoplasma spp. causing witches' broom disease of acid lime (*Citrus aurantifolia*) in India. Journal of Plant Biochemistry and Biotechnology. 2013;**22**(3):343-347. DOI: 10.1007/s13562-012-0160-z

[40] De Boer SH, López MM. New grower-friendly methods for plant pathogen monitoring. Annual Review of Phytopathology. 2012;**50**(1):197-218. DOI: 10.1146/annurev-phyto-081211-172942

[41] Rad F, Mohsenifar A, Tabatabaei M, Safarnejad MR, Shahryari F, Safarpour H, et al. Detection of *Candidatus* Phytoplasma aurantifolia with a quantum dots fret-based biosensor. Journal of Plant Pathology. 2012;**94**(3):525-534. DOI: 10.4454/JPP.FA.2012.054

[42] Whelan JA, Russell NB, Whelan MA. A method for the absolute quantification of cDNA using real-time PCR. Journal of Immunological Methods. 2003;**278**(1):261-269. DOI: 10.1016/S0022-1759(03)00223-0

[43] R Foundation for Statistical Computing. R: A Language and Environment for Statistical Computing; 2018

[44] Wang X, Eijkemans MJC, Wallinga J, Biesbroek G, Trzciński K, Sanders EAM, et al. Multivariate approach for studying interactions between environmental variables and microbial communities. PLoS One. 2012;**7**(11):e50267. DOI: 10.1371/journal.pone.0050267

[45] Oksanen J, Blanchet FG, Kindt R, Legendre P, Minchin PR, O'hara RB, et al. Vegan: Community ecology package. R Packag Version 2 4-6. 2018. Available from: https://cran.r-project.org/package=vegan

[46] Burden JP, Nixon CP, Hodgkinson AE, Possee RD, Sait SM, King LA, et al. Covert infections as a mechanism for long-term persistence of baculoviruses. Ecology Letters. 2003;**6**(6):524-531. DOI: 10.1046/j.1461-0248.2003.00459.x

[47] Mollayi S, Zadali R, Farzaneh M, Ghassempour A. Metabolite profiling of Mexican lime (*Citrus aurantifolia*) leaves during the progression of witches' broom disease. Phytochemistry Letters. 2015;**13**:290-296. DOI: 10.1016/j.phytol.2015.07.010

[48] Mollayi S, Farzaneh M, Ghanati F, Aboul-Enein HY, Ghassempour A. Study of catechin, epicatechin and their enantiomers during the progression of witches' broom disease in Mexican lime (*Citrus aurantifolia*). Physiological and Molecular Plant Pathology. 2016;**93**:93-98. DOI: 10.1016/j.pmpp.2015.12.002

[49] Perring TM, Gruenhagen NM, Farrar CA. Management of plant viral diseases through chemical control of vectors. Annual Review of Entomology. 1999;**44**:457-481. DOI: 10.1146/annurev.ento.44.1.457

[50] Fereres A, Moreno A. Behavioural aspects influencing plant virus transmission by homopteran insects. Virus Research. 2009;**141**(2):158-168. DOI: 10.1016/j.virusres.2008.10.020

[51] Bosque-Pérez NA, Eigenbrode SD. The influence of virus-induced changes in plants on aphid vectors: Insights from luteovirus pathosystems. Virus Research. 2011;**159**(2):201-205. DOI: 10.1016/j.virusres.2011.04.020

[52] Rajabaskar D, Ding H, Wu Y, Eigenbrode SD. Different reactions of potato varieties to infection by potato Leafroll virus, and associated responses by its vector, *Myzus persicae* (Sulzer). Journal of Chemical Ecology. 2013;**39**(7):1027-1035. DOI: 10.1007/s10886-013-0311-2

[53] Jiménez-Martínez ES, Bosque-Pérez NA. Variation in barley yellow dwarf virus transmission efficiency by *Rhopalosiphum padi* (Homoptera: Aphididae) after acquisition from transgenic and nontransformed wheat genotypes. Journal of Economic Entomology. 2009;**97**(6):1790-1796. DOI: 10.1603/0022-0493-97.6.1790

[54] Blua MJ, Perring TM. Effects of zucchini yellow mosaic virus on colonization and feeding behavior of *Aphis gossypii* (Homoptera: Aphididae) alatae. Environmental Entomology. 1992;**21**(3):578-585. DOI: 10.1093/ee/21.3.578

[55] Heil M, Bostock RM. Induced systemic resistance (ISR) against pathogens in the context of induced plant defences. Annals of Botany. 2002;**89**(5):503-512. DOI: 10.1093/aob/mcf076

[56] Phytoalexins KJ, Metabolism S. Stress metabolism, and disease resistance in plants. Annual Review of Phytopathology. 2003;**33**:275-297

[57] Lamb C, Dixon RA. The oxidative burst in plant disease resistance. Annual Review of Plant Physiology and Plant Molecular Biology. 2002;**48**:251-275. DOI: 10.1146/annurev.arplant.48.1.251

[58] van Loon LC, Rep M, Pieterse CMJ. Significance of inducible defense-related proteins in infected plants. Annual Review of Phytopathology. 2006;**44**:135-162. DOI: 10.1146/annurev.phyto.44.070505.143425

[59] Graham JH, Colburn GC, Chung KR, Cubero J. Protection of *Citrus* roots against infection by *Phytophthora* spp. by hypovirulent *P. nicotianae* is not related to induction of systemic acquired resistance. Plant and Soil. 2012;**358**:39-49. DOI: 10.1007/s11104-011-1119-x

[60] Li J, Trivedi P, Wang N. Field evaluation of plant defense inducers for the control of *Citrus* Huanglongbing. Phytopathology. 2015;**106**:37-47. DOI: 10.1094/phyto-08-15-0196-r

[61] Zhang X, Francis MI, Dawson WO, Graham JH, Orbović V, Triplett EW, et al. Over-expression of the *Arabidopsis* NPR1 gene in *Citrus* increases resistance to *Citrus* canker. European Journal of Plant Pathology. 2010;**128**(1):91-100. DOI: 10.1007/s10658-010-9633-x

[62] Rojas EI, Rehner SA, Samuels GJ, Van Bael SA, Herre EA, Cannon P, et al. *Colletotrichum gloeosporioides* s.l. associated with *Theobroma cacao* and other plants in Panamá: Multilocus phylogenies distinguish host-associated pathogens from asymptomatic endophytes. Mycologia. 2010;**102**(6):1318-1338. DOI: 10.3852/09-244

[63] Pérez-Cañamás M, Blanco-Pérez M, Forment J, Hernández C. *Nicotiana benthamiana* plants asymptomatically infected by *Pelargonium* line pattern virus show unusually high accumulation of viral small RNAs that is neither associated with DCL induction nor RDR6 activity. Virology. 2017;**501**:136-146. DOI: 10.1016/j.virol.2016.11.018

[64] Peyraud R, Cottret L, Marmiesse L, Gouzy J, Genin S. A resource allocation trade-off between virulence and proliferation drives metabolic versatility in the plant pathogen *Ralstonia solanacearum*. PLoS Pathogens. 2016;**12**(10):e1005939. DOI: 10.1371/journal.ppat.1005939

Chapter 8

# Emerging Bacterial Disease (Leaf Scald) of Sugarcane in China: Pathogenesis, Diagnosis, and Management

*Muralidharan Govindaraju, Yisha Li and Muqing Zhang*

## Abstract

Sugarcane is the major industrial crop grown in tropical and sub-tropical regions in China. More than 100 sugarcane diseases are identified around the globe; half have been reported in China. Many varieties of sugarcane were replaced due to the infection of new pathogenic disease. Recently, leaf scald was found in China, which is one of the major sugarcane diseases also seriously affecting growth of sugarcane. Several isolates were recovered and identified using ELISA and PCR assays from the symptomatic leaf samples in Guangxi, China. The genomes of our isolates from *X. albilineans* were re-sequenced and revealed that rpf gene encoded regulation of pathogenicity factors mainly involved in the pathogenesis of sugarcane. The disease is mainly transferred through seed cane. In the past, hot water treatment was used to manage the disease. Healthy seed cane from resistant cultivars could effectively manage the leaf scald disease in sugarcane.

**Keywords:** sugarcane, leaf scald, *X. albilineans*, pathogenesis, bacterial disease, management

## 1. Introduction

Sugarcane (*Saccharum* spp.) is an industrially important crop of tropical and sub-tropical regions cultivated mainly for production of sucrose, biofuel, and ethanol [1]. China is one of the third largest sugarcane (*Saccharum officinarum* L.)-producing countries, followed by Brazil and India [2]. In the 1980s, Fujian and Guangdong were the two major sugarcane-producing provinces in China. Due to social, economic and environmental factors, major sugarcane-producing areas were moved to Guangxi and Yunnan provinces which accounts for 64 and 24% of total sugarcane-growing regions during 2015/2016. Since then, approximately 60% of the total cane yield is produced in Guangxi [2]. Sugarcane is the host of many serious plant pathogens that can mainly affect cane production and yield. In sugarcane, more than 100 pathogens have been reported to cause disease, Including fungi, bacteria, phytoplasma, and virus [3]. Several of these diseases are considered to be the most severe threat to sugarcane production in Guangxi, especially leaf scald disease. Sugarcane leaf scald was first reported in the 1980s in Taiwan, China [4, 5], and recently found in 2015 in Guangxi, China. The pathogen from the recovered isolates was identified to be *Xanthomonas albilineans*.

## 1.1 Economic influence of leaf scald disease in sugarcane industry

Leaf scald disease (**Figure 1**) is also known as leaf burning disease, and it is caused by *X. albilineans* (Ashby) Dowson [3]. The major host plants mainly include *S. officinarum*, *Zea mays*, *Panicum antidotale*, *Bambusa vulgaris*, *Pennisetum purpureum*, and *Paspalum conjugatum*. The disease is mainly distributed in Australia, the USA, the Philippines, Myanmar, Thailand, Java, Laos, and Vietnam [6, 7]. Now, it is the most important quarantine disease in Taiwan, Guangxi, Guangdong, Yunnan, Fujian, Jiangxi, and Hainan in China [8]. Leaf scald was the reason for major losses in sugarcane at the beginning of the century when noble canes, *Saccharum officinarum*, was cultivated [9]. The major impact of the disease was reduced by the cultivation of interspecific hybrids. The susceptible cultivars were rapidly destroyed. Sugarcane cultivars resistant to leaf scald disease include F156, F160, F170, F173, and NCO310 in Taiwan, China. Other varieties resistant to this disease include Q42, Q50, Q98, Q813, P0J36, POJ2725, CP807, CP29–CP116, Co290, Co301, Co331, Co421, and B34104. The varieties susceptible to leaf scald disease are CP29–CP291, Co281, Co419, Co7301, Q44, Q63, Q66, B34104, B37161, B070, GT 46, GT 06–2081, GT 08–1589, LC 03–1137, and ROC1 [7, 10].

## 1.2 Symptomology

The major characteristic symptoms of leaf scald disease are divided into three phases: latent, chronic, and acute phases.

### *1.2.1 Latent phase*

During this period, infected plants do not show any symptoms that occur in tolerant varieties and under favorable conditions for growth of plant. Stress can activate the infected plant to pass from the phase of latent into chronic or acute phase.

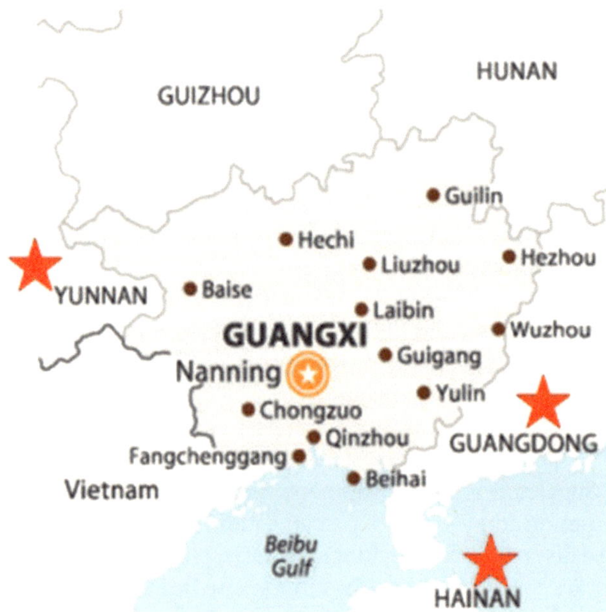


**Figure 1.**
*Major sugarcane areas affected by leaf scald in China.*

### 1.2.2 Chronic phase

The chronic phase is characterized by "white pencil line" stripe 1–2 mm wide and patches of chlorotic tissue on leaves, side shooting and burning of leaf tips. At a later stage, the margins' stripe may become diffuse, and a red pencil line may be formed in the middle of the stripe. In dry weather, the leaf stripes dry out from the leaf apex to the margin, and finally the entire leaf become wilt. Infected plants exhibit shorter internodes, and the node of the stalk produces small tillerings, and a leaf of the tillerings shows white streaks. The disease-infected sections of stalks show reddening, and discolored vessels can pass through the internodes. Necrotic lessons may be noticed in severely affected stalks of plants (**Figure 2**).

### 1.2.3 Acute phase

In the acute phase of the disease, plant dies without showing any major symptoms. The infected stalks section does not show reddening of the vessels and tillerings joined into main stalk (**Figure 3**). It occurs mainly in drought condition of sugarcane growing period. In physiological water shortage condition, the leaves show the chronic streaks on re-tillering of diseased stalks [9].

## 1.3 Field assessment

LSD symptoms were recorded every month in the field. Disease severity was rated according to the procedure described [11]. However, all inoculated sugarcane stalks were rated individually, symptom severity ranging from 0 to 5. The ratings were used to calculate mean disease severity (DS): $DS = [(1 \times FL + 2 \times ML + 3 \times CB + 4 \times N + 5 \times D)/5 \times T]\ 100$. However, FL = number of stalks with one or two pencil-line streaks (rating 1), ML = number of stalks with more than two pencil-line streaks (rating 2),

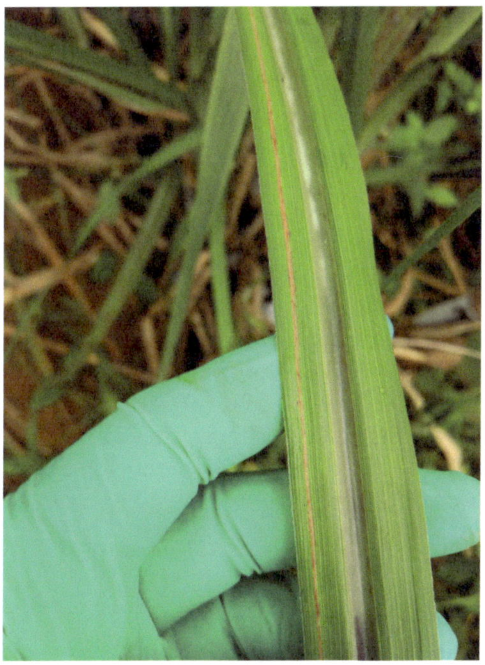

**Figure 2.**
*Chronic phase of infection with pencil line stripe.*

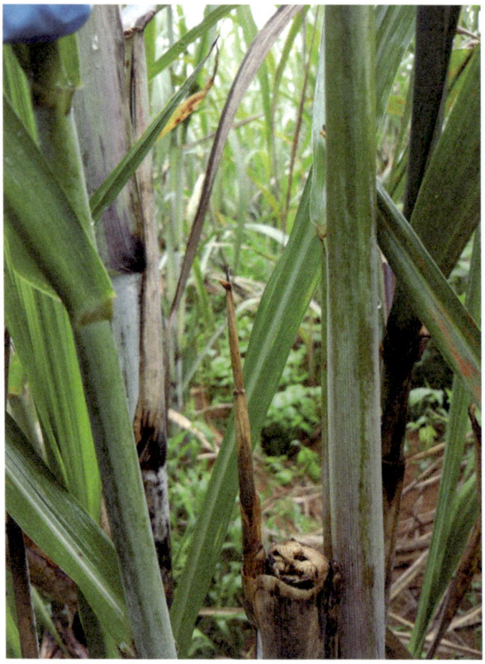

**Figure 3.**
*Acute phase of infected plants leads to death.*

CB = number of stalks with leaf chlorosis or bleaching (rating 3), N = number of stalks with leaf necrosis (rating 4), D = number of dead stalks or stalks with side shooting (rating 5), and T = total number of stalks. The rating of 5 was attributed to stalks with dead inoculated leaves 1 month after inoculation [11].

### 1.4 Phylogenetic

The multilocus sequence analysis (MLSA) of 119 strains of *Xanthomonas* genus is distributed into two uneven groups, with group 2 containing all but five species, namely, *X. albilineans, X. theicola, X. sacchari, X. translucens*, and *X. hyacinthi*, which were clustered into group 1 [12].

Three serovars associated with antigenic variations within *X. albilineans* were detected using three antisera (polyclonal antibodies) method against strains from three different geographical locations [13]. Serovars of 215 strains from 28 locations worldwide are affected by sugarcane leaf scald disease, and the distributed strains are divided into three groups according to serotype: (i) serotype 1 is the largest group, with strains from various geographic locations; (ii) serotype 2 consists of strains from tropical African countries; and (iii) serotype 3 contains strains from Caribbean islands (Fiji and Sri Lanka). This serological characterization of *X. albilineans* strains has been confirmed with monoclonal antibodies of 38 strains from different worldwide locations [14].

## 2. Pathogenesis

The pathogen is limited mainly to the leaf and stalk vascular bundles that are often partly or completely blocked with a gum-like substance. The organism may invade the parenchyma cells between the vascular bundles and cause reddened pockets of gum. No symptom of sugarcane plants can therefore constitute inoculum sources for crop contamination. In addition, various epidemiological factors play a major role in field contamination. Leaf scald is spread by harvesters, hand knives, and infected setts by planting [9]. The pathogen found in the rhizosphere of infected roots has more possible transmission by root contact [15]. Leaf scald disease can also affect many other grasses which are alternate hosts for the disease. High moisture and temperature are the most favorable condition for the disease transmission.

### 2.1 Genes and diseases

The genome sequence of *X. albilineans* shows that the genes are effectively involved in pathogenesis. These genes include a cluster of genes called regulation of pathogenicity factors (rpf) responsible for the biosynthesis of a small diffusible signaling molecule. Diffusible signaling factor (DSF) encoded by RpfF has more similarities to long-chain fatty acyl CoA ligases [16, 17]. DSF quorum sensing and disruption of gene rpfF resulted in reduced virulence in different xanthomonads (*Xanthomonas spp.*), such as *X. axonopodis* pv. citri, *X. campestris* pv. campestris, and *X. oryzae* pv. oryzae [17, 18]. The rpf genes only control production of biofilm and other mechanisms involved in surface attachment of *X. albilineans*. A core group of genes, including *rpfF*, *rpfC* and *rpf G*, has played broader roles in gene regulation other than the transduction of DSF signals in *X. axonopodis spp.* [19]. The pathogen of leaf scald disease, *X. albilineans*, lacks type III secretion system (T3SS), which is found in most of pathogenic xanthomonads and acts as pathogenicity effectors in plant cells. *X. albilineans* also lacks all genes involved in the formation of biofilm, an important factor in virulence of plant pathogenic bacteria.

TonB-dependent transporters (TBDTs) are the important transporters involved in nutrient uptake [20] and also involved in iron or vitamin B12 uptake. These transporters are to facilitate the uptake of carbohydrates present in low amounts on the leaf surfaces [21, 22]. Genomes of several species of *Xanthomonas* are known to have high representation of TBDT genes, and it is functionally associated with pathogenicity of the bacterium [23].

During phyllosphere colonization, *Xanthomonas* encounters nutrient-limited environment on the leaf surfaces. Due to these conditions, TBDT has transported sucrose available in the phyllosphere [24]. Similarly, the genome of *X. albilineans* has 35 putative TBDT genes, and it is involved in the transport of plant cell wall derived nutrients like maltose, xylan, pectin, etc. [24–26].

### 2.2 Albicidin production and pathogenicity

Albicidin is a major phytotoxic compound specifically synthesized by the Gram-negative bacteria *X. albilineans* and plays an important role in pathogenicity [27]. It causes leaf scald in sugarcane [28]. The molecular target of albicidin is DNA gyrase (topoisomerase II) which is essential for DNA replication in bacteria. In planta, albicidin acts as a potent DNA gyrase inhibitor, thus blocking plastid development [29]. Albicidin (**Figure 4**) also has potent antibacterial activity which inhibits the growth of several positive and negative bacteria at nanomolar range with low minimal inhibitory concentration (MIC), e.g., *Escherichia coli* (0.063 μg $mL^{-1}$) [30], *Salmonella enteritidis* (0.5 μg $mL^{-1}$), and *Staphylococcus aureus* (4.0 μg $mL^{-1}$) [31]. Albicidin gives greater advantage to *X. albilineans* against other bacteria within the xylem vessels of sugarcane.

However, the entire 49-kb albicidin biosynthesis gene cluster was cloned and sequenced from *X. albilineans* (Xa23R1) [28]. This cluster is included in a genomic region of XALB1, and it contains three polyketide synthase (PKS) and non-ribosomal peptide synthase (NRPS) genes, as well as several putative modifying resistance and regulatory genes. Two additional 3-kb genomic regions of *X. albilineans* strain Xa23R1, namely, XALB2 and XALB3, were found to be involved

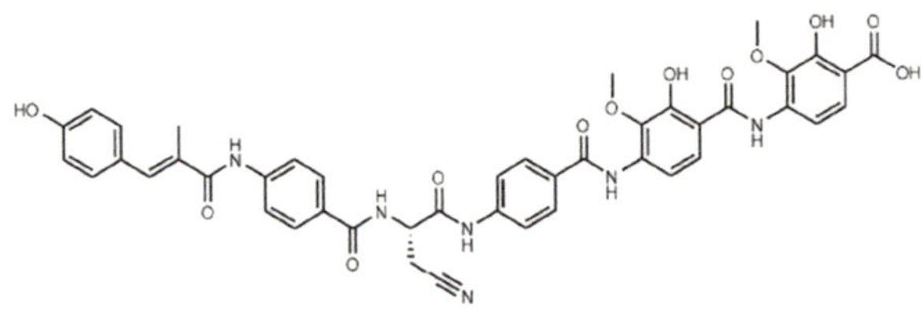


**Figure 4.**
*Structure of albicidin.*

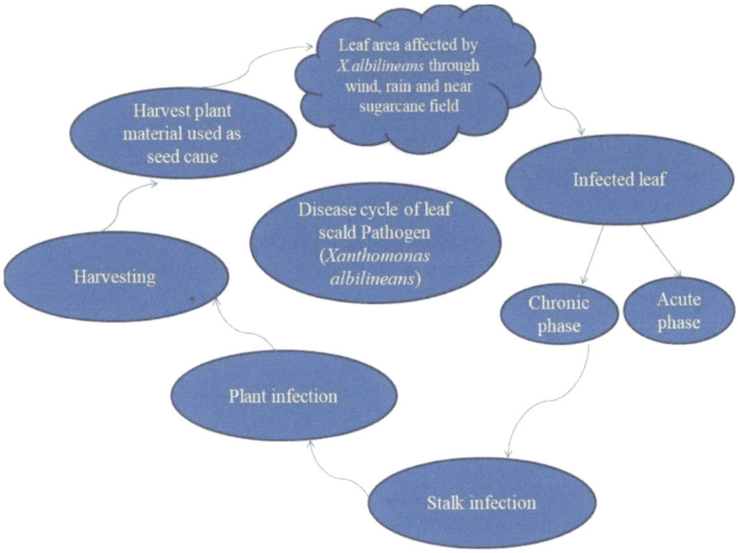


**Figure 5.**
*Infection cycle of leaf scald pathogen.*

in albicidin production. XALB2 has a single gene coding for a phosphopantetheinyl transferase required for posttranslational activation of PKS or NRPS enzymes [32]. XALB3 has a single gene coding for protein (HtpG) in albicidin production, which has not been elucidated [33].

### 2.3 Disease cycle

*Xanthomonas albilineans* can spread from inoculum sources to contaminated field of sugarcane and affect healthy sugarcane under the impact of various climatic conditions (**Figure 5**) [34]. The pathogen then colonizes the surface of the leaf, enters through the stomata, and progresses within the xylem, and symptoms may appear in infected plants. Pathogen can move into the stalk and then infect the stool showing scalding from the leaves [35]. The pathogen can be transmitted mechanically by harvesting equipment (harvesters) and the infected cane setts.

## 3. Diagnosis

### 3.1 Immunoassay

Various diagnostic methods are employed for detection of *X. albilineans*, including isolation on selective media and biochemical, immunological, and molecular assays. ELISA was the most sensitive method and resulted in the detection of bacteria at the low titer [36]. Although isolation of *X. albilineans* with selective media is more time-consuming than other methods, it has proven to be very efficient in detecting the pathogen in symptomless and diseased plants [37]. DAC-ELISA and dot blot techniques were standardized to detect the bacterium in infected canes [38].

### 3.2 Molecular method

Polymerase chain reaction (PCR) protocols have been developed to detect *X. albilineans* in diseased stalks. The primer sets Ala4/L1 [39] and PGBL1/PGBL2 [40] were designed based on ITS region between the 16S and 23S rRNA genes of *X. albilineans*. PCR-based detection was further improved by *X. albilineans* specific amplification of the region between the 16S rRNA-tRNAaIa -tRNAiIe - 23S rRNA gene by a nested PCR reaction [41]. Loop-mediated isothermal amplification (LAMP) was also employed for the detection of *X. albilineans* [42, 43]. It is an auto-cycling strand displacement DNA synthesis technique that involves the use of large fragment of DNA polymerase and a set of six primers [44], and it enables the synthesis of larger amounts of both DNA and by-products, e.g., hydroxy naphthol blue (HNB) [45, 46]. Quantitative PCR (qPCR) is a highly effective and accurate method for the detection of leaf scald disease [47].

## 4. Management strategy

### 4.1 Hot water treatment

Most of sugarcane diseases can be controlled through the use of disease-free seed cane. Hot-water treatments are used to disinfect planting material (seed cane). Before planting, soaking in ambient-temperature running water for 40 h followed by 3–4 h at 50°C is used to manage leaf scald bacteria, and it can provide 95% control efficacy [10].

### 4.2 Molecular approach

This approach is mainly developed to target factors that are responsible for pathogenicity other than toxins. The molecular modification in the host provides them resistance to pathogenicity factors and the factor inactivates by binding of hormones and enzymes. However, foreign genes' inactivation was carried out by gene silencing, nucleases, and coating proteins [48, 49]. The production of host cell surface components interferes with identification of the host and attachment to host cells by the pathogen.

CRISPR-Cas systems are involved in phage and plasmid defense, thus limiting HGT. The genome sequence of *X. albilineans* strain (GPE PC73) unveils the presence of two different systems named CRISPR-1 and CRISPR-2 [50]. The CRISPR-2 is associated with six cas genes (cas1, cas3, csy1, csy2, csy3, and csy4) and contains 28-bp repeats. CRISPR-2 is shared by the four strains (GPEPC73 and Xa23R1 from *X. albilineans*, GPE 39 and MUS 060 from *X. pseudalbilineans*) [50, 51]. Although, CRISPR-2 nucleic acid sequences of the repeats are 100% identical among the four strains, thus confirming the common origin of this locus [52].

Different resistant mechanisms on albicidin have been reported, including the nucleoside transporter Tsx, for which mutations have been described to import albicidin, or the endopeptidase AlbD from Pantoea dispersa [53–55], which cleaves albicidin into two inactive fragments [56]. Another strategy is drug binding that counteracts the antibacterial effect of albicidin tetracycline-binding protein (TetR family) [57] or thiostrepton-binding protein (MerR family) [58]. The albicidin-binding protein AlbA from *Klebsiella oxytoca* [59] and AlbB from *Alcaligenes denitrificans* [60] provide protective effects for survival of the host strains. However, far-ultraviolet (UV) spectroscopy has indicated a mostly α-helical structure for AlbA [61], and amino acid residue His125 has played a vital role in albicidin binding [61, 62].

### 4.3 Genetic approach

The most potent method to prevent or manage leaf scald disease is the development and planting of resistant cultivars [3]. However, accurate determination of the resistant level of genotype against *X. albilineans* is most important in the cultivar selection program for leaf scald by artificial inoculation tests. The erratic symptom expression failed to accurately detect susceptibility, and thus multiple field trials utilizing inoculation are needed. Under this scenario, the marker-assisted selection (MAS) breeding technique, which uses DNA marker(s) linked to useful trait(s), has greater advantage in selecting clones resistant to leaf scald disease [63]. The transgenic sugarcane plants against *Xanthomonas albilineans* were produced by mediating albicidin detoxification (*albD*) gene through microprojectile bombardment [64].

### 4.4 Alternative control

#### *4.4.1 Chemotherapy method*

Spray of antibiotics such as streptomycin + tetracycline (60 g/ha/500 l water) at 2-week intervals was found to efficiently manage the pathogen in the field at 2 months after planting [65]. In preliminary stage, spraying of these antibiotics reduces the severity of leaf scald.

#### *4.4.2 Biocontrol method*

*G. diazotrophicus* may play a major role in defense against pathogens of sugarcane. It inhibited in vitro growth of leaf scald pathogen *Xanthomonas albilineans* [66, 67]. In addition, *G. diazotrophicus*-inoculated sugarcane stems were resistant to infection by *X. albilineans* [68]. Lactic acid bacteria (LAB) may be a biological alternative approach for leaf scald disease in sugarcane, and it produces antimicrobial peptides called bacteriocins and other substances, such as hydrogen peroxide, lactic acid, and reuterin, which are effective against several Gram-positive and Gram-negative bacteria. Antimicrobial peptides are alternatives for conventional pesticides and antibiotics, which are also used to treat against *X. albilineans* [69].

### 4.5 Farmer service program

Since 2000, healthy seed cane program has been developed by a government agency to protect the sugarcane diseases in China, further following recommendation to control or manage leaf scald disease.

1. The Pest and Disease Department plays a vital role by ensuring to provide disease-free parent seed material.

2. The government agency should arrange training program for farmers and take care of harvesting, transportation, and processing.

3. The crop agronomist should employ to cover aspects of growing the crop, such as soils, fertilizer, and herbicides and also to monitor the performance of new varieties.

4. The Inspection Department for all growers' fields should ensure that disease levels are acceptable and that remedial action is implemented where required. The monitoring of fields for pest damage is also important.

5. The efforts should be made to enhance awareness among the sugarcane farmers and strict vigilance by the quality control and regulatory authorities.

## 5. Conclusion

The leaf scald disease is becoming one of the serious threats to sugar industries in China. The infected plants should be removed completely to eliminate the seed cane carrying this disease in the field. Healthy seed cane was used from pathogen-free tissue culture plantlets (PTC). Better fertilization and irrigation practices may reduce the occurrence of this disease. A strict phytosanitary measure is needed to manage exchange of materials of sugarcane (seed cane) and propagation of disease.

## Author details

Muralidharan Govindaraju, Yisha Li and Muqing Zhang*
Guangxi Key Laboratory of Sugarcane Biology, Guangxi University, Nanning, China

*Address all correspondence to: mqzhang@ufl.edu

## References


[1] Lam E, Shine J Jr, Da Silva J, Lawton M, Bonos S, Calvino M, et al. Improving sugarcane for biofuel: Engineering for an even better feedstock. GCB Bioenergy. 2009;**1**(3):251-255

[2] Zhang M, Govindaraju M. Sugarcane production in China. Sugarcane–Technology and Research, Intech. 2018. pp. 49-68. http://dx.doi.org/10.5772/intechopen.73113

[3] Rott P, Davis MJ. Leaf scald In: Rott P, Bailey RA, Comstock JC, Croft BJ, Saumtally AS, editors. A Guide to Sugarcane Diseases. Paris: CIRAD-ISSCT; 2000

[4] Wang JM. Sugarcane Cultivation in China. Beijing: China Agriculture Press; 1985

[5] Huang HN. Distribution and classification of sugarcane diseases and control of main diseases in Guangdong province. Sugarcane and Cane Sugar (In Chinese). 1987;**5**:50-52

[6] Saumtally A, Dookun-Saumtally A, Rao GP, Saumtally AS, Rott P. Leaf scald of sugarcane: A disease of worldwide importance. In: Sugarcane Pathology: Bacterial and Nematode Diseases. New Hampshire: Science Publishers; 2004. pp. 65-76

[7] Zhang R, Shan H, Li W, Cang X, Wang X, Yin J, et al. First report of sugarcane leaf scald caused by *Xanthomonas albilineans* in the province of Guangxi, China. Plant Disease. 2017;**101**(8):1541

[8] Li WF, Huang YK. Diagnosis Detection and Control Technology of Modern Sugarcane Diseases. Beijing: China Agriculture Press; 2012

[9] Ricaud C, Egan B, Gillaspie A, Hughes C. Diseases of Sugarcane: Major Diseases. Amsterdam, The Netherlands: Elsevier Science Publishers B.V.; 1989

[10] Huang Y, Li W. Colored Atlas of Control on Diseases, Insect Pests and Weeds of Modern Sugarcane. Beijing: China Agriculture Press; 2016

[11] Rott P, Mohamed IS, Klett P, Soupa D, de Saint-Albin A, Feldmann P, et al. Resistance to leaf scald disease is associated with limited colonization of sugarcane and wild relatives by *Xanthomonas albilineans*. Phytopathology. 1997;**87**:1202-1213

[12] Young JM, Park DC, Shearman HM, Fargier E. A multilocus sequence analysis of the genus *Xanthomonas*. Systematic and Applied Microbiology. 2008;**31**:366-377

[13] Rott P, Davis MJ, Baudin P. Serological variability in *Xanthomonas albilineans* causal agent of leaf scald disease of sugarcane. Plant Pathology. 1994;**43**:344-349

[14] Alvarez AM, Schenck S, Benedict AA. Differentiation of *Xanthomonas albilineans* strains with monoclonal antibody reaction pattern and DNA fingerprints. Plant Pathology. 1996;**45**:358-366

[15] Klett P, Rott P. Inoculum sources for the spread of leaf scald disease of sugarcane caused by *Xanthomonas albilineans* in Guadeloupe. Journal of Phytopathology. 1994;**142**(3):283-291

[16] Barber C, Tang J, Feng J, Pan M, Wilson T, Slater H, et al. A novel regulatory system required for pathogenicity of *Xanthomonas campestris* is mediated by a small diffusible signal molecule. Molecular Microbiology. 1997;**24**(3):555-566

[17] Dow M. Diversification of the function of cell-to-cell signaling in

regulation of virulence within plant pathogenic xanthomonads. Science Signaling. 2008;**1**(21):23

[18] Chatterjee S, Almeida RPP, Lindow S. Living in two worlds: The plant and insect lifestyles of *Xylella fastidiosa*. Annual Review of Phytopathology. 2008;**46**:243-271

[19] Guo Y, Zhang Y, Li JL, Wang N. Diffusible signal factor mediated quorum sensing plays a central role in coordinating gene expression of *Xanthomonas citri* subsp. citri. Molecular Plant-Microbe Interactions. 2012;**25**:165-179

[20] Delmotte N, Knief C, Chaffron S, Innerebner G, Roschitzki B, Schlapbach R, et al. Community proteogenomics reveals insights into the physiology of phyllosphere bacteria. Proceedings of the National Academy of Sciences of the United States of America. 2009;**106**:16428-16433

[21] Lindow SE, Brandl MT. Microbiology of the phyllosphere. Applied and Environmental Microbiology. 2003;**69**:1875-1883

[22] Vorholt JA. Microbial life in the phyllosphere. Nature Reviews. Microbiology. 2012;**10**:828-840

[23] Rott P, Fleites L, Marlow G, Royer M, Gabriel DW. Identification of new candidate pathogenicity factors in the xylem invading pathogen *Xanthomonas albilineans* by transposon mutagenesis. Molecular Plant-Microbe Interactions. 2011;**24**:594-605

[24] Blanvillain S, Meyer D, Boulanger A, Lautier M, Guynet C, Denance N, et al. Plant carbohydrate scavenging through TonB-dependent receptors: A feature shared by phytopathogenic and aquatic bacteria. PLoS One. 2007;**2**:e224

[25] Pieretti I, Royer M, Barbe V, Carrere S, Koebnik R, Couloux A, et al. Genomic insights into strategies used by *Xanthomonas albilineans* with its reduced artillery to spread within sugarcane xylem vessels. BMC Genomics. 2012;**13**:658

[26] De Bernonville TD, Noel LD, SanCristobal M, Danoun S, Becker A, Soreau P, et al. Transcriptional reprogramming and phenotypical changes associated with growth of *Xanthomonas campestris* pv. Campestris in cabbage xylem sap. FEMS Microbiology Ecology. 2014;**89**:527-541

[27] Birch RG. *Xanthomonas albilineans* and the anti-pathogenesis approach to disease control. Molecular Plant Pathology. 2001;**2**(1):1-11

[28] Royer M, Costet L, Vivien E, Bes M, Cousin A, Damais A, et al. Albicidin pathotoxin produced by *Xanthomonas albilineans* is encoded by three large PKS and NRPS genes present in a gene cluster also containing several putative modifying, regulatory, and resistance genes. Molecular Plant-Microbe Interactions. 2004;**17**(4):414-427

[29] Birch RG, Patil SS. Evidence that an albicidin-like phytotoxin induces chlorosis in sugarcane leaf scald disease by blocking plastid DNA replication. Physiological and Molecular Plant Pathology. 1987;**30**(2):207-214

[30] Kretz J, Kerwat D, Schubert V, Grätz S, Pesic A, Semsary S, et al. Total synthesis of albicidin: A lead structure from *Xanthomonas albilineans* for potent antibacterial gyrase inhibitors. Angewandte Chemie, International Edition. 2015;**54**(6):1969-1973

[31] Rostock L, Driller R, Grätz S, Kerwat D, von Eckardstein L, Petras D, et al. Molecular insights into antibiotic resistance-how a binding protein traps albicidin. Nature Communications. 2018;**9**(1):3095

[32] Huang G, Zhang L, Birch RG. Albicidin antibiotic and phytotoxin biosynthesis in *Xanthomonas albilineans* requires a phosphopantetheinyl transferase gene. Gene. 2000;**258**:193-199

[33] Vivien E, Megessier S, Pieretti I, Cociancich S, Frutos R, Gabriel DW, et al. *Xanthomonas albilineans* HtpG is required for biosynthesis of the antibiotic and phytotoxin albicidin. FEMS Microbiology Letters. 2006;**251**:81-89

[34] Champoiseau P, Rott P, Daugrois J-H. Epiphytic populations of *Xanthomonas albilineans* and subsequent sugarcane stalk infection are linked to rainfall in Guadeloupe. Plant Disease. 2009;**93**(4):339-346

[35] Daugrois JH, Edon-Jock C, Bonoto S, Vaillant J, Rott P. Spread of sugarcane yellow leaf virus in initially disease-free sugarcane is linked to rainfall and host resistance in the humid tropical environment of Guadeloupe. European Journal of Plant Pathology. 2011;**129**(1):71-80

[36] Autrey L, Dookun A, Saumtally S. Improved Serological Methods for Diagnosis of the Leaf Scald Bacterium Xanthomonas albilineans. In: Proceedings of the International Society of Sugar Cane Technologists. Sao Paulo, Brazil: Tropical Plant Pathology; 1989

[37] Davis MJ, Rott P, Baudin P, Dean J. Evaluation of selective media and immunoassays for detection of *Xanthomonas albilineans*, causal agent of sugarcane leaf scald disease. Plant Disease. 1994;**78**(1):78-82

[38] Viswanathan R, Ramesh SA. Isolation and production of antiserum to *Xanthomonas albilineans* and diagnosis of the pathogen through serological techniques. Journal of Mycology and Plant Pathology. 2004;**34**:797-800

[39] Pan YB, Grisham M, Burner D. A polymerase chain reaction protocol for the detection of *Xanthomonas albilineans*, the causal agent of sugarcane leaf scald disease. Plant Disease. 1997;**81**(2):189-194

[40] Pan YB, Grisham M, Burner D, Legendre B, Wei Q. Development of polymerase chain reaction primers highly specific for *Xanthomonas albilineans*, the causal bacterium of sugarcane leaf scald disease. Plant Disease. 1999;**83**(3):218-222

[41] Honeycutt RJ, Sobral BW, McClelland M. tRNA intergenic spacers reveal polymorphisms diagnostic for *Xanthomonas albilineans*. Microbiology. 1995;**141**(12):3229-3239

[42] Garces F, Gutierrez A, Hoy J. Detection and quantification of *Xanthomonas albilineans* by qPCR and potential characterization of sugarcane resistance to leaf scald. Plant Disease. 2014;**98**(1):121-126

[43] Dias VD, Fernandez E, Cunha MG, Pieretti I, Hincapie M, Roumagnac P, et al. Comparison of loop-mediated isothermal amplification, polymerase chain reaction, and selective isolation assays for detection of *Xanthomonas albilineans* from sugarcane. Tropical Plant Pathology. 2018;**43**:351-359

[44] Nagamine K, Hase T, Notomi T. Accelerated reaction by loop-mediated isothermal amplification using loop primers. Molecular and Cellular Probes. 2002;**16**:223-229

[45] Fischbach J, Xander NC, Frohme M, Glökler JF. Shining a light on LAMP assays—A comparison of LAMP visualization methods including the novel use of berberine. Biotechnology Techniques. 2015;**58**:189-194

[46] Goto M, Honda E, Ogura A, Nomoto A, Hanaki K. Colorimetric

detection of loop mediated isothermal amplification reaction by using hydroxy naphthol blue. Biotechnology Techniques. 2009;**46**:167-172

[47] Ginzinger DG. Gene quantification using real-time quantitative PCR: An emerging technology hits the mainstream. Experimental Hematology. 2002;**30**(6):503-512

[48] Beachy RN. Mechanisms and applications of pathogen-derived resistance in transgenic plants. Current Opinion in Biotechnology. 1997;**8**(2):215-220

[49] Matzke M, Mette M, Matzke A. Transgene silencing by the host genome defense: Implications for the evolution of epigenetic control mechanisms in plants and vertebrates. Plant Molecular Biology. 2000;**43**(2-3):401-415

[50] Pieretti I, Royer M, Barbe V, Carrere S, Koebnik R, Cociancich S, et al. The complete genome sequence of *Xanthomonas albilineans* provides new insights into the reductive genome evolution of the xylem-limited *Xanthomonadaceae*. BMC Genomics. 2009;**10**:616

[51] Bogdanove AJ, Koebnik R, Lu H, Furutani A, Angiuoli SV, Patil PB, et al. Two new complete genome sequences offer insight into host and tissue specificity of plant pathogenic *Xanthomonas* spp. Journal of Bacteriology. 2011;**193**:5450-5464

[52] Pieretti I, Cociancich S, Bolot S, Carrère S, Morisset A, Rott P, et al. Full genome sequence analysis of two isolates reveals a novel *Xanthomonas* species close to the sugarcane pathogen *Xanthomonas albilineans*. Genes. 2015;**6**(3):714-733

[53] Birch RG, Pemberton JM, Basnayake WV. Stable albicidin resistance in Escherichia coli involves an altered outer-membrane nucleoside uptake system. Journal of General Microbiology. 1990;**136**:51-58

[54] Fsihi H, Kottwitz B, Bremer E. Single amino acid substitutions affecting the substrate-specificity of the *Escherichia coli* K-12 nucleoside-specific Tsx channel. The Journal of Biological Chemistry. 1993;**268**:17495-17503

[55] Zhang L, Birch RG. The gene for albicidin detoxification from *Pantoea dispersa* encodes an esterase and attenuates pathogenicity of *Xanthomonas albilineans* to sugarcane. Proceedings of the National Academy of Sciences of the United States of America. 1997;**94**:9984-9989

[56] Vieweg L et al. The albicidin resistance factor AlbD is a serine endopeptidase that hydrolyzes unusual oligoaromatic-type peptides. Journal of the American Chemical Society. 2015;**137**:7608-7611

[57] Ramos JL et al. The TetR family of transcriptional repressors. Microbiology and Molecular Biology Reviews. 2005;**69**:326-356

[58] Kahmann JD et al. Structural basis for antibiotic recognition by the TipA class of multidrug-resistance transcriptional regulators. The EMBO Journal. 2003;**22**:1824-1834

[59] Walker MJ, Birch RG, Pemberton JM. Cloning and characterization of an albicidin resistance gene from *Klebsiella oxytoca*. Molecular Microbiology. 1988;**2**:443-454

[60] Basnayake WVS, Birch RG. A gene from Alcaligenes denitrificans that confers albicidin resistance by reversible antibiotic binding. Microbiology. 1995;**141**:551-560

[61] Weng LX et al. Molecular and conformational basis of a specific and high affinity interaction between AlbA and albicidin phytotoxin. Applied

and Environmental Microbiology. 2005;**71**:1445-1452

[62] Weng LX, Xu JL, Li O, Birch RG, Zhang LH. Identification of the essential histidine residue for high-affinity binding of AlbA protein to albicidin antibiotics. Microbiology. 2003;**149**:451-457

[63] Costet L, Cunff L, Royaert S, Raboin LM, Hervouet C, Toubi L, et al. Haplotype structure around Bru1 reveals a narrow genetic basis for brown rust resistance in modern sugarcane cultivars. Theoretical and Applied Genetics. 2012;**125**:825-836

[64] Birch R, Bower R, Elliott A, Hansom S, Basnayake S, Zhang L. Regulation of transgene expression: Progress towards practical development in sugarcane, and implications for other plant species. Plant genetic engineering: towards the third millennium. In: Proceedings of the International Symposium on Plant Genetic Engineering; 6-10 December; Havana. Cuba: Elsevier Science Publishers; 1999, 2000

[65] Viswanathan R, Padmanaban P. Hand Book on Sugarcane Diseases and their Management. Coimbatore: Sugarcane Breeding Institute; 2008

[66] Blanco Y, Blanch M, Piñón D, Legaz ME, Vicente C. Antagonism of *Gluconacetobacter diazotrophicus* (a sugarcane endosymbiont) against *Xanthomonas albilineans* (pathogen) studied in alginate-immobilized sugarcane stalk tissues. Journal of Bioscience and Bioengineering. 2005;**99**(4):366-371

[67] Piñón D, Casas M, Blanch MA, Fontaniella B, Blanco Y, Vicente C, et al. *Gluconacetobacter diazotrophicus*, a sugar cane endosymbiont, produces a bacteriocin against *Xanthomonas albilineans*, a sugar cane pathogen. Research in Microbiology. 2002;**153**(6):345-351

[68] Arencibia AD, Vinagre F, Estevez Y, Bernal A, Perez J, Cavalcanti J, et al. *Gluconacetobacter diazotrophicus* elicitate a sugarcane defense response against a pathogenic bacteria *Xanthomonas albilineans*. Plant Signaling and Behavior. 2006;**1**(5):265-273

[69] Keymanesh K, Soltani S, Sardari S. Application of antimicrobial peptides in agriculture and food industry. World Journal of Microbiology and Biotechnology. 2009;**25**(6):933-944

Section 3

# Management of Plant Disease

Chapter 9

# Choosing an Adequate Pesticide Delivery System for Managing Pathogens with Difficult Biologies: Case Studies on *Diplodia corticola*, *Venturia inaequalis* and *Erwinia amylovora*

*Srđan G. Aćimović, Danielle K.H. Martin, Richard M. Turcotte, Christopher L. Meredith and Isabel A. Munck*

## Abstract

With the challenges that negatively impact tree-based agriculture, landscapes and forests, such as climate change, plant pathogen and insect range expansion, invasive species and limited new pesticides, it is important to introduce new and effective tree protection options. In the last 20 years, pathogens that invade wood i.e. vascular tissues of trees causing wilt, yellowing, premature defoliation, cankers and tree death, have been on the rise. *Diplodia corticola* causes Bot canker of oak species which can kill trees diminishing the valuable ecological services they provide and reducing profits from wood and cork production. Since this and similar pathogens have difficult biologies because they reside in wood and cause severe internal damage and tree death, their management is difficult or inefficient with classical pesticide application methods that cannot reach and distribute the active ingredient in vascular wood tissues. As practical management options for this and other vascular tissue pathogens of trees are limited, we evaluated efficacy of several trunk injected fungicides in control of *D. corticola* and compared it with the efficacy of trunk injection of similar compounds for control of *Venturia inaequalis* and *Erwinia amylovora*, as two well-studied apple tree pathogens with different or partially similar lifestyles to *D. corticola*, respectively.

**Keywords:** trunk injection of pesticides, tree disease management, *Diplodia corticola*, *Venturia inaequalis*, *Erwinia amylovora*

## 1. Introduction

Agricultural, urban, and natural tree stands have been the focus of extensive plant pathogen diagnostic and disease management research in recent decades [1–16] which recorded an increase in the number of new fungal and bacterial pathogens and their detrimental impact on agroecosystems, ecosystems, and the human society. The economic effects of these pathogens are reflected in lost fresh fruit produce [17–19], reduced yields and quality of fruit or wood and cork products [20, 21], diminished ecological tree services, and death of whole trees, stands, and forest regions or decimation of fruit industries [19, 22].

If left unmanaged, apple scab fungus *Venturia inaequalis*, a subcuticular leaf and fruit pathogen can cause 70–100% reduction in marketable fruit yield in each year [23, 24]. A pathogenic fungus *Diplodia corticola*, the causal agent of Bot canker of oak which invades tree xylem is the most widely distributed and virulent fungal pathogen causing canker and decline of cork oak (*Quercus suber*) forests in Europe [25, 26] and of southern live oak (*Q. virginiana*), coast live oak (*Q. agrifolia*), and canyon live oak (*Q. chrysolepis*) in the United States [3, 27]. Recently, there has been a rising incidence of this pathogen in the Unites States on northern red oak, *Q. rubra* [5, 8], black oak, *Q. velutina* [7], white oak, *Q. alba* [28], and bur oak (*Q. macrocarpa*) [29]. Other Botryosphaeriaceae, like *Neofusicoccum australe*, *N. luteum*, *N. parvum* and *N. mediterraneum* infect woody and green plant tissues and are destructive canker pathogens of avocado [1], grapevine, olive, pistachio and ash [30–33] and are recently reported as very virulent pathogens of coast redwood leading to severe decline in urban stands of California [9]. The Blue stain fungi *Grosmannia clavigera* and *Leptographium longiclavatum* are the plant pathogenic insect symbionts vectored by the mountain pine beetle *Dendroctonus ponderosae* [13]. They infect xylem and have led to death of millions of pine trees from 1990 to 2013 and decimation of pine forests in western North America [22, 34, 35]. Under favorable weather conditions during apple bloom and shoot growth, a destructive fire blight bacterium *Erwinia amylovora* inhabits and infects apple flowers and shoots and after spreading through xylem and causing cankers on wood it can kill whole trees. The resulting losses can range from $3.8 to 100 million due to removal of as much as 450,000 apple trees in only one or two years [17, 18, 36, 37]. Fire blight severely reduced both pear and quince production primarily in continental climate regions of the world. Asiatic citrus canker caused by *Xanthomonas axonopodis* pv. *citri* invades leaf mesophyll tissue and is estimated to cause yield losses and cost of disease management of $342 million per year [38]. The citrus greening or Huanglongbing disease is caused by a bacterium *Candidatus Liberibacter asiaticus* which proliferates and is limited to phloem vascular tissue of citrus trees. This pathogen led to $4.5 billion negative economic impact in just 5 years after introduction in the United States [19]. These devastating internal tree pathogens further create a barrier in international trade of fresh fruit and wood products in an attempt to prevent their introduction to new regions [39, 40].

The biology of majority of these microorganisms, excluding *V. inaequalis* and *X. axonopodis* pv. *citri*, has three key shared traits: (1) they invade, reside, and spread in xylem or phloem of woody host tissues, where a significant part of pathogenesis and internal host damage is taking place, and (2) due to specific lifestyle depicted in impacting the internal wood tissues, these pathogens successfully evade exposure to the contact, local-systemic, and green-tissue systemic pesticides applied to plant surfaces, and (3) their management is extremely difficult or inefficient with the classical pesticide delivery methods. Therefore, any pesticide active ingredient in a formulated form needs to distribute in these vascular tissues to reach pathogen propagules at an effective concentration and move systemically to all the uninfected or infected tissue parts to achieve an efficient preventive or curative control, respectively.

Tree injection, often referred to as trunk or stem injection, is a method of target precise delivery or application of pesticides, plant resistance activators and fertilizers into the xylem vascular tissue of a tree with the aim to protect trees from insect pests and pathogens or to provide tree nutrition and/or correction of micronutrient deficiencies. It primarily harnesses the transport capacity of the tree's vascular system driven by transpiration stream of water in these tissues to translocate and distribute the active compounds into the trunk, branches, canopy and roots where protection or nutrition is needed. Tree injection as a plant protection method is viewed as environmentally safer alternative for pesticide application because it secures significant reduction of non-target exposure of water, soil, air and wildlife to pesticides and fertilizers in landscapes and urban greening areas. The active ingredients are delivered within the tree, thus providing selective exposure to plant pests, with limited negative effect of weather conditions like rain or sun radiation on the injected compound and with creating no immediate pesticide residue losses outside the tree.

Trunk injection relies significantly on tree physiology processes related to water transport, xylem and phloem tissue functions, and the weather conditions that influence these specific plant processes. To achieve delivery of an effective pesticide dose, its distribution and expected management of plant detrimental organism or nutrient deficiency, there are several key factors which should be monitored by an applicator as they influence success of trunk injection for these purposes. Besides the plant pathogen biology, ecology, and epidemiology, several factors play a key role in success of trunk injection efficacy: the time of application in relation to detrimental organism establishment and symptom occurrence [11], the season and time of the day of application [41], the chemical properties of pesticide active ingredient and its formulation [42], the injected volume or dose of a pesticide, and the type of tree injection device or technology. For example, a more effective management of plant disease or insect infestation can be achieved by the preventive injections of pesticides in comparison to the therapeutic pesticide applications after the disease or infestation has already occurred. Tree injection of active compounds is much faster and easier during spring and early summer months in comparison to the late or mid-summer, late fall and winter, because water in the soil is abundant and the green leaf canopy is facilitating intensive transpiration pull and flow of water through the xylem tissue in hardwood trees, starting from the roots and branches to the leaves [41]. The three key properties of injected active ingredient that determine its mobility or binding in xylem of the tree are organic carbon-water partitioning coefficient (ml/g or μg/g) or carbon adsorption coefficient ($K_{o/c}$), water solubility, and formulation type. $K_{o/c}$ expresses the level of adhesion or adsorption of pesticide active ingredient to the carbon rich compounds in certain environments such as soil or xylem and is defined as a ratio of mass of a chemical that is adsorbed in a certain environment per unit mass of organic carbon in that environment per the equilibrium chemical concentration in a solution. Active ingredients that have high $K_{o/c}$ values will strongly bind to the organic compounds present in soil, sap or xylem and reduce their systemic movement i.e. translocation, accumulation and distribution in the canopy, thus reducing the efficacy in pathogen or pest control. In contrast, the ingredients with low or moderate $K_{o/c}$ values move and distribute fast after tree injection and distribute well in the canopy, securing good pest or pathogen control. Pesticide formulation is a form of a pesticide active ingredient ready for use or which quite often requires dilution in water prior to application. Formulation is made by adding different inactive ingredients with the aim to improve the properties of an active ingredient such as solubility, surface adhesion, distribution, effectiveness, shelf life, stability, handling or application (e.g. solvents, emulsifiers, surfactants and other adjuvants). Formulation of a pesticide or a fertilizer determines the properties and residue stability of an active ingredient and can modulate its mobility in xylem of phloem after tree injection for pest or plant management [12, 42]. Finally, trunk injection devices can loosely be divided into the ones using drill- or needle-based technology [43]. In case of the first one, access to xylem for pesticide delivery device is enabled by drilling into the trunk or root flare wood, removing a small part of the wood, and sealing of the opened injection port with an inserted plastic plug or not (plug contains an injection valve with a one-way silicone septum) [44]. For the injection application to be faster and hence economical in urban tree care, this system uses compressed air or hydraulic pressure to force-inject the pesticide solution into the wood. The second technology uses a knife-like or a flat, screwdriver-like needle with a lenticular profile, which is inserted into the wood by a hammer thus separating the wood fibers and creating a crevice while the delivery of a pesticide solution is conducted through the needle and infused into the wood [45]. This system can use force of hydraulic or compressed air pressure to deliver the pesticide solution into the xylem or is solely relying on the Venturi effect (vacuum) created by a transpiration stream in xylem to infuse the pesticide solution into the wood [45–47]. This injection technology requires longer time for injection solution delivery, especially when transpiration is limited, and thus is often less economical in urban tree care.

Tree injection was initially developed for pesticide and fertilizer application on large size trees in proximity of urban areas where ground- and air-spray applications are impractical due to substantial pesticide losses through drift, lack of proper canopy coverage, or are prohibited due to possible human and domestic animal exposure. The second driver for development of tree injection and its more frequent use in recent decades has been the destructive nature and an increasing need for effective management options for invasive tree pathogens like *Ophiostoma* fungi that cause Dutch elm disease, *Bretziella fagacearum* fungus that causes oak wilt, and insects pests like Emerald ash borer, *Agrilus planipennis* and Hemlock Wooly Adelgid, *Adelges tsugae*. Because of the unique biology of these organisms which leads to severe internal damage of wood and ultimately causes tree death, their management is extremely difficult or inefficient with classical pesticide application methods like topical spraying. Therefore, the goal of trunk injection to deliver the plant protective materials into the xylem or phloem vascular tissues of trees matches the specific pathogen or pest biologies and pesticide exposure requirements for the most effective management of these detrimental organisms.

Due to a demonstrated ability of single trunk injection to increase the efficacy of injected pesticides over multiple years, a possibility to reduce the of number of topical spray applications [10, 12, 48] and a rising incidence of woody plant pathogens and insect pests in the environment [31, 33, 49–51], this approach has recently been investigated in agriculture where topical pesticide applications for plant food production is intensive. The most investigated tree fruit crops and their pathogens and insect pests are citrus (e.g. *Candidatus* Liberibacter asiaticus) [14, 15], avocado (e.g. avocado thrips, *Scirtothrips perseae*; *Phytophthora* root rot, *Phytophthora cinnamomi*) [49, 50], apple (e.g. fire blight, *Erwinia amylovora*; apple scab, *V. inaequalis* [11, 12]; oblique banded leaf roller, *Choristoneura rosaceana* [10, 52]), and grapevine (e.g. grapevine downy mildew, *Plasmopara viticola* [53]; powdery mildew, *Uncinula necator* [54]). Domesticated apple, *Malus pumila* is an important research model in continental climate because management of *V. inaequalis* in humid regions requires intensive spray programs with as many as 15–22 spray applications of fungicides in one growing season [55]. Since this research is novel for tree disease management in contemporary agriculture, the proof of concept experiments on cultivated trees are conducted by using the trunk injection devices primarily designed for delivering pesticides and fertilizers for tree protection purposes in landscapes and urban forestry [10, 44, 52, 56]. Besides the smaller tree sizes in orchards in comparison to the urban landscapes as an obvious advantage driving the investigation of efficacy of pesticides delivered with this method [52, 57, 58], some of the key researched topics are efficacy and its lasting [10, 11], application timing optimization for season- and two-seasons-long control [12, 50, 59], trunk wounding by injection ports i.e. points [43], pesticide residue accumulation in fruit, nectar, and leaves [12, 59, 60] and their spatial and temporal distribution in the tree [61]. Even though tree injection originated from widely present needs for pest and disease control and plant nutrition in urban forestry, it holds an important potential for use in tree fruit agriculture where in the last 30 or so years there has been an increase of public pressure on apple producers to reduce pesticide use, while maintaining a high level of fruit quality [62]. Since the tree injection of pesticides and nutrients as a delivery approach is currently gaining more popularity in urban greening, landscapes and forestry management [13, 48, 63–65], we predict intensification of research for insect pest and pathogen control in tree-based agriculture and silviculture in the near future.

While trunk injection for pesticide delivery is a relatively new technology investigated in tree-based agriculture for managing diseases like citrus greening [14–16, 66–68] or fire blight [11, 44], research in agricultural engineering will first need to design or invent an application system/s that allow scalability, i.e. achieving simultaneous trunk injection of large number of trees in a short period of time. Besides this end goal many other key questions arising from research outlined above will need to be addressed through experimental work before tree injection is used in agriculture, even in limited fashion. The first steps are providing enough evidence i.e. providing proof of concept that injected pesticides are effective in tree pathogen and insect management and that injected materials have minimal negative effect on fresh fruit consumer and beneficial orchard fauna. Because effective management options for Bot canker and decline of different *Quercus* species caused by *D. corticola* and other aforementioned plant pathogens of vascular tissues are limited or lacking, we evaluated the efficacy of trunk injected fungicides for *D. corticola* control and compared it to the efficacy of similar active ingredients for management of *V. inaequalis* and *E. amylovora* which are more intensively studied models in continental climate. Our goal was to present new disease management data that argues in favor of a hypothesis that for plant pathogens with difficult biologies, i.e. for those that impact internal wood tissues, it is necessary to select appropriate pesticide delivery system/s such as trunk injection to achieve the maximum disease control through increasing pathogen exposure and thus efficiency of applied pesticides. We present efficacy data of trunk-injected pesticides in management of these three woody plant pathogens with different or partially similar lifestyles to elucidate and promote the translation of tree injection as a target precise delivery system for plant protection in agriculture and silviculture of the future.

## 2. Trunk injection delivery of pesticides for management of three important plant pathogens in continental climate

### 2.1 Biology of *Diplodia corticola*, *Venturia inaequalis* and *Erwinia amylovora*

#### *2.1.1 Diplodia corticola*

In the binomial nomenclature of fungi, Bot canker pathogen *D. corticola* is a commonly found asexual stage of an ascomycete *Botryosphaeria corticola*, a sexual stage of this fungus [69]. Asexual stage forms white to dark olive-green aerial mycelium with a dark green to black underside [5]. During 24 weeks after the host plant infection, the fungus forms dark brown to black, circular or flask-shaped fruiting bodies called pycnidia, that are up to 1 mm in diameter and emerge through the dead bark of oak. Pycnidia can form on all above ground tree parts and are visible on bark as black masses of fungal tissue called stromata. Pycnidia have multiple chambers or locules in them, each 200–300 μm in diameter, in which spores called conidia are produced for around 2 years and serve as source of inoculum for new infections [69]. When pycnidia are mature they are partially erumpent through the host bark and form a circular opening on the top called ostiole serving for conidia release. Conidia are oval-shaped to cylindrical, straight, with both ends rounded, usually translucent and single-celled, but with aging rarely become brown and with multiple cells [69]. Inside, conidia are usually without an oil vesicle called guttule but can form one in the center. The sexual stage *B. corticola* forms spores called ascospores. Eight ascospores arranged in two rows form in one sac called ascus and multiple asci are formed in the dark brown to black fruiting bodies called pseudothecia [69]. Pseudothecia are up to 1 mm in diameter, circular and partially erumpent on the host bark when mature. Each pseudothecium has multiple chambers or locules 200–300 μm in diameter [69]. For release of ascospores, pseudothecia form a circular opening on the top called ostiole. Ascospores are spindle-shaped to rhomboid and translucent, one-celled, or rarely becoming light brown and with age two- or three-celled [69].

Because *D. corticola* has been described only recently [69], its life cycle describing how this pathogen reaches and colonizes oak species as a primary host is not fully known. Based on the other pathogenic and opportunistic pathogen members of the family Botryosphaeriaceae, *D. corticola* can probably infect through wounds and maybe plant natural openings. Once infection is established it spreads within the host via xylem to large distances with xylem sections exhibiting black streaking and cankers can form intermittently on the bark of trunk or branches [5, 8, 28, 29]. Some trees with xylem necrosis do not always exhibit visible external cankers [7]. With time, crown sections of infected trees show wilting and eventually host can die [5, 8]. It is assumed that conidia and ascospore production on cankers and germination are favored by moisture and high relative air humidity. Recently, in a study analyzing aerial fungal spore samples collected by the air spore traps and passive rain collectors, *D. corticola* was detected in 16 of the 32 sampled locations in Canada by a highly specific molecular detection method which targets a pathogen-specific DNA region [70]. This data indicates that *D. corticola* has aerial disseminated spores. It is reported that conidia of *D. corticola* are dispersed by wind [71], water and/or insect vectors [26]. A pest of oak wood, oak pinhole borer (*Platypus cylindrus*), acts as a vector of *D. corticola* spores as this fungus was detected in the insects gut and mycangia (structures in the insect body adapted for transport of spores of insect-symbiotic fungi) [72]. The invasive insects *Xyleborus affinis* and *Xylosandrus crassiusculus* in Florida have also been found to vector *D. corticola* as this fungus was frequently isolated from their mycangia [73]. Even though the knowledge on timing of seasonal spore release and relative inoculum abundance is limited [71], under natural infection pressure originating from a declining cork oak forest, *D. corticola* was found to infect cork oak seedlings at two infections peaks, in May and in September [71]. The role of *B. corticola* ascospores and their importance in pathogen dissemination have not been discussed in literature so far and much about epidemiology of this pathogen is unknown.

Majority of evidence indicates that *D. corticola* is a true pathogen of *Quercus* species [5, 8, 28, 29]. *D. corticola* was isolated from northern red oak trees in an urban stand where no obvious signs of environmental or other biotic stresses were visible, aside of the Bot canker occurrence [5]. It is not clear how environmental and biotic factors that can stress oak trees favor *D. corticola* infections and their severity, but it is possible they could worsen the disease. In the northeastern USA, this fungus has been isolated from infected black oak trees (*Quercus velutina*) which were at the same time infested with a damaging gall wasp, *Zapatella davisae* [7]. However, in support of the true pathogen lifestyle, the inoculation tests with isolated *D. corticola* strains conducted on young, healthy, naturally established trees of black oak clearly demonstrated the pathogenicity of *D. corticola*. In a similar case in California, closely related Botryosphaeriaceae fungi *Neofusicoccum australe*, *N. luteum*, *N. parvum*, *N. mediterraneum* and *Botryosphaeria dothidea* have been isolated from declining coast redwood trees (*Sequoia sempervirens*) in the urban stands, which were severely drought stressed [9]. However, the inoculation tests with the isolates of these fungal species on potted healthy young trees of coast redwood clearly showed that *Neofusicoccum* species were true and very virulent pathogens, while *B. dothidea* was an opportunistic pathogen that did not cause severe infection on healthy trees [9]. The other members of Botryosphaeriaceae family, such as *B. dothidea* [23, 74, 75] or *Diplodia sapinea* [76], are well-known opportunistic pathogens that dwell on the tree asymptomatically for months or even years, until the plant becomes weakened through any number of abiotic or biotic stresses (e.g. drought or insect infestation), and then infect it [9, 77–81]. The stressed plant host is the key conducive condition for these pathogens to establish infection and express the disease symptoms. Future experiments, similar to the drought contribution studies done for *B. dothidea* infection [9, 74, 77–79], should demonstrate which role the different plant stresses play in predisposing the oak species to *D. corticola* infection in continental and other climate types of the world where this pathogen is also widely present.

### *2.1.2 Venturia inaequalis*

The sexual stage of an ascomycete fungus *V. inaequalis* (Cooke) Winter, 1875, a cause of apple scab disease, starts by sexual reproduction in fall which results in formation of round initials of fungal fruiting bodies called pseudothecia. These bodies are embedded in a stroma or dense mat of fungal mycelia inside the mesophyll tissue of dead apple leaves. Late in winter and the beginning of spring, pseudothecia mature, gain pear-like shape and form sexual spores called ascospores. There are eight ascospores arranged linearly in each of the 50–100 elongated cylindrical sacs called asci that form in each pseudothecium. Ascospores are translucent to brown, two-celled, with one cell always larger than the other giving them a typical shape of a shoe "footprint". Mature pseudothecia form a circular opening or ostiole at the top of the pseudothecium, which protrudes through the surface of the dead apple leaves and allows ascospore release. There is only one cycle of ascospore production in spring of each year and they cause primary scab infections. The asexual stage *Spilocaea pomi* (Fr.) (syn. *Fusicladium dendriticum*) forms a translucent mycelium below the cuticle of the infected green apple tissues. With time, mycelia become dark gray to black, forming a dense mycelial mat that gives rise to asexual spores called conidia. Conidia are dark green, teardrop-shaped, i.e. pointed at one end and rounded on the other, single-celled or rarely two-celled. Conidia cause secondary infections during the apple growing season. There can be many cycles of conidia production and thus secondary infections, sometimes even more than 20 [82].

Depending on the substrate it colonizes over the year, the life cycle of apple scab fungus has the saprophytic and the parasitic phase in its development. The saprophytic phase starts with apple leaf drop in autumn. *V. inaequalis*, the sexual stage of apple scab fungus, overwinters in the dead fallen leaves and fruit debris of apple on the orchard floor as initials of fruiting bodies called pseudothecia. Fungus rarely overwinters as *S. pomi* in the form of mycelium on twig lesions or in the inner bud tissues [23, 83, 84]. After winter rest, pseudothecia mature in early spring and release ascospores that enable first or the primary infections on newly developing green apple tissues. Hence, ascospores in the leaf litter and debris are prime inoculum sources in spring. With each wetting from rain of heavy dew [85], pseudothecia absorb water, swell and asci expand through the ostiole, allowing forcible ascospore discharge. Ejected ascospores can reach a height of about 5–30 mm above the ostiole and are further disseminated by air currents, wind and rain aerosol [86]. They germinate only in water droplets or film coating the plant surfaces and their germination ends the saprophytic phase of pathogen's life cycle. Depending on region, the period of ascospore discharge triggered by wetting events can last from 3 to 9 weeks during late March and over April, May and mid-June. Ascospores are airborne and can reach at least 45 m away from the inoculum source [87]. *Spilocaea pomi* as the asexual stage of this fungus begins with ascospore germination and infection of the newly developing green tissues of apple leaves, flowers and fruit. The infection of current season's apple growth starts the parasitic phase of the pathogen's life cycle. Fungal mycelium penetrates below the waxy cuticle and grows between the outer cell wall of host's epidermal cells and the cuticle covering them. If the primary infections with ascospores are successful, after incubation period the plant cuticle of infected organ ruptures due to pressure created by thickening mycelium and masses of asexual spores of *S. pomi* called conidia. The infections are first visible as light chlorotic spots on leaves against the light, then gradually turn into pale olive to dark gray and ultimately black, velvety apple scab lesions. Infections on flower pedicel lead to flower drop. Infected leaves senesce and drop, while young fruit become deformed and fall off. Conidia cause new or often known secondary infections during the season and are dislodged and dispersed primarily with the help of rain water and dew. Their dispersal allowing more new infections is occurring primarily within the tree because very few conidia can reach 10 m or more from the inoculum source [88].

During the time after spores of apple scab fungus land on the susceptible plant surface, while they germinate, and up to 72 h after they penetrate below the cuticle on green tissue, they are vulnerable to spray-applied contact and systemic fungicides, respectively. However, once the infection is established by formation of mycelium under the cuticle, almost all fungicides applied to green plant surfaces have no efficacy in eradicating these infections and eventually lesions with conidia, or their effect is minimal. Furthermore, continued post-infection scab management with spray applications of fungicides that aim to prevent new infections on green tissues is complicated by large populations of conidia, which if exposed to fungicides with specific modes of action might increases the potential for fungicide resistance selection in this devastating pathogen. Because of the specific lifestyle of *S. pomi* to reside in subcuticular spaces of green tissues during the parasitic phase of the life cycle, successful management of the apple scab is crucially dependent on preventive fungicide applications that are delivered to leaves and fruit before the major infection periods occur. To time fungicide spray applications, several epidemiological models based on pathogen ecology and biology have been developed and can predict discharge of *V. inaequalis* ascospores and the infection occurrence by using the weather forecast for up to 10 days (NEWA, RIMpro) [89–92]. They are used in all the major apple growing regions.

### 2.1.3 *Erwinia amylovora*

Fire blight is caused by a Gram-negative bacterium *Erwinia amylovora* (Burrill 1882) Winslow et al. [93] in the family Enterobacteriaceae. The bacterial cells are rod-shaped, 0.3 × 1–3 μm in size and occur as single cells or pairs and sometimes short chains. They are motile by 2–7 peritrichous flagella per cell [94]. The pathogen cells are not visible to the naked eye. On infected hosts, pathogen is visible in the form of droplets or smears of bacterial ooze which are opaque white, amber or orange. Ooze is a sticky mixture of bacterial cells and exopolysaccharides which plays a major role in pathogen dissemination within and between the apple trees and orchards [95, 96]. In humid conditions, ooze exudes from the cracks on infected wood tissues with fire blight cankers and through stomata and lenticels on green, succulent parts of infected flowers, immature fruit, and shoots. In low humidity conditions, fire blight bacteria can survive in dry ooze for more than a year [97]. In the laboratory, *E. amylovora* forms domed, circular, mucoid colonies on microbiological media that contain sucrose nutrient agar [98, 99] which differ in color depending on specific contents of agar medium, ranging from red to orange, yellow white, and light blue opalescent [100]. This pathogen has a wide range of cultivated, landscape or forest plant hosts from Rosaceae family: apple, crabapple (*Malus*), pear, Asian pear, Callery pear (*Pyrus*), quince (*Cydonia*), raspberry (*Rubus*), as well as hawthorn (*Crataegus*), firethorn (*Pyracantha*), mountain ash (*Sorbus*), serviceberry (*Amelanchier*), *Cotoneaster*, loquat (*Eriobotrya*), flowering quince (*Chaenomeles*), etc.

*E. amylovora* survives through the winter in the bark around the canker edge and below the fire blight cankers initiated after pathogen progression from flower and shoot infections established in the previous years. Bacterial cells can also overwinter in asymptomatic host buds or as latent infections in asymptomatic wood [101]. It is possible that cells of this pathogen are in a viable but non-culturable physiological state in asymptomatic tissues [102, 103]. With warm spring weather, pathogen cells multiply and emerge in bacterial ooze exuding on the edges of overwintered cankers. On apple, this process usually occurs during late bloom and petal fall growth stages. Every single droplet of ooze may contain up to 1 billion cells of *E. amylovora* [95]. The ooze protects bacteria from unfavorable weather conditions and bacteria are disseminated from ooze to flowers, shoots and injured tissues by rain, wind, birds and presumably insects that touch or feed on ooze [95, 96, 104, 105]. For example, in experimental conditions, *E. amylovora* was found to survive and can be transmitted for up to 8 days in the digestive tract of Mediterranean fruit fly *Ceratitis capitata* and up to 28 days on its surface [106]. Insects that might vector *E. amylovora* are still investigated, but it is probable that the insect vectors will vary depending on the region of the world. Recent investigation shows that flies are attracted to feed on ooze and can acquire from 100 to 100,000 viable *E. amylovora* cells per fly individual [96]. It appears that honeybees do not visit ooze droplets on cankers in spring and might not spread the bacteria from cankers to flowers. It is assumed that in low humidity conditions, dry ooze strings or particles exuded through lenticels or stomata on the bark can break off and reach or settle on nearby susceptible flowers or shoots after carried by wind or insects. The closer the fire blight cankers are to any open flowers or shoots, the higher is the chance for *E. amylovora* cells to reach the flower surfaces by previously mentioned pathways. The period of apple susceptibility to *E. amylovora* infection lasts from the day when the first flowers open in the orchard and ends when the last terminal buds set on shoots. However, risk for severe infections becomes lower after flowering ends because the number of flowers as entry points for the pathogen significantly declines. Shoots initiate growth just before flowering ends and are susceptible until their growth stops. Terminal bud set is an apple growth stage when the current year vegetative growth stops, and a bud is formed at the top of the shoot. In continental climate, this usually occurs during July, varying somewhat among different apple cultivars. After this stage, risk from fire blight infections is negligent due to age-related resistance, unless a hail injury occurs on trees providing new entry points for fire blight infections (trauma blight).

Once *E. amylovora* bacteria reach the apple flower surfaces, they multiply rapidly on the surfaces of nutrient-rich flower stigmas if temperatures are favorably warm [107]. After colonizing young, just opened flowers [108], bacteria require achieving necessary population size and presence of moisture for infection establishment. The bacteria only have few days to grow their numbers on young flowers to reach at least 100,000 and up to 1 million live cells before a possible infection event can be triggered by rain, dew, or hail. During this time and before the moisture becomes available to allow infection, honeybees could spread the bacteria from contaminated flowers to newly opened flowers [109, 101]. This pollinator-facilitated spreading continues the necessary pathogen population increase. Flower surfaces of many other species of Rosacease family, except European plum *Prunus domestica*, which are not susceptible to fire blight were found to be potential sites for population increase of *E. amylovora* during their periods of bloom [110]. With a wetting event in the form of rain, dew or hail, the pathogen is washed down from stigmas to the nectar glands located in the floral cup where pathogen enters the host and causes the infection. Infection of succulent green shoots occurs either via (1) internal pathogen spread through green tissues from the infected flowers to the base of the nearby shoots, (2) direct transfer of the pathogen from cankers or contaminated plant or tool surfaces to the shoots, or (3) by pathogen dispersal from contaminated or infected flowers to the shoot tips and leaves. Insects might play a vector role in these three pathways. For limited amount of time, *E. amylovora* cells can survive on other healthy surfaces of leaves and branches. However, population growth on these surfaces does not occur. Pathogen enters and colonizes the cortical parenchyma through stomata on the leaves or green stem, or through the microinjuries i.e. punctures and tears caused by wind, wind-carried soil particles, hail, friction of plant parts, or sucking or chewing insects [111]. During the time before infections take place, the lifestyle of *E. amylovora* involves inhabiting and growing on the plant surfaces and is influenced by the temperature and moisture from the environment and by nutrients on the plant host. This is known as epiphytic phase of *E. amylovora* biology during which successful management of fire blight is achieved by preventive spray applications of antibiotics that are delivered to flowers, before or up to 24 h after the predicted rain event/s that would trigger the infection/s. Several fire blight epidemiological models have been designed based on environmental and biological requirements of *E. amylovora* and can predict infection events by using the weather forecast for up to 10 days in advance to calculate the near-future infection risks (NEWA's EIP, Maryblyt, RIMpro, Cougarblight).

During the incubation, i.e. usually sometime around 10 – 14 days before the first conspicuous blossom or shoot blight symptoms are visible, small white, amber or orange droplets of bacterial ooze can emerge and drip from the infected green tissues (flower pedicels, floral cup, sepals, immature fruit and shoots). With more wetting events and insect activity, ooze can spread to new flowers and actively growing shoots across the whole orchard. Since blossom and shoot blight symptoms are not yet visible, this dissemination of ooze allows secondary infections and can propel a fire blight outbreak into an epidemic, especially if the antibiotic spray application/s were not conducted during bloom. Once incubation is over, blossom blight is visible as dead, black or brown flower clusters with more droplets of bacterial ooze developing if weather conditions are humid. Shoot blight and immature fruit infections are visible as black or brown "flags" or "strikes" and brown to black shriveled fruitlets, respectively. Blighted shoot tips often bend in the typical shape of Shepherd's crook. Fire blight cankers on branches, trunk and rootstock are formed by pathogen's progress via xylem or the cortical parenchyma from the established infections on flowers, shoots and suckers, into the wood bark tissues.

When *E. amylovora* enters the succulent tissues of flowers or shoots, it begins the pathogenic phase of its lifestyle when it causes the disease and acquires moisture and nutrients from the host and can migrate to other close or far host tissues and organs. During this phase, pathogen colonizes the cortical parenchyma tissue and xylem vessels and can continue with systemic migration and distribution in the plant [112–114]. Fire blight bacteria migrate internally via xylem of symptomless branch and trunk tissues and ahead of the visible blight or canker symptoms, thus reaching uninfected plant parts and apple rootstocks and causing infection far from the visible infections in the canopy [115]. On susceptible rootstocks, the resulting infections can express as cankers, often causing tree death due to trunk or rootstock girdling, or can remain latent i.e. as a symptomless infections of trunk or rootstock. Rootstock or trunk infections can also be initiated by *E. amylovora* migration from the externally infected rootstock suckers (shoot growth from the root system or rootstock stem) or water sprouts (shoot growth from the trunk or thick branches). When *E. amylovora* resides as an endophyte in an apparently healthy plant tissues of branches, rootstock or budwood, this lifestyle is referred to as an endophytic phase of its biology. Finally, in nurseries, *E. amylovora* cells which survive on bark surfaces can infect rootstock or scion when either are bruised or injured during the processes of vegetative material harvest, transport, or grafting.

## 2.2 Materials and methods

### *2.2.1 Trunk injection of pesticides for Diplodia corticola management*

To test the effect of injected fungicides and activators of plant systemic acquired resistance (SAR) [11] for reduction of Bot canker caused by *D. corticola* we conducted experiments on potted northern red oak trees (*Q. rubra*) with fully developed canopy. We evaluated trunk-injected fungicides and application rates listed in **Table 1**, which were selected based on the EPA labels of pesticides for landscape use (**Table 1**) and the preliminary fungicide screenings *in vitro* for suppression of *D. corticola* colonies on fungicide-amended Petri of plates with potato dextrose agar medium (Aćimović et al. unpublished data). Since in year one of the experiment Phosphojet at 1.5 ml dose caused phytotoxicity on tree trunks, we reduced the dose to 0.75 ml in year two repetition of the experiment (**Table 1**).

| | Year one | | |
|---|---|---|---|
| **Treatment** | **Active ingredient** | **Dose and dilution** | **Total volume** |
| Propizol | Propiconazole 14.3% (Propizol, Arborjet Inc.) | 1.5 ml + 1.5 ml water | 3 ml |
| Arbotect | Thiabendazole 20% (Arbotect 20-S, Syngenta) | 0.06 ml + 2.94 ml water | 3 ml |
| Phosphojet | Mono- and di-potassium salts of phosphorous acid[x] 45.8% (Phosphojet, Arborjet Inc.) | 1.5 ml + 1.5 ml | 3 ml |
| Water control | - | 3 ml | 3 ml |
| | **Year two** | | |
| **Treatment** | **Active ingredient** | **Dose** | **Total volume** |
| Propizol | Propiconazole 14.3% (Propizol, Arborjet Inc., Woburn, MA) | 1.5 ml + 1.5 ml water | 3 ml |
| Arbotect | Thiabendazole 20% (Arbotect 20-S, Syngenta) | 0.06 ml + 2.94 ml water | 3 ml |
| Phosphojet | Mono- and di-potassium salts of phosphorous acid 45.8% (Phosphojet, Arborjet Inc.) | 0.75 ml + 2.25 ml water | 3 ml |
| Water control | - | 3 ml | 3 ml |

[x] Commonly called potassium phosphites

**Table 1.**
*Trunk injected fungicide treatments evaluated for management of Bot canker fungus Diplodia corticola on northern red oak trees, Quercus rubra.*

One injection point i.e. port per trunk of each potted tree, positioned ca. 5–7 cm above the ground level, was created by drilling 7–10 mm into the xylem tissue with a 4.3 mm diameter drill attached to a cordless drill. To inject the protective liquid solutions listed in **Table 1**, we used a Stinger needle for plugless trunk injection assembled on an individual feed line attached to the Tree IV air/hydraulic microinjection system, which operated at 60 psi air pressure (Arborjet Inc., Woburn, MA). The Stinger needles are used for injection of trees when trunk injection ports of large diameter (9.5 mm) are of concern or should be avoided and for injection of trunks with small diameters. The diameter of injection port for inserting a Stinger needle is smaller and does not require sealing with an Arborplug. In year one, the injected potted oak trees had trunk diameter at 5 cm height averaging 1.3 cm and ranging from 1 to 2.1 cm. In year two, a new set of injected trees had the diameter at 5 cm height averaging 1.5 cm and ranging from 1.1 to 2.2 cm. Trunk injection were conducted on 12 June in year one and on 16 August in year two.

Trees were inoculated with *D. corticola* on 21 June and on 25 August, i.e. 9 days after injection of fungicides. Trunk bark on the opposite side from the injection port and 10 cm above the port was cut at three sides of rectangle to create a sleeve which was peeled longitudinally. A PDA plug 5 mm in diameter from 10-day-old colony of *D. corticola* isolate from our previous work [8] was placed in the sleeve on each injected tree and wrapped with parafilm (**Table 1**). Once the first symptoms of canopy wilt were observed, trees were destructively examined by stripping the bark off above and below the inoculation point. The necrosis length (cm) and width (cm) of Bot canker in xylem of the oak trunks were measured on 10 July in year one and on 27 September in year two. Xylem necrosis area ($cm^2$) was calculated by multiplying the length and width for each individual tree and treatment mean was calculated from six replicate trees.

Statistical analysis was done with MIXED procedure in SAS Studio software (SAS Institute Inc. 2017, Cary, NC) using the xylem necrosis areas ($cm^2$). If the fungicide effect was found to be statistically significant ($p < 0.1$ in year one; $p < 0.05$ in year two), treatment comparisons were done with LSD test. We presented the fungicide management results as percent reduction of Bot canker necrosis area, also known as percent disease control, calculated as: percent reduction of necrosis area = [percent necrosis area in water control – percent necrosis area in specific treatment] × 100/percent necrosis area in water control.

### *2.2.2 Trunk injection of pesticides for Venturia inaequalis management*

With the goal to optimize timing and number of fungicide injections for management of apple scab fungus *V. inaequalis*, we conducted two experiments. In the experiment 1, we trunk-injected fungicides listed in **Table 2** on 29-year-old 'Mac Spur' apple trees four times, with the first injection applied in the fall of year one and the next three injections conducted in the spring of next, year two. In the experiment 1, the injection on 11 April was conducted at 50% apple bloom (**Table 2**). In the experiment 2, we injected 29-year-old 'Mac Spur' apple trees with fungicides only one to two times in total, but by delivering them at different seasons i.e. in fall or spring, as per schedule listed in **Table 2**. In the experiment 2, the injection on 21 April was conducted at the silver tip growth stage of apple (**Table 2**).

On each trunk injection date with fungicides listed in **Table 2**, a separate set of four cardinally-oriented trunk injection ports per each tree of 'Mac Spur' was created by drilling 25 mm into the xylem with a 9.5 mm diameter drill bit attached to a cordless drill. The first set of four injection ports was positioned ca. 25 cm above the ground level. The subsequent sets of four injection port were positioned ca. 5 cm above and between the lower four-port sets. Every port was sealed with Arborplug no. 4 (Arborjet

| EXPERIMENT 1 | | | | |
|---|---|---|---|---|
| **Treatment** | **Active ingredient** | **Dose** | **Dates of injections or sprays** | |
| | | | **Year one** | **Year two** |
| Phosphojet low F[u] + 3S[v] | Mono- and di-potassium salts of phosphorous acid[w] 45.8% (Phosphojet, Arborjet Inc.) | 2.59 ml / 2.5 cm of DFH[x] | 15 October | 11 April, 11 May, 8 June |
| Phosphojet high F + 3S | | 5.17 ml / 2.5 cm of DFH | 15 October | 11 April, 11 May, 8 June |
| Alamo low F + 3S | Propiconazole 14.3% (Alamo, Arborjet Inc.) | 8.3 ml / 2.5 cm of DFH | 15 October | 11 April, 11 May, 8 June |
| Alamo high F + 3S | | 16.6 ml / 2.5 cm of DFH | 15 October | 11 April, 11 May, 8 June |
| Water control | - | 8.3 ml / 2.5 cm of DFH | 15 October | 11 April, 11 May, 8 June |
| Spray standard | Mancozeb 75%, (Penncozeb 75 DF, Cerexagri Inc.) + Fenarimol 12% (Rubigan EC, Dow AgroSciences LLC) | 2.7 kg / 0.405 ha + 354.9 ml / 0.405 ha | | 27 March; 3, 13, 18[y] April; and 1 May 2012 |

| EXPERIMENT 2 | | | | | |
|---|---|---|---|---|---|
| **Treatments** | **Active ingredient** | **Dose** | **Dates of injections or sprays** | | |
| | | | **Year one** | **Year two** | |
| Phosphojet F | Mono- and di-potassium salts of phosphorous acid 45.8% (Phosphojet, Arborjet Inc.; Agrifos, Agrichem PTY.) | 5.17 ml / 2.5 cm of DFH | 11 October | - | - |
| Phosphojet F + S[z] | | 5.17 ml / 2.5 cm of DFH | 11 October | 21 April | - |
| Phosphojet S | | 5.17 ml / 2.5 cm of DFH | - | 21 April | - |
| Phosphojet S + S | | 5.17 ml / 2.5 cm of DFH | - | 21 April | 22 May |
| Agrifos sprays | | 1,892.7 ml / 0.405 ha | 1, 8, 16, 21, 31 May and 5, 11, 19, 26 June 2013 | | |
| Inspire Super F | Difenoconazole 8.4% + Cyprodinil 24.1% (Inspire Super EW, Syngenta) | 7 ml/ tree | 11 October | - | - |
| Inspire Super F + S | | 3.5 ml/ tree | 11 October | 21 April | |
| Inspire Super S | | 7 ml/ tree | - | 21 April | - |
| Inspire Super S + S | | 7 ml/ tree | - | 21 April | 22 May |
| Inspire Super sprays | | 354.8 ml/ 0.405 ha | 1, 8, 16, 21, 31 May 2013 | | |
| Water control | - | 500 ml/ tree | 11 October | 21 April | 22 May |

[u] F - one fall injection
[v] 3S - three spring injections
[w] Commonly called potassium phosphites
[x] DFH - trunk diameter at one-foot height (30.5 cm)
[y] Date with single fenarimol application
[z] S - one spring injection

**Table 2.**
*Fungicide treatments trunk-injected across two seasons and sprayed for management of apple scab fungus Venturia inaequalis on 'Mac Spur' apple trees.*

Inc., Woburn, MA) positioned just below the bark level to allow port closure with cambium callus [44]. To inject the fungicides, we used the Quik-jet microinjection system (Arborjet Inc.) operating at hand-generated hydraulic pressure to deliver low volumes of liquid for injection, thus allowing faster application times, and the Tree IV air/hydraulic microinjection system (Arborjet Inc.) operating at up to 60 psi of air pressure to deliver large solution volumes of liquid for injection (≥600 ml). In the experiment 1 (**Table 2**), we injected all the treatments listed for 15 October in year one with Quik-jet (**Table 2**). On 11 April in year two, we injected propiconazole using the Viper air/hydraulic microinjection system set at 90 psi air pressure (Arborjet Inc.). At the later dates, we injected Alamo using the Tree IV and Phosphojet using the Quik-jet. In the experiment 2, we injected Phosphojet with Quik-jet and cyprodinil + difenoconazole with Tree IV. The needle/s of each of the used injection devices was inserted through the Arborplugs allowing the total liquid volume per tree, at one injection time, to be divided and delivered equally among the four ports.

All the experiments were conducted under naturally high infection pressure during the primary season of *V. inaequalis* ascospore release in spring. In the experiment 1, we rated percent incidence of apple scab only on leaves, since fruits were lost due to spring frosts. In the experiment 2, we rated percent incidence of scab on leaves and fruit. A total of chose 20 spurs and 20 terminal shoots per tree were selected, with about five from each crown quadrant, and rated for leaf scab incidence. The fruit scab incidence was rated by selecting and rating 100 fruits per tree, with about 25 per crown quadrant, and if less was found we rated all the fruits per tree. The data were analyzed using MIXED procedure in SAS 9.3 (SAS Institute, Cary, NC). The tree was the subject of repeated measures. If the main effects or their interactions were found to be statistically significant ($p < 0.05$),

| Treatment | Active ingredient | Dose |
|---|---|---|
| *For control of blossom and shoot blight incidence on 'Gala' apple trees* | | |
| Actigard 1 | Acibenzolar-S-methyl 50% (Actigard, Syngenta) | 1 x 0.34 g/tree |
| Actigard 2 | | 2 x 0.34 g/tree |
| Phosphojet | Mono- and di-potassium salts of phosphorous acid[x] 45.8% (Phosphojet, Arborjet Inc.) | 2 x 22.5 ml/tree |
| Agrimycin | Streptomycin 17% (Agrimycin, Nufarm Ltd.) | 2 x 1.82 g/tree |
| Water control | - | 2 x 520 ml/tree |
| *For control of shoot blight severity on 'Jonathan' apple trees* | | |
| Arborbiotic | Oxytetracycline hydrochloride 39.6% (Arborbiotic™, MFG Scientific Inc.) | 1 x 0.28 g + 2.52 ml water / each 25.4 mm of DFH[y] |
| Water control | - | 2.52 ml water / each 25.4 mm of DFH |

[x] Commonly called potassium phosphites
[y] DFH - trunk diameter at one-foot height (30.5 cm)

**Table 3.**
*Trunk-injected treatments of bactericides and SAR-activators for management of fire blight bacterium Erwinia amylovora on flowers and shoots of 'Gala' and 'Jonathan' apple trees.*

examination, i.e. slicing of interactions within main effects was performed, $F$-tests conducted and pairwise or specific time or treatment comparisons were done with $t$-tests ($\alpha = 0.05$). We presented the fungicide management results as percent of disease reduction, also known as percent disease control, calculated as: percent reduction of disease incidence = [percent disease incidence in water control – percent disease incidence in specific treatment] $\times$ 100/percent disease incidence in water control.

### *2.2.3 Trunk injection of pesticides for Erwinia amylovora management*

#### *2.2.3.1 Treatments for reducing blossom and shoot blight incidence*

To test the effect of injected bactericides and activators of plant systemic acquired resistance (SAR) for blossom and shoot blight incidence reduction, the orchard experiments were conducted over 2 years (**Table 3**). The early spring injections in year one (26 March) were conducted with Viper air/hydraulic micro-injection system® at under 110 psi of air pressure and late spring injections (23 April) were done with Tree IV® air/hydraulic micro-injection system, at 60 psi air pressure (Arborjet Inc., Woburn, MA). In the year two, trunk injections on 1 and 22 May were applied using Tree IV® air/hydraulic micro-injection system at 60 psi of air pressure. The injection needles of these devices were inserted through the one-way valve silicone septum in the Arborplugs® which allowed delivery of protective solutions into he drilled injection ports. In each injection, the total injected volume per tree was divided equally among the four ports (**Table 3**). Four injection ports per each apple per tree, positioned ca. 10–15 cm above the ground level, were cardinally oriented and created by drilling 25 mm into the xylem tissue using a 9.5 mm diameter drill bit attached to a cordless drill. Each port was sealed with Arborplug® no. 4, by pushing the plug with a specialized screwdriver-like tapper hit with a hammer (Arborjet Inc., Woburn, MA, USA). The plug was positioned just below the bark level to allow port closure with cambium callus.

In the year one, we used 14-year-old 'Gala' apple trees which were trunk-injected using the compounds and dosages listed in **Table 3**. Injections were performed at the tight cluster growth stage in apples (26 March), or 21 days before 80% bloom, and at petal fall growth stage (23 April). In the year two, experiments were conducted on a new set of 21-year-old 'Gala' apple trees, injected with the same doses in **Table 3**. Injections were applied at early tight cluster growth stage (1 May) or 13 days before 80% bloom and at petal fall (22 May). The treatment

Actigard 1 was injected only on the first date in both years (**Table 3**). Each dose in every treatment, except the Phosphojet, was diluted and injected with 520 ml of water per tree. The doses per tree were chosen according to the four rules: (1) the dose was equivalent to the US EPA pesticide label rate for a maximum amount per 0.405 ha with 250 planted apple trees; (2) the dose was one half of the maximum US EPA label rate allowed per one season; (3) the dose was equal to a rate delivered in one spray application treatment per 0.405 ha with 250 apple trees; or (4) the dose was selected based on previous research with trunk injection of similar pesticides [116]. Trees injected with water and the non-injected non-inoculated trees served as negative controls for efficacy comparisons. In year one, each treatment was replicated on four trees arranged in a randomized complete block design, where blocking controlled the variable crown tree sizes (large, medium, medium-small, and small) [117]. In the year two, we used the same number of replicate trees per treatment but arranged in a completely randomized design (CRD).

In year one, on 16 April at 80% bloom, apple flowers of all experimental trees were inoculated with a suspension of *E. amylovora* strain in distilled water using a hand-sprayer ($5.4 \times 10^6$ CFU/ml; CFU—colony forming units). In year two, on 14 May at 80% bloom, flowers were inoculated with *E. amylovora* ($0.7 \times 10^6$ CFU/ml). In year one, we evaluated blossom blight incidence 22, 29 May and 5 June, and in year two on 11, 18, and 25 June. Rating of blossom blight incidence consisted of random selection of flower clusters to form a 100-cluster sample per tree and calculating the percent of diseased and healthy blossom clusters in that sample. Shoot blight incidence was evaluated on 29 May and 5 June in year one and in year two on 11, 18, and 25 June. After randomly selecting enough shoots to form a sample of 100-shoots per tree, shoot blight incidence percent was calculated for each tree from the number of blighted and healthy shoots. Mean percent of blossom and shoot blight incidences for each treatment were calculated from the disease incidences on four replicate trees. For clarity, presented means consist of four replicate trees averaged across two or three time points i.e. dates listed above when fire blight incidences on flowers or shoots were rated.

We analyzed the data with MIXED procedure in SAS 9.3 (SAS Institute, 2012). The main effect of treatments on blossom and shoot blight incidence were analyzed using *F* test ($\alpha = 0.05$) and if found significant, pairwise treatment comparisons were done using *t*-tests ($\alpha = 0.05$). We presented the fire blight management results as percent of disease reduction, also known as percent disease control, calculated as: percent reduction of blossom or shoot blight incidence = [percent blossom or shoot blight incidence in water control – percent blossom or shoot blight incidence in specific treatment] × 100/percent blossom or shoot blight incidence in water control.

#### *2.2.3.2 Treatments for reducing shoot blight severity*

To test the reduction of shoot blight severity with bactericide oxytetracycline hydrochloride (Arborbiotic, MFG Scientific Inc., EPA Reg. No 88482-1; Arbor-OTC® Injectable Tree Antibiotic, Arborjet Inc., Reg No. 74578-7), apple trunk injections were performed in a similar fashion described above, but by using a Quik-jet® micro-injection system instead (Arborjet Inc., Woburn, MA, USA). This device relies solely on hand-generated hydraulic pressure to inject the necessary pesticide solution volume in each port. The injection ports were created and sealed with Arborplugs (Arborjet Inc.) in the same way as described above and injected volume per tree was divided equally among the four ports. The experiments were conducted in 2 years. In year one, at petal fall growth stage (23 April) mature 12-year-old apple trees of cv. 'Jonathan' were trunk-injected with Arborbiotic using dose in **Table 3** diluted at 10% in water. The total dose per tree was calculated based on the unique trunk diameters at 30 cm height using the EPA label instructions. In year two, the same apple trees injected in year one were re-injected at petal fall (22 May) using the same dose in **Table 3** delivered via a fresh set of drilled injection ports above the previous year's set of injection ports. In both years, Arborbiotic treatment as well as water control were replicated on four trees arranged in a CRD.

A total of 10 terminal shoots per each tree were inoculated on 7 May in year one and on 30 May in year two. We used a previously reported inoculation method [114]. In brief, the upper third of leaf blade of the second or the third youngest leaf on each shoot tip was cut perpendicular to the leaf midvein with scissors dipped in *E. amylovora* suspension (year one: $4.7 \times 10^7$ CFU/ml; year two: $5 \times 10^8$ CFU/ml). An additional 10 shoots per each tree were wounded with scissors dipped in distilled water and used as an in-per-tree negative control. When the disease started developing on inoculated shoots, the length of shoot blight lesion (necrosis) and the total shoot length was measured for each inoculated shoot and the shoot blight severity percent was calculated by comparing the ratio of necrotic lesion length and the total shoot length (cm). Only the total shoot length was measured for negative control shoots. The shoot necrosis lesions and total shoot lengths were measured at 7-day intervals after inoculation and were ceased when terminal bud set on shoots occurred (year one: 14, 21, and 28 May and 4, 11, and 18 June; year two: 10, 17, and

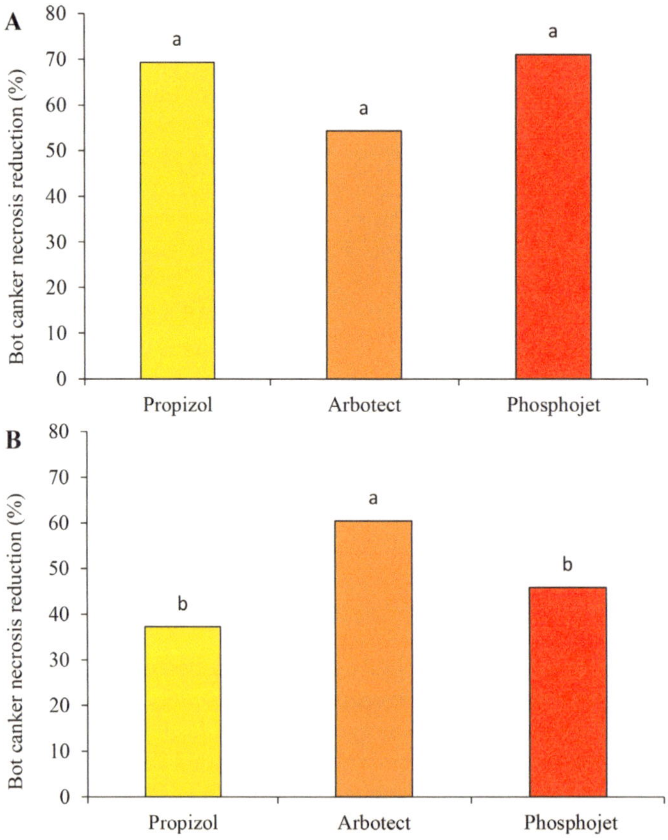


**Figure 1.**
*Percent reduction i.e. control of Bot canker necrosis area in trunk xylem in relation to water control on Quercus rubra trees in year one (A) and year two (B) achieved with trunk injections of fungicides Propizol (propiconazole), Arbotect (thiabendazole) and Phosphojet (potassium phosphites). Means followed by different letters are significantly different (A: $p < 0.1$, LSD test; B: $p < 0.05$, LSD test). In year one (A), the area of Bot canker necrosis in trunk xylem in water control was 5.15 $cm^2$ and in year two (B) 5.8 $cm^2$. Each mean consists of six replicate trees.*

24 June and 1, 8, and 15, 2013 July). The mean of shoot blight severity percent in per tree basis was calculated from the 10 shoot replicates. For each time point when the disease was rated, the average shoot blight severity was calculated from the four tree replicate means. For clarity, presented means consist of four replicate trees averaged across five or six time points i.e. dates listed above when fire blight severity on shoots was rated.

We analyzed the data using MIXED procedure in SAS 9.3 (SAS Institute, 2012). If the main effect of treatment on shoot blight severity was found significant (*F* test, $\alpha = 0.05$), comparison to water control was conducted using re *t*-tests ($\alpha = 0.05$). We presented the fire blight management results as percent of disease reduction, also known as percent disease control, calculated as: percent reduction of shoot blight severity = [percent shoot blight severity in water control – percent shoot blight severity in specific treatment] × 100/percent shoot blight severity in water control.

## 3. Results

### 3.1 Trunk injection of pesticides for *Diplodia corticola* management

All the three fungicides trunk-injected preventively provided significant reduction of Bot canker caused by *D. corticola* for 37.2–71.1% (**Figure 1**). Phosphojet at 1.5 ml per tree gave the best disease control when averaged across both years (58.5%) but caused phytotoxicity on four out of six tree replicates in year one and these trees died before the disease was rated. In year two, Phosphojet rate was reduced to 0.75 ml and this negative effect was not detected again. Averaged across both years, Arbotect provided the second-best control of 57.5%, followed by Propizol with 53.3% (**Figure 1**).

### 3.2 Trunk injection of pesticides for *Venturia inaequalis* management

In the experiment 1, fungicides injected four times in total, once in fall and then three additional times in spring, during the primary scab infection period, provided significant reduction of apple scab incidence on spur and shoot leaves (**Figure 2A**). On spur leaves, the best scab reduction of 45.5% was achieved with injected Phosphojet high, but this control was not better in comparison to 78.6% in spray standard applied in spring during the primary scab season (**Figure 2A**). In contrast, control with injected Phosphojet high on shoots outperformed the spray standard with 73.6 vs. 62.9% in scab reduction (**Figure 2A**). Similarly, Alamo performed better on shoot leaved than on spur leaves (**Figure 2A**).

In the experiment 2, fungicides injected 1–2 times in total, across or within two seasons of fall and spring, revealed that the injected Inspire Super treatments largely did not significantly reduce disease incidence on spur and shoot leaves when compared to the water control. In contrast, all the injected Phosphojet treatments and Agrifos sprays did. Comparisons among these treatments clearly demonstrated that on all the three rated apple organs (**Figure 2B**), Phosphojet trunk injections provided statistically better apple scab reduction i.e. control in comparison to all the Inspire Super trunk injections. On spur leaves, two Phosphojet trunk injections, fall plus spring, was the best treatment among injections by providing 46.3% control which was similar to the Inspire Super sprays (**Figure 2B**). On shoot leaves, two Phosphojet trunk injections both done in spring, provided the best scab control of 66.5% similar to nine sprays of Agrifos (**Figure 2B**). On fruit, scab control was the best in Phosphojet trunk injection done once or twice in spring, and in fall plus

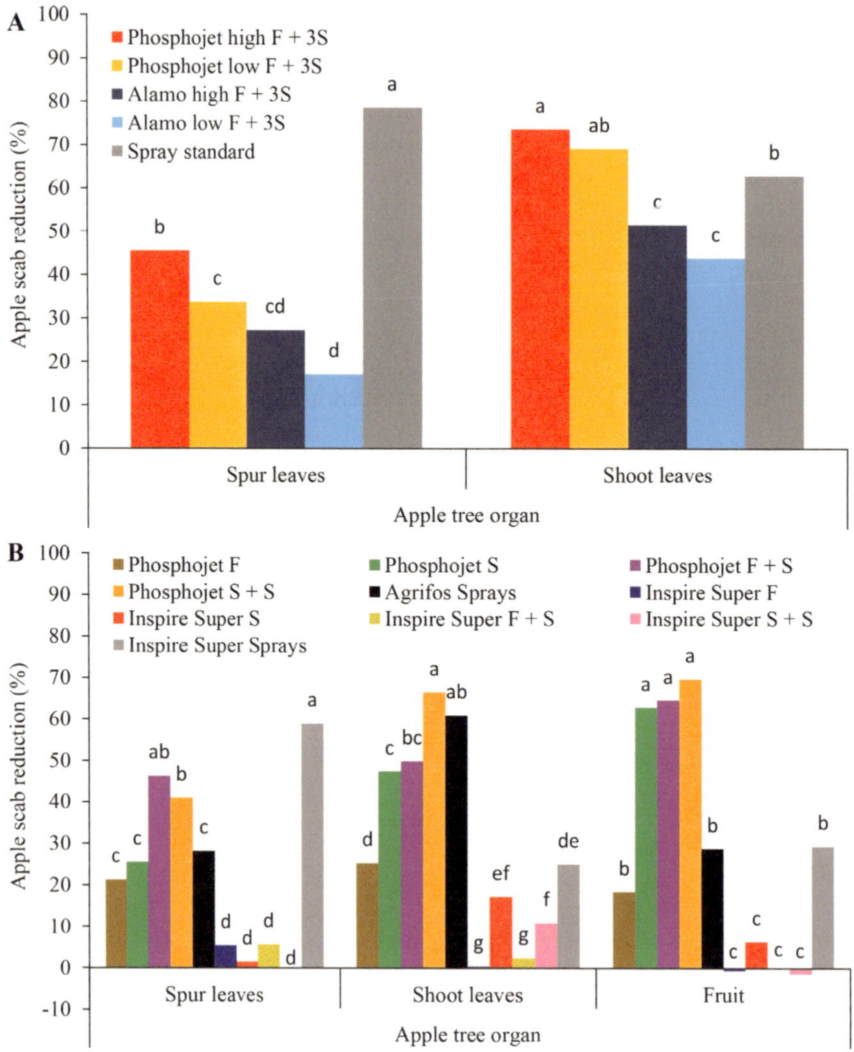


**Figure 2.**

*Percent reduction i.e. control of apple scab in relation to water control on 'Mac Spur' trees after in experiment 1 (A) and experiment 2 (B) achieved with trunk injections and sprays of potassium phosphites (Phosphojet, Arborfos) and of difenoconazole + cyprodinil (Inspire Super). Means within each graph section i.e. apple organ followed by different letters are significantly different (t-test, $p < 0.05$). F - one fall injection; 3S - three spring injections; S - one spring injection. In experiment 1 (A), scab incidences in water control on spur and shoot leaves were 72.2 and 54%. In experiment 2 (B) scab incidences in water control on spur leaves, shoot leaves and fruit were 88.3, 94.4 and 95.5%, respectively. Each mean consists of six replicate trees.*

spring: 62.8, 69.7 and 64.6%, significantly outperforming both the Agrifos and the Inspire Super sprays (**Figure 2B**).

## 3.3 Trunk injection of pesticides for *Erwinia amylovora* management

### *3.3.1 Treatments for reducing blossom and shoot blight incidence*

In both year one and year two, all the trunk-injected bactericides (Agrimycin) and SAR-activators (Actigard, Phosphojet) provided significant reduction of

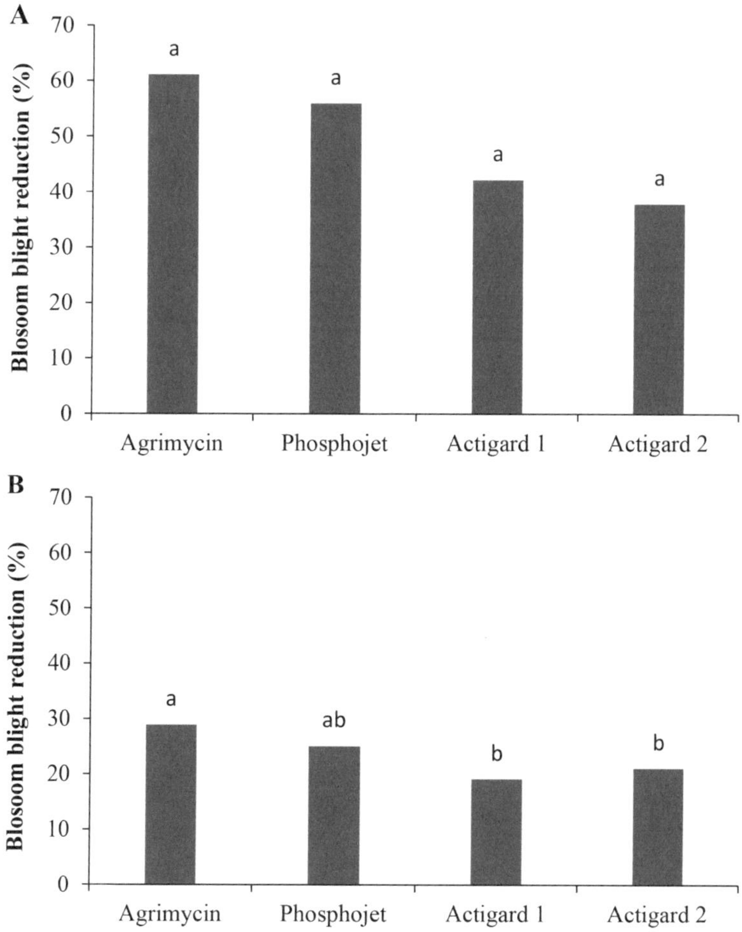


**Figure 3.**
*Percent reduction i.e. control of blossom blight incidence in relation to water control on 'Gala' apple trees in year one (A) and year two (B) achieved with one to two trunk injections of 'Gala' apple trees with Agrimycin (streptomycin), Phosphojet (potassium phosphites) and Actigard (acibenzolar-S-methyl). Means within each graph followed by different letters are significantly different (t-test, $p < 0.05$). Blossom blight incidence in water control in year one was 47.2% (A) and in year two 72.9% (B). Each mean consists of four replicate trees averaged across three time points when disease was rated.*

blossom blight incidence in comparison to the water control (**Figure 3**). In year one, which had low disease pressure (**Figure 3A**), there was no significant difference among all the treatments in disease reduction i.e. control (37.9–61.1%). In year two, with high infection pressure, Agrimycin was the best providing 28.9% blossom blight control (**Figure 3B**). Averaged across both years, Agrimycin and then Phosphojet were the best treatments with 45 and 40.5% achieved control, respectively (**Figure 3**).

In year one, none of the trunk-injected products provided significant reduction of shoot blight incidence in comparison to the water control, hence did not differ among each other (**Figure 4A**). In year two, under high disease pressure, all the injected products significantly reduced shoot blight incidence for 23.4–36.5% in comparison to the water control, but when compared they did not significantly differ between each other (**Figure 4B**). If averaged across both years, Agrimycin and then Phosphojet achieved the best control of 53.5 and 42.8%, respectively (**Figure 4**).

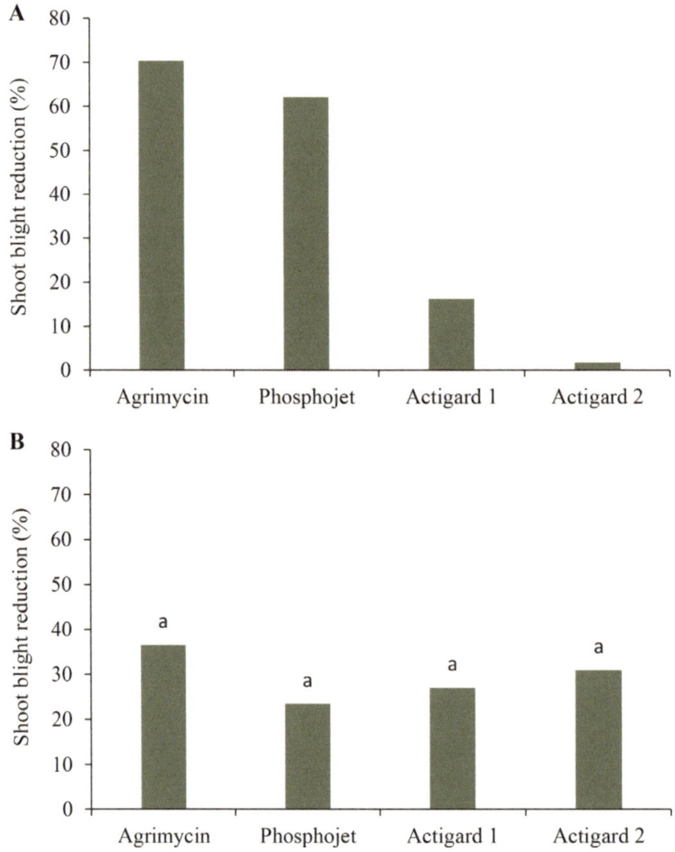


**Figure 4.**
*Percent reduction i.e. control of shoot blight incidence in relation to water control on 'Gala' apple trees in year one (A) and year two (B) achieved with one to two trunk injections of Agrimycin (streptomycin), Phosphojet (potassium phosphites) and Actigard (acibenzolar-S-methyl). (A) In year one, the injected treatments did not significantly reduce shoot blight incidence relative to water control. (B) Means followed by different letters are significantly different (t-test, $p < 0.05$). Soot blight incidence in water control in year one was 22.4% (A) and in year two 68.5% (B). Each mean consists of 4 replicate trees averaged across two time points in (A) and three time points in (B) when disease was rated.*

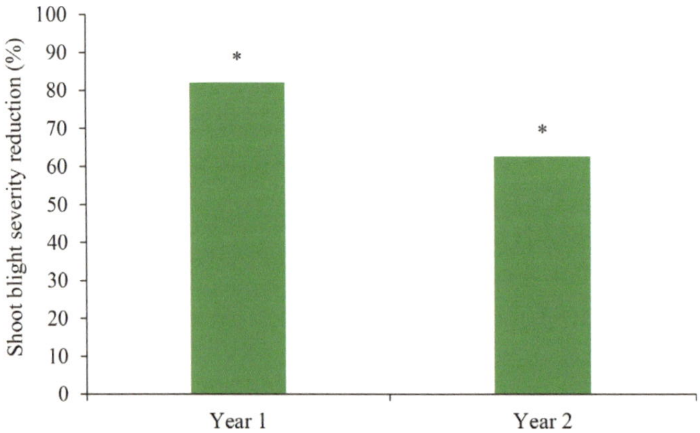


**Figure 5.**
*Percent reduction i.e. control of shoot blight severity relative to water control achieved from a single trunk injection of 'Jonathan' apple trees with Arborbiotic (oxytetracycline hydrochloride) in each year. Means with an asterisk indicate significant reduction of shoot blight severity (year one: Tukey's HSD test; year two: t-test, $p < 0.05$). Each mean consists of four replicate trees averaged across five time points in year 1 and six time points in year 2 when disease was rated.*

#### *3.3.2 Treatments for reducing shoot blight severity*

In both years Arborbiotic provided significant reduction i.e. control of shoot blight severity in comparison to the water control (**Figure 5**). When averaged across both years, the control of shoot blight severity reached 72.4% (**Figure 5**).

## 4. Discussion

### 4.1 *Diplodia corticola*

We present the first data on management of *D. corticola* on northern red oak using fungicides thiabendazole, propiconazole and potassium phosphites delivered by trunk injection as an alternative pesticide application method which offers selective exposure of this and other wood pathogens to the injected compounds. Since this fungus invades and spreads via tree xylem on different oak species as hardwood trees and causes necrosis and vascular occlusion [7, 8], ultimately killing the tree, trunk injection of fungicides seems as the most suitable fungicide delivery method for this pathogen's biology and likely more effective for managing the resulting Bot canker disease. The achieved levels in control of Bot canker in xylem ranged from 37.2 to 71.1% with an overall average of 56.4% across all the fungicides we trunk injected. Phosphojet provided control of 58.5%, but the most reliable fungicides and across-years consistent were Arbotect (thiabendazole) and Propizol (propiconazole) which achieved control of 57.5 and 53.3%. A higher efficacy was not achieved probably because of the short time between fungicide injection and inoculation with *D. corticola* which could have reduced the uniformity in distribution of these fungicides in xylem, thus hampering the efficacy. On the debarked cork oak trees and under moist conditions, the canker length caused by *D. corticola* is reduced for 25.8–98.5% by preventive spray applications of thiophanate-methyl and/or copper-calcium sulphate, delivered immediately after the cork peeling [20]. On average, across different test locations, Bot canker control in this study was 64.7% with thiophanate-methyl and/or copper-calcium sulphate [20].

The organic carbon-water partitioning coefficient ($K_{o/c}$) for thiabendazole is moderate to high and ranges from 1104 to 4680 ml/g, while water solubility is 50 mg/L at pH 7 and 38 mg/ml at pH 2 [118]. These parameters indicate on low to no mobility of thianbendazole in xylem as a carbon rich environment. The $K_{o/c}$ of propiconazole is 1086–1817 ml/g which is moderate to high [119, 120] and water solubility is low, 100–150 mg/L [121]. This could have contributed to slow and reduced uniformity in distribution of injected fungicides in xylem. However, both Arbotect and Propizol are fungicides formulated for trunk injection on hardwood trees and if properly diluted and delivered preventively they can accumulate sufficiently to secure the internal control of specific plant diseases (e.g. Dutch elm disease caused by *O. ulmi* and *O. novo-ulmi*; sycamore/London plane anthracnose caused by *Apiognomonia veneta*).

In the future studies, we predict that the efficacy of preventive fungicide applications against *D. corticola* via trunk injection delivery can be increased: (1) with more time allowed between injection and infection with *D. corticola*, (2) with more injections per season, and (3) a larger dose per tree. These factors should allow continued and better distribution of these fungicides in the wood xylem and canopy and probably secure the higher fungicide efficacy in Bot canker control, especially on larger trees.

### 4.2 *Venturia inaequalis*

We evaluated the similar fungicides on apple, *M. pumila*, another hardwood tree species. When Phosphojet and Inspire Super, where the latter one contains a DMI (demethylation inhibitor) fungicide difenoconazole from the same class as Alamo or Propizol (propiconazole), were trunk-injected for management of apple scab fungus *V. inaequalis*, the best control was achieved with Phosphojet and then by Alamo.

The efficacy against this subcuticular pathogen that infects just below the waxy layer on leaves and fruit, clearly depended on the apple canopy organ and the time/s of fungicide injection/s. Namely, on spurs which hold much fewer leaves in total in comparison to the shoots, the best leaf scab incidence reduction was 45.5 and 46.3%. In contrast, scab reduction on shoot leaves with Phosphojet reached 66.5 and 73.6%. On apple fruit, scab reduction reached up to 62.8, 64.6 and 69.7%. These efficacy patterns clearly demonstrate the differential influences of the tree's yearly and organ-specific physiology, the properties of injected compound, and the injection timing on the accumulation of fungicides in the canopy. Since the major water transport in xylem, occurs in spring, at least one to two injections of phosphites in early spring gave a good disease control, depending on the canopy organ. The best scab control with injected phosphites was achieved on the shoot leaves, followed by apple fruit, and then on the spur leaves. The injected phosphites probably accumulated more in the shoot leaves than in the spur leaves and they accumulate more in fruit than in spur leaves. This can be explained by the variable rates of transpiration from these organs, which influences the speed and abundance of fungicide accumulation after trunk injection. The total leaf area on shoots is larger in comparison to spurs. The fewer leaves on spurs, which are first to develop in spring and early reach their full size, have fewer total number of stomata on them in comparison to more numerous shoot leaves. Additionally, from petal fall up until terminal bud set, shoots keep growing and developing more leaves on the tips. Hence, apple shoots hold the higher number of stomata in total, thus allowing much higher transpiration intensity, abundant accumulation of injected fungicides and thus scab control. Similarly, apple scab control was lower on fruit than on shoots which could be explained by the fact that apple fruit hold 10- to 100-fold lower frequency of stomata on their epidermis in comparison to the apple leaves [122].

The chemical properties of different active ingredients impact their distribution and accumulation in the canopy. For example, potassium phosphites have higher water solubility of 500 g/L in comparison to propiconazole and difenoconazole which have low to very low water solubilities of 100–150 mg/L and 13 mg/L, respectively [121, 123]. Potassium phosphites have low organic carbon-water partitioning coefficient ($K_{o/c}$) from 228 to 587 ml/g in comparison to moderate to high of propiconazole, 1086–1817 ml/g, and of difenoconazole, 3870–11,202 ml/g, respectively [119, 120]. This difference likely allowed phosphites to move faster in xylem [124] and accumulate more in leaves and fruit than the other injected fungicides. At the same time, propiconazole and difenoconazole were probably bound to the organic phase of xylem symplast and apoplast, thus lowering their accumulation in leaves and fruit and reducing their effect on scab incidence [65]. This is often referred to as a reservoir effect and $K_{o/c}$ as is an important property of a pesticide that can explains its limited or abundant accumulation in the canopy [65, 125]. Besides the $K_{o/c}$ and water solubility, the inactive components of the Inspire Super pesticide formulation we injected (stickers, emulsifiers, surfactants, etc.) could reduce the abundant accumulation of difenoconazole and a better scab control. Fungicides have to be formulated for injection to secure their upward translocation in xylem and often diluted prior to trunk injection to reduce the impact of $K_{o/c}$ effect. Once the high solubility, low $K_{o/c}$

and injectable formulation are possible for one active ingredient, a rapid and desired control effect on plant pathogen or insect pest can be expected [42, 45, 126].

The reduction of apple scab and our prior work on analyzing the residues of injected pesticides on apple leaves and fruit [12, 61] indicates that accumulation of trunk-injected fungicides in the wood and canopy is a time-demanding process chiefly shaped by the tree physiology and tissue resistance points [127, 128]. Trunk injection is an opposite process to the immediate deposition of fungicide solution on the tree canopy by foliar spray applications. However, even though the injected dose per tree of phosphites in Phosphojet was 1.6–2 times higher than in the Agrifos sprays, the fact that just two injections secured better control of scab on fruit and spur leaves in comparison to nine Agrifos sprays demonstrated better persistence of injected Phosphojet. This shows that trunk injection is a superior delivery method for phosphites as it enhances their activity for 1–2 growing seasons [12].

### 4.3 *Erwinia amylovora*

The fire blight bacterium *E. amylovora* is a pathogen of apple trees with a unique and complicated biology involving several lifestyles: (1) *in planta* overwintering in fire blight cankers on bark or asymptomatically in host buds or as latent infections in asymptomatic wood [101], (2) residing on different plant surfaces and colonizing flower surfaces before their infection, and (3) migration after infection to other close or far host tissues and organs through colonizing the cortical parenchyma and xylem vessels. Therefore, it seems that for the stages of pathogen overwintering in wood or bark and especially for migration via xylem, the use of trunk injection delivery of compounds active against *E. amylovora* might be the most suitable way to control this pathogen. Overall, our trunk injection experiments with antibiotic bactericides, Phospojet and Actigard, both known SAR-activators [11], demonstrated good to poor fire blight incidence reduction in years with low and high infection pressures, respectively.

The best control i.e. reduction of blossom blight incidence across both trial years was achieved with two trunk injections of Agrimycin (45%) and of Phosphojet (40.5%). However, under high and low infection pressures in the two trial years, the levels of control with these materials (28.9, 61.1%, 25.1, 55.9) were far from comparable to 92–99% control often achieved and expected with preventive flower spray application of Agrimycin and Kasugamycin in commercial apple orchards [129, 130]. In the case of injected Phosphojet and Actigard, the achieved blossom blight reduction probably originated from an SAR effect triggered in the nearby spur leaves by these compounds, as the SAR effect in flowers was inconsistent [11]. SAR is a defense plant response which is activated after localized plant exposure to a pathogen or after a spray applications of a synthetic or natural compound, known as an SAR-inducer or activator [131]. Our 1–2 trunk injections of Actigard reduced blossom blight incidence for only 19–42%, indicating that this delivery method cannot not improve the SAR-effect of Actigard on flowers to combat blossom blight successfully. Namely, different sources report from 3 to 91% of blossom blight control with foliar sprays of Actigard on other apple cultivars [132–134].

Vegetative flowers parts in *Malus* species and later fruit have 10- to 100-fold lower frequency of stomata on epidermis when compared to the epidermis of leaves [122]. Flowers also have a considerably smaller green tissue volume. This leads to a conclusion that due to a very low transpiration footprint of green flower parts with lower number of stomata in comparison to the leaves and fruit, accumulation of injected compounds in these parts was weaker and slow thus reducing their efficacy. Second, it is possible that the injected antibiotics could not reach the surface of stigmas where *E. amylovora* multiplies to reduce its populations as successfully as after the topical spray application, or that they do reach stigma surfaces but at a too low of a dose or too late for a better reduction. The reached levels of control with the injected Agrimycin probably originated from the limited accumulation i.e. presence of a suboptimal dose of this antibiotic in the green flower tissues. This only partially stopped the progress of the infection once *E. amylovora* entered the flower tissues. Therefore, the injected compounds aiming to reduce blossom blight should be formulated to translocate and accumulate faster in flower green tissues to reach a potentially higher efficacy. Otherwise, these should be injected much earlier in comparison to our injection dates, probably in fall of the previous year, to increase the time for compound accumulation and ultimately improve the disease reduction. A process of optimizing the trunk injection timing/s is a common topic research on agricultural tree crops to maximize the effect in pathogen or pest control [10, 12, 50, 56]. It appears that higher dose of injected compounds might be necessary for longer-lasting control of fire blight on both flowers and shoots.

Even though reduction of shoot blight incidence was not statistically significant in year one, which was characterized with low infection pressure, it indicated that trunk-injected Agrimycin and Phosphojet might have potential to perform better than Actigard treatments. However, in year two, under the heavy infection pressure, this was not the case as all the injected treatments were similar. Overall, it seems that the reduction of shoot blight incidence with injected Agrimycin and Phosphojet across both years of 53.5 and 42.8%, was slightly better than the reduction of blossom blight incidence with the same materials of 45 and 40.5%, respectively. Shoots obviously have much higher green tissue area and transpiration rate in comparison to the flowers. Shoots likely accumulate higher amounts of trunk injected compounds in comparison to the green flower parts, which allowed slightly better disease reduction early after injection. Still, the shoot blight incidence reduction was far from the expected control with spray applied antibiotics in commercial apple orchards. In a trial with trunk injection of Arborfos (45.8% mono- and di-potassium salts of phosphorous acid, Mauget Inc., Arcadia, CA, USA), shoot blight was reduced for 67% on inoculated 'Paulared' apple trees [116]. The same dose per tree which we delivered in two injections of Phosphojet, achieved shoot blight incidence reduction of 23.4–62.1%. Since we have split the dose delivery temporally, this weakened shoot blight incidence reduction by Phosphojet and probably by Actigard too. In shoot inoculated trials multiple Actigard sprays achieved shoot blight reduction between 2.8 and 50.7% [135, 136] while by trunk injection we achieved only 1.7–30.9% of shoot blight reduction. Hence, the two-time trunk injection does not improve shoot blight reduction by Actigard.

The reduction of shoot blight severity with Arborbiotic (MFG Scientific Inc., USA) was excellent and reached up to 82%. Such an effect with oxytetracycline hydrochloride demonstrates that this active ingredient is readily soluble in water and that the formulation we used is designed for trunk injection. Our results indicated that the trunk injected Arborbiotic limits i.e. stops systemic spread of *E. amylovora* in xylem of apple shoots [11]. Even though oxytetracycline hydrochloride is a bacteriostatic, when we delivered it via trunk injection in apple trees only one time per year, it demonstrated prolonged effectiveness that was higher in comparison to spray applications [44, 137, 138]. Trunk injection delivery enhanced the efficacy of oxytetracycline hydrochloride in control of shoot blight severity. Finally, in our prior work we also showed that the injected Arborbiotic at a dose of 0.31 g + 2.52 ml water per each 2.5 cm of trunk diameter at 30.5 cm height, can achieve a formidable reduction of blossom and shoot blight incidence for 60.6 and 60.7%, respectively [44]. This indicates that this bactericide in this formulation and probably at a slightly higher dose is the best candidate to achieve satisfactory accumulation inside and deposition on the susceptible apple plant tissues and surfaces to secure the higher efficacy.

## 5. Conclusion

Our results on management of three different pathogens with partially similar or different biologies, where *D. corticola* and *E. amylovora* invade and spread in xylem while *V. inaequalis* does not and infects subcuticularly, indicate that trunk injection of pesticides that are formulated for xylem translocation can be more-less similar in control of these three pathogens. However, the interaction of chemical properties of the active ingredient, the injected dose per tree, as well as the transpiration footprint of plant organs, played the key roles that determined the achieved levels of efficacy.

In the biology i.e. life cycle of *D. corticola*, it seems that the dominant phase is the invasion and necrosis of xylem, leading to vascular occlusion, canopy wilting and canker development on wood before it kills oak trees. Hence the logical approach to prevent this disease is trunk injection delivery of fungicides. In our two-year experiments on potted trees, the injected potassium phosphites (Phosphojet) achieved levels of Bot canker control in xylem of up to 71.1%. Averaged across both years, potassium phosphites achieved disease reduction of 58.5%, but the more consistent results were achieved with fungicides thiabendazole (Arbotect) and propiconazole (Propizol) which reduced xylem necrosis for 57.5 and 53.3% on average. The maximums in reduction in individual years for these two fungicides were of 60.5 and 69.3%, respectively. We predict that higher efficacy with these fungicides can be achieved with optimization of preventive fungicide injection which would increase the uniformity of distribution of these fungicides in xylem, thus increasing their efficacy.

In the case of *V. inaequalis*, for which the injected fungicides would need to translocate the farthest via xylem to reach and accumulate in and on the epidermal cells of green plant surfaces in tree canopy, the most efficient apple scab reduction of 45.5–73.6% was achieved with potassium phosphites (Phosphojet). Unlike this readily mobile compound, scab control with propiconazole that is much less xylem mobile ranged from 17.1 to 51.5%, while the least xylem mobile difenoconazole underperformed with only up to 10.8% apple scab control. It is assumed that the injected potassium phosphites secured its efficacy against *V. inaequalis* through a strong plant defense response in the tissues called SAR [11, 139], as apparently it is not directly toxic to this pathogen [140]. We speculate that better efficacy with other systemic fungicides active against apple scab might be achieved if their formulations were re-designed for trunk injection i.e. to facilitate easier and faster translocation in xylem, thus securing higher accumulation in tissues exposed to infection.

Finally, there is the case of a complex biology of *E. amylovora* which combines life stages of inhabiting and multiplying on plant surfaces, migrating through internal host tissues after infecting, dwelling and overwintering asymptomatically in host buds or wood, and overwintering in fire blight cankers on bark. The injected compounds active against this pathogen would need to translocate and distribute in in xylem and phloem, reach in and onto the stigma surfaces of flowers and accumulate at effective doses in these and green tissues of the apple tree canopy. Based on presented research, it seems that these multiple difficult tasks in this and our previous study [44] were best achieved with oxytetracycline hydrochloride—both on the apple flowers [44] and on shoots [11]. Overall the injected antibiotic streptomycin (Agrimycin) formulated for foliar application gave the best reduction of blossom blight ranging from 28.9 to 61.1% and of shoot blight from 36.5 to 70.4%. The shoot blight severity reduction with Arboriotic, the injectable formulation of oxytetracycline hydrochloride, reached an excellent 82%. Hence, the effect depended on the plant organ, bactericide active ingredient, injected dose and formulation. The SAR-activating potassium phosphites (Phosphojet) were the second best to antibiotics with 25.1 and 55.9% of blossom blight reduction and 23.4 and

62.1% of shoot blight reduction. Actigard underperformed with blossom blight reduction of 19 and 42% and shoot blight reduction of only 1.7 and 30.9%.

## Acknowledgements

The work on *Diplodia corticola* was funded by the USDA-APHIS PPQ grant awards USDA-APHIS-10025-PPQS&T00-18-0155 to DKHM and USDA-APHIS-18PPQS&T00-C11-0SGA to SGA for the project "Evaluation of the origin, epidemiology, and fungicide use in controlling *Diplodia corticola*, a new pathogen of red oak." We thank Peter Jentsch, Director of Cornell University's Hudson Valley Research Laboratory in Highland NY for supporting this research with injection equipment.

The work on *Venturia inaequalis* was supported by the grant awards to JCW by the Michigan Apple Research Committee for the project "Trunk Injection of Fungicides and Bio-pesticides for Apple Scab Control" and the IR-4 Project "Enhancing Performance of Phosphorous Acid Salts for Apple Scab Management through Trunk Injection Delivery."

The fire blight work was funded by USDA-NIFA Pest Management Alternatives grant MICL05066 in 2012 and continuation grant MICL07748 in 2013–2014 to JCW for project "Trunk Injection: A Discriminating Delivery System for Tree Fruit IPM". The work with evaluating Arborbiotic in reduction of fire blight severity was funded by Arborjet Inc., Woburn, MA, USA.

We thank Joseph J. Doccola, director of research and development at Arborjet Inc. and John J. Aiken, regional technical manager, for donating injection equipment and chemicals used in apple scab and fire blight experiments. For assistance in conducting or facilitating experiments, we thank research staff of at Michigan State University's Trevor Nichols Research Center (TNRC) in Fennville, MI, Anthony VanWoerkom, Gail Ehret, Jerri Gillett, Jason Seward, Laura Lamb and Kyle Coffindaffer. We acknowledge Dr. Annemiek Schilder, Dr. Brad Day, Dr. Jianjun Hao, Dr. Jim Miller and Dr. Randolph Beaudry for generously sharing their laboratory resources at Michigan State University in support of this research.

## Conflict of interest

All authors declare that the research was conducted without any commercial or financial relationships that could be interpreted as a potential conflict of interest.

## Author details

Srđan G. Aćimović[1]*, Danielle K.H. Martin[2], Richard M. Turcotte[2], Christopher L. Meredith[1] and Isabel A. Munck[3]

1 Plant Pathology and Plant Microbe Biology Section, Cornell University, Hudson Valley Research Laboratory, Highland, New York, USA

2 USDA Forest Service, Forest Health Protection, Northeastern Area State and Private Forestry, Morgantown, West Virginia, USA

3 USDA Forest Service, Northeastern Area State and Private Forestry, Durham, New Hampshire, USA

*Address all correspondence to: acimovic@cornell.edu

## References


[1] McDonald V, Lynch S, Eskalen A. First report of *Neofusicoccum australe, N. luteum, and N. parvum* associated with avocado branch canker in California. Plant Disease. 2009;**93**:967-967

[2] Lynch SC, Eskalen A, Zambino P, et al. First report of bot canker caused by *Diplodia corticola* on coast live oak (*Quercus agrifolia*) in California. Plant Disease. 2010;**94**:1510-1510

[3] Dreaden TJ, Shin K, Smith JA. First report of *Diplodia corticola* causing branch cankers on live oak (*Quercus* virginiana) in Florida. Plant Disease. 2011;**95**:1027-1027

[4] Eskalen A. First report of a *Fusarium sp*. and its vector tea shot hole borer (*Euwallacea fornicatus*) causing Fusarium dieback on avocado in California. Plant Disease. 2012;**96**:1070

[5] Aćimović SG, Harmon CL, Bec S, et al. First report of *Diplodia corticola* causing decline of red oak (*Quercus* rubra) trees in Maine. Plant Disease. 2015;**100**:649. DOI: 10.1094/PDIS-09-15-0994-PDN

[6] Munck IA, Livingston W, Lombard K, et al. Extent and severity of Caliciopsis canker in New England, USA: An emerging disease of eastern white pine (*Pinus strobus* L.). Forests. 2015;**6**:4360-4373

[7] Munck IA, Wyka SA, Bohne MJ, et al. First report of *Diplodia corticola* causing bleeding cankers on black oak (*Quercus velutina*). Plant Disease. 2016;**101**:257

[8] Martin DKH, Turcotte RM, Miller TM, et al. First report of *Diplodia corticola* causing stem cankers and associated vascular occlusion of northern red oak (*Quercus rubra*) in West Virginia. Plant Disease. 2017;**101**:380

[9] Aćimović SG, Rooney-Latham S, Albu S, et al. Characterization and pathogenicity of Botryosphaeriaceae Fungi associated with declining urban stands of coast redwood in California. Plant Disease. 2018;**102**:1950-1957. DOI: 10.1094/PDIS-02-18-0339-RE

[10] VanWoerkom AH, Aćimović SG, Sundin GW, et al. Trunk injection: An alternative technique for pesticide delivery in apples. Crop Protection. 2014;**65**:173-185. DOI: 10.1016/j.cropro.2014.05.017

[11] Aćimović SG, Zeng Q, Mcghee GC, et al. Control of fire blight (*Erwinia amylovora*) on apple trees with trunk-injected plant resistance inducers and antibiotics and assessment of induction of pathogenesis-related protein genes. Frontiers in Plant Science. 2015;**6**:16. DOI: 10.3389/fpls.2015.00016

[12] Aćimović SG, VanWoerkom AH, Garavaglia T, et al. Seasonal and cross-seasonal timing of fungicide trunk injections in apple trees to optimize management of apple scab. Plant Disease. 2016;**100**:1606-1616. DOI: 10.1094/PDIS-09-15-1061-RE

[13] Wyka SA, Doccola JJ, Strom BL, et al. Effects of *Grosmannia clavigera* and *Leptographium longiclavatum* on Western white pine seedlings and the fungicidal activity of Alamo®, Arbotect®, and TREE-age®. Arboriculture & Urban Forestry. 2016;**42**:84-94

[14] Hu J, Wang N. Evaluation of the spatiotemporal dynamics of oxytetracycline and its control effect against citrus huanglongbing via trunk injection. Phytopathology. Epub ahead of print 2 August 2016. DOI: 10.1094/PHYTO-02-16-0114-R

[15] Hu J, Jiang J, Wang N. Control of citrus Huanglongbing via trunk injection of plant defense activators and antibiotics. Phytopathology. 2017;**108**:186-195

[16] Li J, Li L, Pang Z, et al. Developing citrus Huanglongbing (HLB) management strategies based on the severity of symptoms in HLB-endemic citrus-producing regions. Phytopathology. 2018;**109**:582-592

[17] Longstroth M. The fire blight epidemic in Southwest Michigan. Compact Fruit Tree. 2001;**34**:16-19

[18] Fatmi M, Yaich M, Bougsiba M, et al. Fire blight (*Erwinia amylovora* [Burrill] Winslow) in Morocco: Importance, geographical distribution and characterization. Phytopathologia Mediterranea. 2011;**50**:212-227

[19] Neupane D, Moss CB, van Bruggen AH, Ariena HC. Estimating Citrus Production Loss Due to Citrus Huanglongbing in Florida. 2016; Proceedings of Southern Agricultural Economics Association (SAEA) Annual Meeting, San Antonio, Texas, February, 6-9, 2016

[20] Serrano MS, Romero MA, Jiménez JJ, et al. Preventive control of Botryosphaeria canker affecting *Quercus suber* in southern Spain. Forestry: An International Journal of Forest Research. 2015;**88**:500-507

[21] Costa JC, Martín A, Fernández R, et al. Dehesas de Andalucía: Caracterización ambiental. Cons Medio Ambiente Junta Andal. Sevilla: A.G. Novograf, S.L. ISBN: 84-96329-81-X

[22] Rosner H. Pine beetle epidemic—The bug That's eating the woods. National Geographic. April 2015;**227**:96-115. https://www.nationalgeographic.com/magazine/2015/04/pine-beetles-forest-destruction-canada-rockies/ [Accessed: 01 July 2019]

[23] Sutton TB, Aldwinckle HS, Agnello AM, et al. Compendium of Apple and Pear Diseases and Pests. 2nd ed. St. Paul MN: Am Phytopath Society; 2014

[24] MacHardy WE. Apple Scab: Biology, Epidemiology, and Management. St. Paul MN: American Phytopathological Society (APS Press); 1996

[25] Linaldeddu BT, Sirca C, Spano D, et al. Physiological responses of cork oak and holm oak to infection by fungal pathogens involved in oak decline. Forest Pathology. 2009;**39**:232-238

[26] Moricca S, Linaldeddu BT, Ginetti B, et al. Endemic and emerging pathogens threatening Cork oak trees: Management options for conserving a unique Forest ecosystem. Plant Disease. 2016;**100**:2184-2193

[27] Úrbez-Torres JR, Peduto F, Rooney-Latham S, et al. First report of *Diplodia corticola* causing grapevine (Vitis vinifera) cankers and trunk cankers and dieback of canyon live oak (*Quercus chrysolepis*) in California. Plant Disease. 2010;**94**:785-785

[28] Reed SE, English JT, Lalk SR, et al. First report of *Diplodia corticola* causing stem and branch cankers on white oak (*Quercus alba*) in Missouri, U.S.A. Plant Disease. 2018;**102**:2657

[29] Smith DR, Stanosz GR. Occurrence of *Diplodia corticola*, including new oak host records, in Wisconsin, USA. Forest Pathology. 2018;**48**:e12427

[30] Chen SF, Morgan DP, Michailides TJ. Botryosphaeriaceae and Diaporthaceae associated with panicle and shoot blight of pistachio in California, USA. Fungal Diversity. 2014; **67**:157-179

[31] Moral J, Muñoz-Díez C, González N, et al. Characterization and pathogenicity of Botryosphaeriaceae species collected from olive and other hosts in Spain and California. Phytopathology. 2010;**100**: 1340-1351

[32] Moral J, Ahimera N, Felts DG, et al. Effects of wound size, amount of sap,

and number of blighted nuts on infection of pistachio organs by *Neofusicoccum mediterraneum*. Plant Disease. 2017;**101**:2027-2033

[33] Úrbez-Torres JR, Peduto F, Gubler WD. First report of grapevine cankers caused by *Lasiodiplodia crassispora* and *Neofusicoccum mediterraneum* in California. Plant Disease. 2010;**94**:785-785

[34] Ono H. The mountain pine beetle: Scope of the problem and key issues in Alberta. In: Mountain Pine Beetle Symposium: Challenges and Solutions. Natural Resources Canada, Canadian Forest Service, Information Report BC-X-399; Kelowna, British Columbia. 2003. pp. 62-66

[35] Carroll AL, Taylor SW, Régnière J, et al. Effect of climate change on range expansion by the mountain pine beetle in British Columbia. In: Shore TL et al., editor Mountain Pine Beetle Symposium: Challenges and Solutions; Oct. 30-31, 2003; Kelowna BC. Victoria: Natural Resources Canada, Infromation Report BC-X-399; 2003. pp. 223-232

[36] Douglas SM. Fire blight. Conn Agric Exp Stn PP0299 503R. 2006;**5**:1-8

[37] Norelli JL, Jones AL, Aldwinckle HS. Fire blight management in the twenty-first century: Using new technologies that enhance host resistance in apple. Plant Disease. 2003;**87**:756-765

[38] Gottwald TR, Graham JH, Schubert TS. Citrus canker: The pathogen and its impact. Plant Health Progress. 2002;**3**:15

[39] Park DH, Lee Y-G, Kim J-S, et al. Current status of fire blight caused by *Erwinia amylovora* and action for its management in Korea. Journal of Plant Pathology. 2017;**99**:59-63

[40] Fatmi M, Cox KD. Chapter 40: Detection of *Erwinia amylovora* in asymptomatic budwood of pear, apple, and quince. In: Detection of Plant-Pathogenic Bacteria in Seed and Other Planting Material. 2nd ed. St. Paul, MN: The American Phytopathological Society. pp. 295-301

[41] Fleancu M. Diurnal and seasonal changes in the transpiration rate of apple trees. Annals of the University of Oradea, Fascicula Biologie. 2005;**XII**: 147-157

[42] Doccola JJ, Wild PM. Tree injection as an alternative method of insecticide application. In: Soloneski S, Larramendy M, editors. Insecticides—Basic and Other Applications. Croatia: InTech; 2012. pp. 61-78

[43] Aćimović SG, Cregg BM, Sundin GW, et al. Comparison of drill- and needle-based tree injection technologies in healing of trunk injection ports on apple trees. Urban Forestry & Urban Greening. 2016;**19**:151-157. DOI: 10.1016/j.ufug.2016.07.003

[44] Aćimović SG, Mcghee GC, Sundin GW, et al. Evaluation of trunk-injected bactericides and prohexadione-calcium for environmentally friendly control of fire blight (*Erwinia amylovora*) in apples. In: Proceedings of the 7th Congress on Plant Protection. Zlatibor, Serbia: Plant Protection Society of Serbia & International Organization for Biological Control EPRS and WPRS; 2015. pp. 129-134

[45] Montecchio L. A venturi effect can help cure our trees. Journal of Visualized Experiments. Epub ahead of print 1 October 2013. DOI: 10.3791/51199

[46] Montecchio L. Bite—Blade for Infusion of Trees, International Patent by University of Padova, Italy. Padova, Italy: 2011

[47] Dal Maso E, Cocking J, Montecchio L. Efficacy tests on commercial fungicides against ash dieback in vitro and by trunk injection. Urban Forestry

& Urban Greening. 2014;**13**:697-703. DOI: 10.1016/j.ufug.2014.07.005

[48] Smitley DR, Doccola JJ, Cox DL. Multiple-year protection of ash trees from emerald ash borer with a single trunk injection of emamectin benzoate, and single-year protection with an imidacloprid basal drench. Journal of Arboriculture. 2010;**36**:206

[49] Byrne FJ, Urena AA, Robinson LJ, et al. Evaluation of neonicotinoid, organophosphate and avermectin trunk injections for the management of avocado thrips in California avocado groves. Pest Management Science. 2012; **68**:811-817

[50] Byrne FJ, Krieger RI, Doccola J, et al. Seasonal timing of neonicotinoid and organophosphate trunk injections to optimize the management of avocado thrips in California avocado groves. Crop Protection. 2014;**57**:20-26

[51] Castle SJ, Byrne FJ, Bi JL, et al. Spatial and temporal distribution of imidacloprid and thiamethoxam in citrus and impact on *Homalodisca coagulata* populations. Pest Management Science. 2005;**61**:75-84

[52] Coslor CC, Sundin GW, Wise JC. The efficacy of trunk injections of emamectin benzoate and phosphorous acid for control of obliquebanded leafroller and apple scab on semi-dwarf apple. Crop Protection. 2019;**118**:44-49

[53] Düker A, Kubiak R. Stem application of metalaxyl for the protection of *Vitis vinifera* L. ('Riesling') leaves and grapes against downy mildew (*Plasmopara viticola*). Vitis. 2009;**48**: 43-48

[54] Düker A, Kubiak R. Stem injection of triazoles for the protection of '*Vitis vinifera*'L. ('Riesling') against powdery mildew ('*Uncinula necator*'). VITIS— Journal of Grapevine Research. 2011;**50**: 73-79

[55] Jamar L, Cavelier M, Lateur M. Primary scab control using a "during-infection" spray timing and the effect on fruit quality and yield in organic apple production. Biotechnology, Agronomy, Society and Environment. 2010;**14**:423-439

[56] Wise JC, VanWoerkom AH, Aćimović SG, et al. Trunk injection: A discriminating delivering system for horticulture crop IPM. Entomology, Ornithology and Herpetology. 2014;**3**: 126. DOI: 10.4172/2161-0983.1000126

[57] Coslor CC. Refining Trunk Injection Strategies for Control of Foliar Insect Pests and Disease in Michigan Apple Orchards. PhD thesis. Michigan State University. Entomology, East Lansing, MI 48824, USA. 2017

[58] Coslor CC, Vandervoort C, Wise JC. Control of insect pests using trunk injection in a newly established apple orchard. International Journal of Fruit Science. 2018;**0**:1-14

[59] Coslor CC, Vandervoort C, Wise JC. Insecticide dose and seasonal timing of trunk injection in apples influence efficacy and residues in nectar and plant parts. Pest Management Science. 2019; **75**:1453-1463

[60] VanWoerkom AH. Trunk injection: A new and innovative technique for pesticide delivery in tree fruits [thesis]. East Lansing: Michigan State University; 2012

[61] Aćimović SG, VanWoerkom AH, Reeb PD, et al. Spatial and temporal distribution of trunk-injected imidacloprid in apple tree canopies. Pest Management Science. 2014;**70**:1751-1760. DOI: 10.1002/ps.3747

[62] Carisse O, Jobin T, McFadden-Smith W, Meloche C, Lasnier J. Apple scab: Improving understanding for better management. Agriculture and

Agri-Food Canada, 2006; ISBN 0-662-44584-8. pp. 1-22

[63] Doccola JJ, Bristol EJ, Sifleet SD, et al. Efficacy and duration of trunk-injected imidacloprid in the management of hemlock woolly adelgid (*Adelges tsugae*). Arboriculture & Urban Forestry. 2007;**33**:12-21

[64] Doccola JJ, Cruz BI, Wild PM, et al. A New Strategy to Control Hemlock Woolly Adelgid (Adelges tsugae Annand) Using Imidacloprid and an Arboricultural Method to Gauge Hemlock Health. 2008. Proceedings from Fourth symposium on Hemlock Woolly Adelgid in the Eastern United States, USDA Forest Service, West Virginia, Hartford, CT, February 12-14, 2008. pp. 101-110

[65] Doccola JJ, Hascher W, Aiken JJ, et al. Treatment strategies using Imidacloprid in hemlock woolly Adelgid (*Adelges tsugae* Annand) infested eastern hemlock (*Tsuga canadensis* Carrière) trees. Arboriculture & Urban Forestry. 2012;**38**:41-49

[66] McVay J, Sun X, Jones D, et al. Limited persistence of residues and metabolites in fruit and juice following penicillin trunk infusion in citrus affected by Huanglongbing. Crop Protection. Epub ahead of print 20 March 2019. DOI: 10.1016/j.cropro.2019.03.001

[67] Shin K, Ascunce MS, Narouei-Khandan HA, et al. Effects and side effects of penicillin injection in huanglongbing affected grapefruit trees. Crop Protection. 2016;**90**:106-116

[68] Zhang M, Yang C, Powell CA, et al. Field evaluation of integrated management for mitigating citrus Huanglongbing in Florida. Frontiers in Plant Science. 2019:**9**:1890. DOI: 10.3389/fpls.2018.01890

[69] Alves A, Correia A, Luque J, et al. *Botryosphaeria corticola*, sp. nov. on *Quercus* species, with notes and description of *Botryosphaeria stevensii* and its anamorph, *Diplodia mutila*. Mycologia. 2004;**96**:598-613

[70] Bérubé JA, Gagné PN, Ponchart JP, et al. Detection of *Diplodia corticola* spores in Ontario and Québec based on highthroughput sequencing (HTS) methods. Canadian Journal of Plant Pathology. 2018;**40**:378-386

[71] Linaldeddu BT, Maddau L, Franceschini A. Nuove acquisizioni su aspetti epidemiologici del patosistema *Quercus suber*/*Botryosphaeria corticola* in Sardegna. Micologia Italiana. 2010;**39**: 49-57

[72] Inácio ML, Henriques J, Guerra-Guimarães L, et al. Platypus cylindrus Fab. (Coleoptera: Platypodidae) transports *Biscogniauxia mediterranea*, agent of cork oak charcoal canker. Boletin de Sanidad Vegetal Plagas. 2011; **37**:181-186

[73] Kostovcik M, Bateman CC, Kolarik M, et al. The ambrosia symbiosis is specific in some species and promiscuous in others: Evidence from community pyrosequencing. The ISME Journal. 2015;**9**:126-138

[74] Ma Z, Morgan DP, Michailides TJ. Effects of water stress on Botryosphaeria blight of pistachio caused by *Botryosphaeria dothidea*. Plant Disease. 2001;**85**:745-749

[75] Huang Y, Meng L, Liu J, et al. First report of *Botryosphaeria dothidea* causing shoot canker on mulberry in China. Plant Disease. 2019;**103**:1788. DOI: 10.1094/PDIS-01-19-0183-PDN

[76] De Wet J, Burgess T, Slippers B, et al. Multiple gene genealogies and microsatellite markers reflect relationships between morphotypes of *Sphaeropsis sapinea* and distinguish a new species of *Diplodia*. Mycological Research. 2003;**107**:557-566

[77] Schoeneweiss DF. The role of environmental stress in diseases of woody plants. Plant Disease. 1981;**65**: 308-314

[78] Schoeneweiss DF. A method for controlling plant water potentials for studies on the influence of water stress on disease susceptibility. Canadian Journal of Botany. 1975;**53**:647-652

[79] Wene EG, Schoeneweiss DF. Localized freezing predisposition to Botryosphaeria canker in differentially frozen woody stems. Canadian Journal of Botany. 1980;**58**:1455-1458

[80] Flowers J, Nuckles E, Hartman J, et al. Latent infection of Austrian and scots pine tissues by *Sphaeropsis sapinea*. Plant Disease. 2001;**85**:1107-1112

[81] Flowers J, Hartman J, Vaillancourt L. Detection of latent *Sphaeropsis sapinea* infections in Austrian pine tissues using nested-polymerase chain reaction. Phytopathology. 2003;**93**: 1471-1477

[82] Ivanović MS, Ivanović DM. Mikoze i pseudomikoze biljaka. 2nd ed. Belgrade, Serbia: Poljoprivredni Fakultet, Univerziet u Beogradu, De-eM-Ve, Beograd; 2001

[83] Nichols LP, Petersen DH. Overwintering of *Fusicladium dendriticum*, the imperfect stage of the apple scab fungus, on twigs of flowering crab apples. Plant Disease Report. 1971; **55**:509

[84] Holb IJ, Heijne B, Jeger MJ. Overwintering of conidia of *Venturia inaequalis* and the contribution to early epidemics of apple scab. Plant Disease. 2004;**88**:751-757

[85] Stensvand A, Amundsen T, Semb L, et al. Discharge and dissemination of Ascospores by *Venturia inaequalis* during dew. Plant Disease. 1998;**82**: 761-764

[86] Aylor DE, Anagnostakis SL. Active discharge distance of ascospores of *Venturia inaequalis*. Phytopathology. 1991;**81**:548-551

[87] Holb IJ, Heijne B, Withagen JCM, et al. Dispersal of *Venturia inaequalis* Ascospores and disease gradients from a defined inoculum source. Journal of Phytopathology. 2004;**152**:639-646

[88] González-Domínguez E, Armengol J, Rossi V. Biology and epidemiology of *Venturia* species affecting fruit crops: A review. Frontiers in Plant Science. 2017; **8**:1496. DOI: 10.3389/fpls.2017.01496

[89] Beresford RM, Henshall WR, Palmer JW. A new apple scab risk model that integrates ascospore release, infection risk and susceptible leaf area. New Zealand Plant Protection. 2004;**57**:20

[90] Trapman M, Polfliet M. Management of primary infections of apple-scab with the simulation program RIMpro: Review of four years field trials. IOBC WPRS Bulletin. 1997;**20**: 241-250

[91] Philion V, Mattedi L, Comai M, et al. Validation of the apple scab simulator Rimpro using potted trees. In: Cornell University, editor. Proceedings of the International Epidemiology Congress IE10. Geneva, NY; 2009

[92] Aćimović SG, Wallis AE, Basedow M. Two years of experience with RIMpro apple scab prediction model on commercial apple farms in eastern New York. Fruit Quarterly. 2018;**26**:21-27

[93] Winslow C-EA, Broadhurst J, Buchanan RE, et al. The families and genera of the bacteria final report of the Committee of the Society of American bacteriologists on characterization and classification of bacterial types. Journal of Bacteriology. 1920;**5**:191-229

[94] Paulin J-P. *Erwinia amylovora*: General Characteristics, Biochemistry

and Serology. Wallingfod: Fire Blight CABI Publ; 2000. pp. 87-115

[95] Slack SM, Zeng Q, Outwater CA, et al. Microbiological examination of *Erwinia amylovora* exopolysaccharide ooze. Phytopathology. 2017;**107**:403-411

[96] Boucher M, Cox K, Loeb G. Establishing a Role for Flies in the Disease Cycle of Fire Blight (*Erwinia amylovora*). Fruit Quarterly. **27**:19-22

[97] Hildebrand EM. Studies on fire blight ooze. Phytopathology. 1939;**29**: 142-156

[98] Billing E, LAE B, Crosse JE, et al. Characteristics of English isolates of *Erwinia amylovora* (Burrill) Winslow et al. The Journal of Applied Bacteriology. 1961;**24**:195-211

[99] Bereswill S, Jock S, Bellemann P, et al. Identification of *Erwinia amylovora* by growth morphology on agar containing copper sulfate and by capsule staining with lectin. Plant Disease. 1998;**82**:158-164

[100] Schaad NW, Jones JB, Chun W. Laboratory Guide for Identification of Plant Pathogenic Bacteria. St. Paul, MN: APS Press; 2001

[101] Thomson SV. Epidemiology of fire blight. In: Vanneste JL, editor. Fire Blight: The Disease and its Causative Agent, *Erwinia amylovora*. Hamilton, NZ: CABI Publishing; 2000. pp. 9-35

[102] Santander RD, Català-Senent JF, Marco-Noales E, et al. In planta recovery of *Erwinia amylovora* viable but nonculturable cells. Trees. 2012;**26**: 75-82

[103] Santander RD, Biosca EG. *Erwinia amylovora* psychrotrophic adaptations: Evidence of pathogenic potential and survival at temperate and low environmental temperatures. PeerJ. 2017;**5**:e3931. DOI: 10.7717/peerj.3931

[104] Slack SM, Sundin GW. News on ooze, the fire blight spreader. Fruit Quarterly. 2017;**25**:9-12

[105] Ogawa JM, English H. Diseases of temperate zone tree fruit and nut crops. Agriculture & Natural Resources. 1991. 464 p. ISBN-13: 978-0931876974, ISBN-10: 0931876974

[106] Ordax M, Piquer-Salcedo JE, Santander RD, et al. Medfly Ceratitis capitata as potential vector for fire blight pathogen *Erwinia amylovora*: Survival and transmission. PLoS One. 2015;**10**:e0127560

[107] Cougar Blight Model Overview, Chelan & Douglas Counties, Washington State University. Chelan & Douglas Counties. Available from: https://extension.wsu.edu/chelan-douglas/agriculture/treefruit/pestmanagement/cougarblightmodeloverview/ [Accessed: 23 April 2019]

[108] Pusey PL, Smith TJ. Relation of apple flower age to infection of hypanthium by *Erwinia amylovora*. Plant Disease. 2007;**92**:137-142

[109] Keitt GW, Ivanoff SS. Transmission of fire blight by bees and its relation to nectar concentration of apple and pear blossoms. Journal of Agricultural Research. 1941;**62**:745-753

[110] Johnson KB, Sawyer TL, Temple TN. Rates of epiphytic growth of *Erwinia amylovora* on flowers common in the landscape. Plant Disease. 2006; **90**:1331-1336

[111] Billing E. Fire blight. Why do views on host invasion by *Erwinia amylovora* differ? Plant Pathology. 2011;**60**:178-189

[112] Mohammadi M. Enhanced colonization and pathogenicity of *Erwinia amylovora* strains transformed with the near-ubiquitous pEA29 plasmid on pear and apple. Plant Pathology. 2010;**59**:252-261

[113] Bogs J, Bruchmüller I, Erbar C, et al. Colonization of host plants by the fire blight pathogen *Erwinia amylovora* marked with genes for bioluminescence and fluorescence. Phytopathology. 1998; **88**:416-421

[114] Koczan JM, McGrath MJ, Zhao Y, et al. Contribution of *Erwinia amylovora* exopolysaccharides amylovoran and Levan to biofilm formation: Implications in pathogenicity. Phytopathology. 2009;**99**:1237-1244

[115] Momol MT, Norelli JL, Piccioni DE, et al. Internal movement of *Erwinia amylovora* through symptomless apple Scion tissues into the rootstock. Plant Disease. 1998;**82**:646-650

[116] Spitko R. Efficacy of Microinjected Apogee and ArborFos against Fire Blight Disease Incidence and Shoot Growth of Apple. Arcadia, CA: J.J. Mauget Co.; 2008 [Accessed: 28 October 2011]

[117] Harrell M. Imidacloprid concentrations in green ash (*Fraxinus pennsylvanica*) following treatments with two trunk-injection methods. Arboriculture & Urban Forestry. 2006; **32**:126

[118] National Center for Biotechnology Information. Thiabendazole. PubChem Database. Thiabendazole. 2019. https://pubchem.ncbi.nlm.nih.gov/compound/5430 [Accessed: 27 April 2019]

[119] PPDB. Pesticide Properties DataBase—difenoconazole (Ref: CGA 169374). Pesticide Properties DataBase. 2013. Available from: http://kartofel.org/pesticides_op/difenokonazol.PDF [Accessed: 24 October 2013]

[120] BCP Council. The Pesticide Manual: A World Compendium. Tomlin, CDS: British Crop Protection; 2011

[121] Herner AE, Acock B. USDA-ARS pesticide properties database. In: Encyclopedia of Agrochemicals. John Wiley & Sons, Inc.; 2003 . Available from: http://onlinelibrary.wiley.com/doi/10.1002/047126363X.agr237/abstract [Accessed: 24 October 2013]

[122] Blanke MM, Lenz F. Fruit photosynthesis. Plant, Cell & Environment. 1989;**12**:31-46

[123] Mensink B. Environmental risk limits for difenoconazole. 601716005/2008. Netherlands: National Institute for Public Health and the Environment; 2008 . Available from: http://www.rivm.nl/bibliotheek/rapporten/601716005.pdf [Accessed: 24 October 2013]

[124] EFSA. Conclusion on the peer review of the pesticide risk assessment of the active substance potassium phosphonates, European Food Safety Authority. EFSA Journal. 2012;**10**:1-43

[125] Tanis SR, Cregg BM, Mota-Sanchez D, et al. Spatial and temporal distribution of trunk-injected 14C-imidacloprid in Fraxinus trees. Pest Management Science. 2012;**68**:529-536

[126] Kondo ES. Scope and limitations of carbendazim $H_2PO_4$ injections in Dutch elm disease [*Ceratocystis ulmi*, North America]. Journal of Arboriculture. 1978;**4**:80-86

[127] Coomes DA. Challenges to the generality of WBE theory. Trends in Ecology & Evolution. 2006;**21**:593-596

[128] McCulloh KA, Sperry JS, Adler FR. Water transport in plants obeys Murray's law. Nature. 2003;**421**:939-942

[129] McGhee GC, Sundin GW. Evaluation of Kasugamycin for fire blight management, effect on nontarget bacteria, and assessment of Kasugamycin resistance potential in *Erwinia amylovora*. Phytopathology. 2011;**101**:192-204

[130] Sundin GW, Werner NA, Yoder KS, et al. Field evaluation of biological control of fire blight in the eastern United States. Plant Disease. 2009;**93**: 386-394

[131] Hammerschmidt R. Introduction: Definitions and some history. In: Walters D, Newton A, Lyon G, editors. Induced Resistance for Plant Defence. Hoboken, NJ, USA: Blackwell Publishing; 2007. pp. 1-8

[132] Thomson SV, Gouk SC, Paulin JP. Efficacy of BION®(Actigard®) to control fire blight in pear and apple orchards in USA, New Zealand and France. In: VIII International Workshop on Fire Blight 489. 1998. pp. 589-596

[133] Brisset MN, Cesbron S, Thomson SV, et al. Acibenzolar-*S*-methyl induces the accumulation of defense-related enzymes in apple and protects from fire blight. European Journal of Plant Pathology. 2000;**106**:529-536

[134] Zeller W, Zeller V. Control of fire blight with the plant activator BION®. In: VIII International Workshop on Fire Blight 489. 1998. pp. 639-646

[135] Maxson KL, Jones AL. Management of fire blight with gibberellin inhibitors and SAR inducers. In: IX International Workshop on Fire Blight 590. 2001. pp. 217-223

[136] Maxson-Stein K, He SY, Hammerschmidt R, et al. Effect of treating apple trees with acibenzolar-*S*-methyl on fire blight and expression of pathogenesis-related protein genes. Plant Disease. 2002;**86**:785-790

[137] Johnson KB, Stockwell VO. Management of fire blight: A case study in microbial ecology. Annual Review of Phytopathology. 1998;**36**:227-248

[138] McManus PS, Stockwell VO, Sundin GW, et al. Antibiotic use in plant agriculture. Annual Review of Phytopathology. 2002;**40**:443-465

[139] Deliopoulos T, Kettlewell PS, Hare MC. Fungal disease suppression by inorganic salts: A review. Crop Protection. 2010;**29**:1059-1075

[140] Boneti J da S, Katsurayama Y. Viabilidade do uso de fosfitos no controle da sarna-da-macieira. Agropecuaria Catarinense. 2005;**18**: 51-54

Chapter 10

# Management of the Cacao Swollen Shoot Virus (CSSV) Menace in Ghana: The Past, Present and the Future

*George A. Ameyaw*

## Abstract

This chapter outlines and discusses some of the challenges associated with management of the cacao swollen shoot virus (CSSV) disease in Ghana and its impact on cocoa production. The discussion will bring to the fore some of the factors that has militated against implementation of the recommended management strategies in the past and its consequential effect on the present widespread of the disease across the various cocoa regions in West Africa. The wide variability in the different strains of the virus as manifested in recent molecular studies is highlighted as a possible contributor and explanation for the prevalence and varying virulence of the disease in new infections, especially, in the Western region of Ghana. Current research efforts and strategies aimed at minimizing of CSSV continuous spread and devastation on Ghana's cocoa production is discussed.

**Keywords:** cocoa, swollen shoot virus disease, mealybug vector, CSSVD

## 1. Introduction

The cocoa industry plays critical role in the socioeconomic development of Ghana by providing employment and source of livelihood to many farm families and other stakeholders in the cocoa value chain. Export of cocoa beans and other cocoa products is a major avenue for the generation of the much needed foreign exchange for the economies of Ghana and Cote d'Ivoire. Sustainability of the cocoa industry is therefore critical for the governments and people of these West African nations and other stakeholders in the cocoa business. Cocoa cultivation is however bedeviled with several production problems as the cocoa plant is affected by numerous diseases and pests which accounts for significant yield losses in the various cocoa producing nations across the world (**Tables 1** and **2**). Five major diseases of the cocoa plant (*Theobroma cacao* L.) namely; *Phytophthora* pod rot (black pod), witches broom, cacao swollen shoot virus, vascular streak dieback, and monilia pod rot account for over 40% annual yield loss across the different production regions [1].

The cacao swollen shoot virus disease (CSSVD) which is considered the most economically important cocoa virus disease could account for 15–50% yield loss if the severe strains are involved in infections [2, 3]. Since the discovery of this important disease in Ghana, it has been managed through the "cutting out and replanting

| Type of pathogen | Disease (common name) | Causal pathogen |
|---|---|---|
| Oomycete | Black pod | *Phytophthora palmivora* |
| Oomycete | Black pod | *Phytophthora capsici* |
| Oomycete | Black pod | *Phytophthora citrophthora* |
| Oomycete | Black pod | *Phytophthora heveae* |
| Oomycete | Black pod | *Phytophthora megakarya* |
| Fungus | Black rot | *Rosellinia bunodes* |
| Fungus | Black rot | *Rosellinia pepo* |
| Fungus | Black thread | *Marasmius scandens* |
| Oomycete | Canker | *Phytophthora palmivora* |
| Oomycete | Canker | *Phytophthora megakarya* |
| Oomycete | Canker | *Phytophthora citrophthora* |
| Fungus | Charcoal pod rot | *Lasiodiplodia theobromae,* |
| Fungus | Cushion gall | *Colonectra rigidiuscula* |
| Fungus | Frosty pod | *Moniliophthora roreri* |
| Fungus | Mealy pod | *Trachysphaera fructigena* |
| Fungus | Pink disease | *Corticium salmonicolor* |
| Fungus | Root rot | *Phellinus noxius* |
| Fungus | Thread blight | *Marasmius scandens* |
| Fungus | Warty pod | *Trachysphaera fructigena* |
| Fungus | White thread | *Marasmiu sequicrinis* |
| Fungus | Witches' broom | *Moniliophthora perniciosa* |
| Fungus | Witches' broom | *Moniliophthora crinipellis* |
| Viruses | Cacao swollen shoot virus disease | *Cacao swollen shoot virus* (CSSV) |
| Viruses | Cacao yellow mosaic virus | *Cacao yellow mosaic virus (*CYMV) |
| Viruses | Cacao necrosis virus | *Cacao necrosis nepovirus (*CNV*)* |

**Table 1.**
*Causal pathogens of common cocoa diseases in the world. Source: [48].*

system" with the aim of removing sources of inoculum from affected cocoa plantations and replanting with tolerant cocoa hybrids [3–5]. Nonetheless, reports from many reassessments and disease surveys indicate that the prevalence of the disease is still high with varying virulence across the cocoa regions. This has partly been attributed to the poor implementation of the cutting out program to manage the disease. This chapter highlights some of the past challenges that have bedeviled the "cutting out system" and discusses some of the current strategies being implemented by the various stakeholders and researchers to minimize the continuous spread and impact of the disease on cocoa production in Ghana and Cote d'Ivoire.

| Diseases | Pathogen | Region | Estimated reduction in production and income | |
|---|---|---|---|---|
| | | | (tons x 1000) | ($ millions) |
| Black Pod | *Phytophthora* spp. | Africa/Brazil/ Asia | 450 | 423 |
| Witches' Broom | *Crinipellis perniciosa* | Latin America | 250 | 235 |
| Cocoa Swollen Shoot Virus Disease | CSSV | Africa | 50 | 47 |
| Frosty Pod Rot | *Moniliophthora roreri* | Latin America | 30 | 28 |
| Vascular-streak dieback | *Oncobasidium theobromae* | Asia | 30 | 28 |

**Table 2.**
*Economic losses from some important cocoa diseases across the world. Source: [48].*

## 2. The cacao swollen shoot virus disease (CSSVD)

The *Cacao swollen shoot virus* disease (CSSVD) was first noted in the Eastern Region of Ghana in 1936 by a farmer in a form of cocoa stem swollen conditions [6] but its virus nature was confirmed in 1939 [7]. The disease is considered the most important cocoa viruses in West Africa due to its devastating effect on yield and possibility of causing death of cocoa plants especially when the severe strains are involved in infections [8, 9]. The virus affects all parts of the cocoa plant and the severe strains induce varying leaf symptoms and swellings of the stems and roots. Some of the leaf symptoms include; red vein banding of the immature "flush" leaves [10] (**Figure 1**); chlorotic vein flecking or banding which may occur in angular flecks (**Figure 2**). Stem swellings occur at the nodes, internodes or tips of the stem [2, 10], (**Figures 3** and **4**).

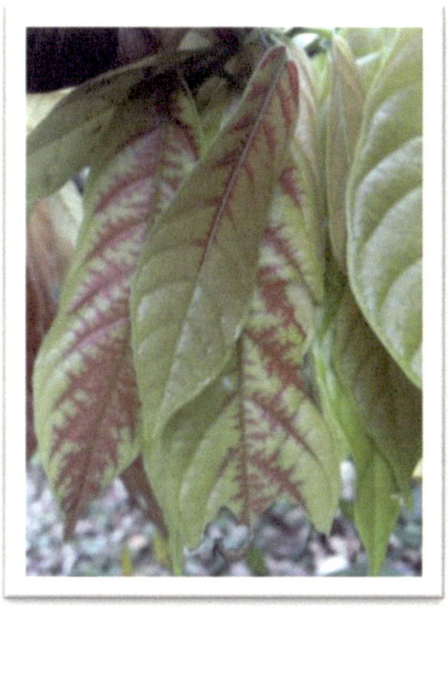

**Figure 1.**
*Red vein banding.*

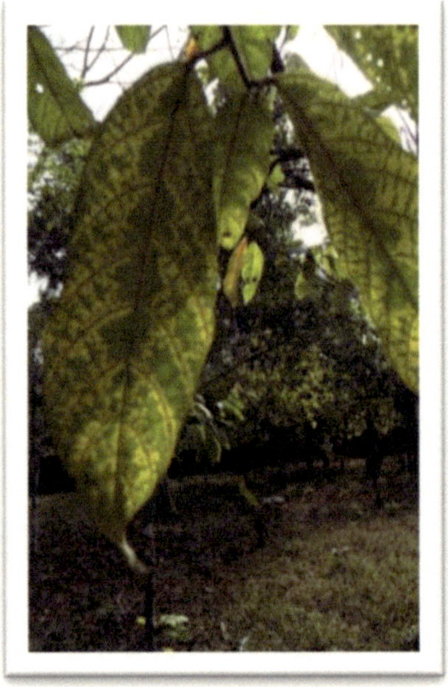

**Figure 2.**
*Chlorotic vein banding.*

Some strains also cause infected pods to change shape and become rounder, smaller and with smoother surfaces [11].CSSV is classified as a member of the plant-infecting pararetroviruses in the genus badnaviridae which are with non-enveloped bacilliform particles that encapsulate a circular double stranded DNA-genome [12–15]. The viral particle of CSSV is identified with length measurements in the range of 121–130 and a width of 28 nm [12]. The genome size ranges from 7.4 to 8.0 kilobase pair depending on strain [16, 17]. The CSSV genome is organized into five putative open reading frames (ORFs 1, 2, 3 X and Y) located on the plus strand of the 7.16 kbp [15].

## 2.1 CSSVD isolates and strains

Generally, isolates of the virus have been designated by naming them according to the nearest town or village where they are first collected and are generally

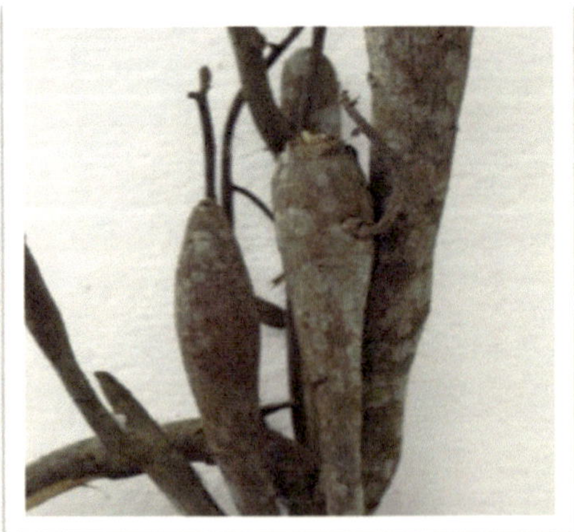

**Figure 3.**
*Tip swelling.*

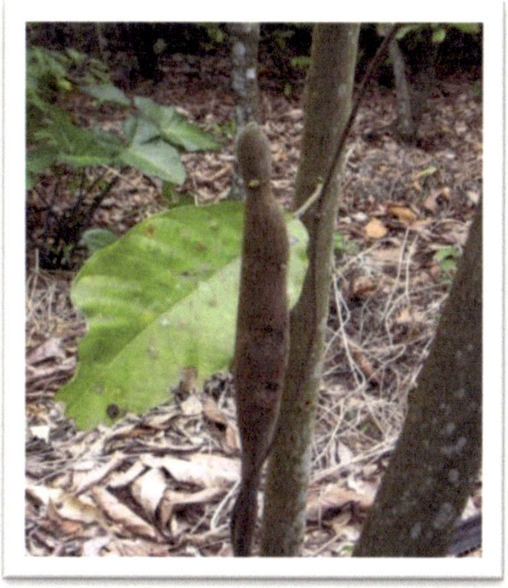

**Figure 4.**
*Shoot swelling.*

grouped according to severity of symptom expression and geographical origin [12–15]. Ghanaian CSSVD isolates are distinguished five groups of through enzyme linked immunosorbent assay (ELISA) and immunosorbent electron microscopy (ISEM) techniques and by using leaf symptoms [18]. Recent molecular studies with the use of advance sequencing methods such Next generation tools have provided the opportunity to further classify CSSV isolates across the West African sub-region into new groups based on their molecular information at the DNA level. Some of these studies have identified wide variability in the strains of the virus and virulence of the disease in new infections especially in the Western region of Ghana [3, 19, 20]. The strains of the virus have now been reclassified based on their molecular diversity into groups A, B, C, D, E, F, G, H, G, J, K. L, M, and N [**Figure 5**].

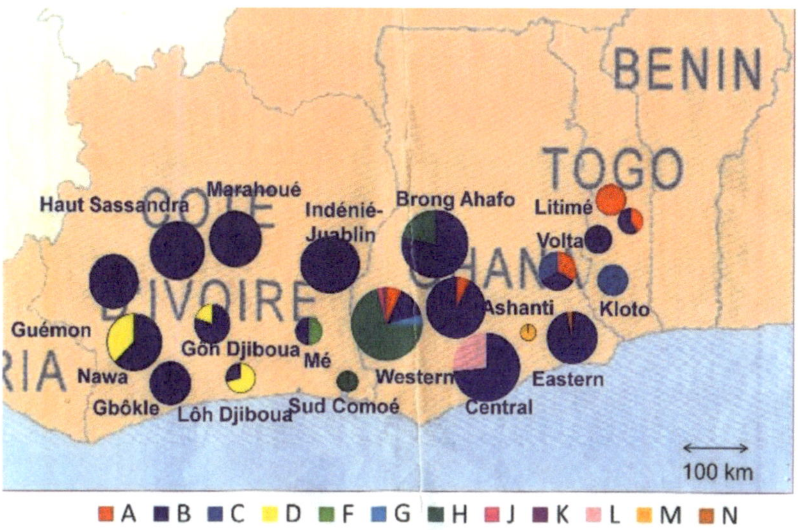


**Figure 5.**
*Molecular diversity of CSSV in West Africa [47].*

### 2.2 CSSVD transmission

CSSV is semi-persistently transmitted by several species of mealybugs (*Pseudococcidae*, *Homoptera*) on cocoa [21, 22]. The vectors feed on all parts of the cocoa tree including flowers, cherelles, pods and leaves. The mealybug species differ in their ability to transmit different strains of the virus. The most efficient mealybug transmitters of the virus include the *Planococcoides njalensis* (Laing), *Planococcus citri* (Rossi) and *Ferrisia virgata* (Okll) specie which are also dominant on cocoa fields in Ghana and Cote d'Ivoire (**Figure 6**). The ages of the mealybugs are also important in the spread of the virus in that only the young adults (nymphs) are very mobile and so are more efficient transmitters than the adults which are most often sedentary [23]. The use of mechanical inoculation procedures to transmit CSSV was made possible in 1960 [24]. Considering the continual spread of the virus to new cocoa plantings, research is still focusing on other insect pests in the cocoa environment to ascertain their vector status regarding CSSV transmission in the field.

### 2.3 CSSVD alternative hosts

The virus is considered to have originated from wild indigenous forest trees within the cocoa environment [25–28]. This suggestion was based on studies in the Western Region of Ghana which showed that some of the CSSV isolates could be found in some forest trees such as *Cola chlamydantha* (K. Schum), trees and the prevalence of the disease was also high in areas where these trees were found. Other tree species that have subsequently been identified as wild alternative hosts of CSSV include *Erythropsis barteri* (Mast), *Sterculia tragacantha* (Lindle), *Sterculia rhinopetala* (K. Schum), *Cola gigantean* var. *glabrescens* (BronnanetKeay), *Adansonia digitata* (L.), *Bombax buonopozense*, and *Ceiba pentandra* (L.), [25]. It is, however, noteworthy to indicate that not all the wild hosts are good sources of the virus and also its availability declines to a low level in the bigger and old trees which sometimes makes the virus not readily available to the mealybug vectors. Mechanically transmission CSSV from some of the wild hosts to cocoa and vice versa was achieved in 1962 [24]. It was therefore recommended that the abovementioned forest trees known to be alternative host plants for the virus be removed as much as possible from cocoa plantations before replanting with new cocoa to prevent early

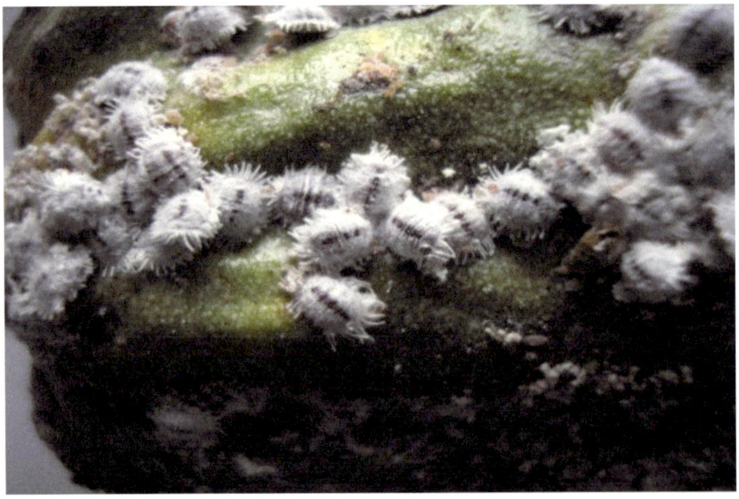

**Figure 6.**
*Mealybug infested cocoa pods.*

reinfection [29]. Currently, research is focusing on other possible alternative host plants of CSSV in the forms of weeds and food crops within the cocoa ecosystem.

### 2.4 CSSVD spread in the field

Generally, the spread of the virus in the field is triggered by several factors such as the size of the initial source of infection, and the age and type of the mealybug population present [8, 9, 29]. Apparently, natural spread of the virus is slow under low inoculum pressure (i.e., presence of few inoculums sources) because it is dependent on the movement of the mealybug vectors infected with the virus. It is also slow within young plantings until the trees become well established and form a continuous canopy of interlocking branches [29]. Nevertheless, virus infected mealybugs are occasionally blown by wind to uninfected trees some distance from the original site of infection resulting in jump spread of the virus to uninfected areas to initiate new outbreaks [30, 31]. New outbreaks of CSSV tended to be concentrated around the periphery of existing outbreaks (infections) or abandoned forests with alternative hosts which then spread slowly to give clearly defined expanding foci [29]. The pattern of spread within outbreaks was noted to be of a circumscribed nature and tended to be high close to source of infection. Existing outbreaks then initiates new "satellite" outbreaks through "jump" spread over wider distance by windblown mealybugs. These new "satellite" outbreaks enlarge and eventually coalesce to form large areas of mass infection. Spread of the disease within outbreaks was however noted to result from movement of mealybugs carrying the virus from infected to healthy trees. It was noted that new outbreaks get bigger close to large sources of infection and diminish further away from them [32].

## 3. CSSVD control strategies

Management of CSSVD in Ghana has over the years been carried out in an integrated manner involving the use of different strategies such; as the cutting out method, mealybug control, removal of alternative hosts, and the use of tolerant planting materials. These control strategies and some of their challenges are discussed below.

### 3.1 The cutting out method

Cutting-out of CSSVD infected cocoa trees together with a ring of nearby apparently healthy cocoa trees have been the main method adopted to control the spread of the virus in Ghana since 1946. The aim of this strategy is to eliminate or reduce the sources of infection (inoculums) within new cocoa plantings. Once the infected cocoa trees are removed, the field is expected to be replanted with CSSVD tolerant cocoa varieties from the seed gardens. This method has gone through several challenges in its implementation thereby resulting in the continuous spread of the virus to new areas [5, 9]. Although most of these challenges are intertwined, notable among them include; late discovery of infections, lack of continuity of the program, non-co-operation of farmers due to issues of compensation payments, land tenure issues, and non-adherence to replanting recommendations after the removal of sources of infection [5, 8, 29].

#### *3.1.1 Late discovery of infections*

The effectiveness of the cutting out procedure depends largely on the efficiency of early detection of infections [9]. The disease identification system whereby trained diseased spotters carry out tree-by-tree inspection for visual symptoms of the virus inevitably means that latently infected trees which have not produced symptoms at the time of inspection are missed. Considering the pattern of CSSVD spread [29] which is mainly limited to adjacent trees around the periphery of existing outbreaks, it can be argued that, the disease spotters follow the virus and are always "one step behind". It is also generally known that CSSVD symptoms tend to be least conspicuous during the dry season when the trees deteriorate and leaves and shoots are shed or damaged by capsids [9]. Considering the common phenomenon of dehydration and less active growth of infected trees during the dry season, it is very likely that disease spotters would miss some infected trees in the field during these periods. There is thus a high possibility that these missed infections could be supporting mealybug population and also transmit the disease even though they may not show conspicuous symptoms [8, 9, 23]. The challenge of lack of efficient detection protocol for the virus at the early stages has therefore generally been considered among the reasons why the disease continues to spread at an increasing rate in Ghana. The need for efficient early detection tools has always been advocated to be one of the means to help in the effective management of the virus.

#### *3.1.2 Lack of continuity of the cutting out program*

National implementation of the cutting out program has been delayed or halted on many occasions for numerous reasons such as; farmer opposition, logistical constraints, lack of funding, and at times political interference [5]. Although, it is known that continuity in the cutting out operation would have been very essential for the control of other viral diseases in other areas it has never been achieved most especially in Ghana. There is always time lag between symptom identification in outbreaks and time to treatment and replanting.

#### *3.1.3 Non-adherence to replanting recommendations*

Replanting of treated cocoa farms according to laid down recommendations could have been successful in rehabilitating devastated cocoa areas. However, it was noted that newly planted farms in most of the cocoa areas, especially, in the Western Region, showed symptoms of re-infection with the virus [4]. This is because farms are replanted very close to the boundary of abandoned cocoa farms containing visible infections, without much attempt to remove the infected trees in the old plantations. The recommendation that replanting should only occur after the complete removal of sources of infected cocoa trees or alternative host plants, have not been applied adequately in the eradication and replanting exercise hence contributing to the prevalence of the disease across cocoa farms.

#### *3.1.4 Presence of alternative hosts in newly replanted farms*

The occurrence of wild alternative host plants of the virus in and around cocoa farms is a contributory factor to spread and early re-infection of new cocoa plantings in Ghana [25]. Even though, removal of wild alternative host trees has been recommended, it is seldom applied. The advice to farmers to leave at least a 15 m barrier with some economic crops such as citrus and oil palm around new cocoa plantings to delay reinfection from old plantations and forest trees have also not been implemented fully. Farmers always want to fully utilize all available space of land for cocoa planting and also use the alternative host trees as a source of natural shade for their cocoa during the early growth period.

#### *3.1.5 Lack of effective control methods for mealybugs*

The use of synthetic chemicals for the control of the mealybug vectors has not been effective over the years. This is attributed to the morphology of the mealybugs having a protective wax covering and also the building of mud tents over them by black ants [33–36]. Attempts by scientists with the use of biological means have also not been successful [37].

#### *3.1.6 Use of resistant cocoa varieties*

Even though it has long be envisaged that planting of cocoa varieties tolerant to CSSVD would be the most effective means to manage the disease [38], most of the available cocoa planting materials has however shown low levels of resistance under field conditions. It is notable that many of the inter-Amazon hybrids developed and recommended by the British Research Team and currently available to farmers [38] have only partial resistance to CSSVD [38–40]. Although partial resistance is beneficial for being able to tolerate the virus to give appreciable yield in the short to medium term, the need for varieties that could offer greater resistance cannot be overemphasized. The continuous search for varieties that could offer long-term resistance that has been going on over the years using modern breeding approaches such as mutation and tissue culture techniques in Ghana and elsewhere is therefore very appropriate [41].

#### *3.1.7 Mild strains cross protection*

Long term field assessment of the mild strain cross protection experiments carried out at the Cocoa Research Institute of Ghana (CRIG) has shown that, the immunity conferred on the healthy cocoa plants from the available mild strains N1 and SS365B eventually breaks down after 20 years [42, 43]. These reports support past works and suggestions that further investigations on the effectiveness of the mild strain phenomenon need to be carried out before its adoption as a management strategy for the virus [44–46].

## 4. Current strategies on CSSVD management

The cutting out and rehabilitation program was re-launched in June 2018 to concurrently cut out CSSVD infected cocoa trees along the borders of Ghana and Cote d'Ivoire. The expectation is to progressively remove about 100,000 ha of infected CSSVD outbreaks across the cocoa regions in Ghana by 2023. The current cutting out activities involves the total removal of CSSVD infected cocoa trees in blocks of outbreaks and replanting with tolerant cocoa varieties. Payment of compensation to farmers and land owners has been incorporated into the program to sustain farmers' livelihood during the periods of cocoa tree removal and replanting. Additionally, farmers would be supported in their cocoa farm establishment and maintenance activities such as provision of temporary and permanent shade plants, farm weeding and fertilizer application. Cutting out activities are to be intensified in high prevalent areas such as the Western and Eastern regions of Ghana.

Scientific research activities to support the program have been strengthened to include development of early detection tools, mealybug vectors control, identification of other alternative hosts and vectors as well as development of resistant cocoa varieties. Characterization of the diversity and virulence of the disease across the West African Sub-region is also to progress to understand the nature of the virus at the molecular level. Diversity studies to classify the virus into distinct groups of strains and isolates as identified in the Western region and adjoining areas of the Brong Ahafo Region is also being aggressively pursued to explain the difference in virulence and symptoms of the disease in different outbreaks.

## 5. Conclusion

The cutting out approach to remove sources of infection from farms still remains the most feasible method to manage the spread of CSSVD in an integrated system with other agronomic practices. Emphasis should therefore be placed on finding the most logical and efficient means of carrying out the program with the support of farmers and other relevant stakeholders. Accordingly, extensive farmer education on the effects of the disease and the rationale behind removal of sources of infection from outbreak areas is very imperative. Additionally, policies and rate of treatment and replanting needs careful coordination both at the District and Regional levels and this should take into consideration the severity of the disease and the availability of adequate manpower and resources to implement the program according to laid down recommendations.

The ineffectiveness of the cutting out strategy as noted in the past should be placed in the appropriate context of the many problems or challenges in its implementation together with the logistical and manpower constraints that have characterized the cutting out scheme from the outset. This chapter highlighted some of the challenges of the cutting out system and still recommends its application in an integrated approach involving the use of different measures in a coordinated manner. The focus for current and future scientific research and topics for consideration include; the use of modern breeding techniques to develop resistant cocoa varieties for CSSV, studies on chemical and biological control of the mealybug vectors, development of early detection tools, and identification of other vectors and hosts of the virus.

## Acknowledgements

The author thanks fellow scientists for reading through the manuscript and for their useful contributions and suggestions. This paper is published with the kind permission of the Executive Director of the Cocoa Research Institute of Ghana (CRIG).

## Author details

George A. Ameyaw
Cocoa Research Institute of Ghana (CRIG), Ghana

*Address all correspondence to: gaakumfi@yahoo.co.uk

## References

[1] Flood J, Guest D, Holmes KA, Keane P, Padi B, Sulistyowati E. Cocoa under attack. In: Flood J, Murphy R, editors. Cocoa Futures: A Source Book of Some Important Issues Facing the Cocoa Industry. Chinchina, Colombia: CABI-FEDERACAFE, USDA. The Commodities Press; 2004. pp. 33-53. ISBN 958-97441-1-7

[2] Posnette AF. Viruses of cocoa in West Africa: 1. Cocoa viruses 1A, 1B, 1C, and 1D. Annals of Applied Biology. 1947;**34**:388-402

[3] Muller E, Ravel S, Agret C, Abrokwah F, Dzahini-Obiatey H, Galyuon I, et al. Next generation sequencing elucidates cacao badnavirus diversity and reveals the existence of more than ten viral species. Virus Research. 2018;**244**:235-251

[4] Dzahini-Obiatey H, Ameyaw GA, Ollennu LA. Control of cocoa swollen shoot disease by eradicating infected trees in Ghana: A survey of treated and replanted areas. Crop Protection. 2006;**25**:647-652

[5] Ameyaw GA, Dzahini-Obiatey HK, Domfeh O. Perspectives on cocoa swollen shoot virus disease (CSSVD) management in Ghana. Crop Protection. 2014;**65**:64-70

[6] Steven WF. Swollen shoot and die-back—A new disease of cocoa. Gold Coast Farmer. 1936;**5**:144

[7] Posnette AF. Transmission of "swollen shoot" disease of cacao. Tropical Agriculture, Trinidad and Tobago. 1940;**17**:98

[8] Owusu GK. The cocoa swollen shoot virus problem in Ghana. In: Plumb RT, Thresh JM, editors. Plant Virus Epidemiology. Oxford: Blackwell Scientific Publications; 1983. pp. 73-83

[9] Thresh JM. Control of cacao swollen shoots disease. A review of the present situation. Technical Bulletin; West African Cocoa Research Institute; No. 4, WACRI, Tafo, Ghana; 1958

[10] Posnette AF. Swollen-shoot virus disease of cacao. Tropical Agricultura. 1941;**18**:87-90

[11] Posnette AF. The diagnosis of swollen shoot disease of cacao. Tropical Agriculture. 1943;**21**:156-158

[12] Brunt AA, Kenten RH, Nixon HL. Some properties of cocoa swollen hoot virus. Journal of General Microbiology. 1964;**36**:303-309

[13] Kenten RH, Legg JT. Varietal resistance of cocoa to swollen shoot disease in West Africa. FAO Plant Protection Bulletin. 1971;**19**:2-12

[14] Adomako D, Lesemann DE, Paul HL, Owusu GK. Improved methods for the purification and detection of cacao swollen shoot virus. Annals of Applied Biology. 1983;**103**:109-116

[15] Muller E, Sackey S. Molecular variability analysis of five new complete cacao swollen shoot virus genomic sequences. Archives of Virology. 2005;**150**:53-66

[16] Lot H, Djiekpor E, Jacquuemond M. Characterization of the genome of cacao swollen shoot virus. Journal of General Virology. 1991;**72**:1735-1739

[17] Hagen LS, Jacquemod M, Lepingle A, Lot H, Tepfer M. Nucleotide sequence and genome organisation of cacao swollen shoot virus. Virology. 1993;**196**:619-628

[18] Sagerman W, Lesemann D-E, Paul HL, Adomako D, Owusu GK. Detection and comparison of some Ghanaian isolates of cocoa swollen shoot virus (CSSV) by enzyme-linked

immunosorbent assay (ELISA) and immunoelectron microscopy (EM) using an antiserum to CSSV strain 1A. Journal of Phytopathology. 1985;**114**:78-89

[19] Nomatter C, Kouakou K, Aka R, Ameyaw G, Gutierrez OA, Herrmann H-W, et al. The proposed new species, cacao red vein virus, and three previously recognized badnavirus species are associated with cacao swollen shoot disease. Virology Journal. 2017;**14**:199-213

[20] Ameyaw GA, Chigandu N, Dzahini-Obiatey HK, Domfeh O, Gutierrez O, Judith K. Brown Variable detection potential of some newly designed primers on Ghanaian CSSV isolates. Lima, Peru: International Symposium on Cocoa Research (ISCR); 13-17 November 2017

[21] Posnette AF, Strickland AH. Virus diseases of cocoa in West Africa. Technique of insect transmission. Annals of Applied Biology. 1948;**35**:53-63

[22] Campbell CAM. The assessment of mealybugs (*Pseudococcidae*) and other Homoptera on mature cocoa trees in Ghana. Bulletin of Entomological Research. 1983;**73**:137-151

[23] Cornwell PB. Effect of wind currents on vector dispersal. Annual Report; West African Cocoa Research Institute; 1956. p. 46

[24] Brunt AA, Kenten RH. The mechanical transmission of cocoa swollen shoot virus to and from cocoa and other hosts. Annals of Applied Biology. 1962;**50**:749-754

[25] Posnette AF, Robertson NF, Todd JM. Virus diseases of cocoa in West Africa. V. Alternative host plants. Annals of Applied Biology. 1950;**37**:229-240

[26] Posnette AF. The role of wild hosts. In: Thresh JM, editor. Pests, Pathogens and Vegetation. London, U.K.: Pitman; 1981. pp. 71-78

[27] Dale WT, Attafuah A. The host range of cocoa viruses. Annual Report of the West African Cocoa Research Institute; 1955/1956. pp. 28-30

[28] Attafuah A, Glendenning DR. Studies on resistance and tolerance to cocoa viruses in Ghana. I. A survey of T17 progeny. The Annals of Applied Biology. 1965;**56**:219

[29] Thresh JM, Owusu GK, Ollennu LAA. Cocoa swollen shoot virus: An archetypal crowd disease. Journal of Plant Diseases and Protection. 1988;**95**:428-446

[30] Cornwell PB. Movements of the vectors of virus diseases of cacao in Ghana. II. Wind movement and aerial dispersal. Bulletin of Entomological Research. 1960;**51**:175-201

[31] Strickland AH. The dispersal of *Pseudococcidae* (*Hemiptera-Homoptera*) by air currents in the Gold Coast. Proceedings of the Royal Entomological society, London. 1950;**25**:1-9

[32] Thresh JM, Lister RM. Coppicing experiments on the spread and control of cacao swollen shoot disease in Nigeria. Annals of Applied Biology. 1960;**48**:65-74

[33] Donald RG. Mealybug studies. Annual Report of West African Cocoa Research Institute; 1953/1954. p. 101

[34] Decker FE. Mealybug studies; biological control of mealybugs. Annual Report of West African Cocoa Research Institute. 1953. p. 23

[35] Hanna AD, Judenko EB, Heatherington W. Systemic insecticides for the control of insects transmitting the swollen shoot virus of cocoa in the Gold Coast. Bulletin of Entomological Research. 1955;**46**:669-710

[36] Hanna AD. Research in the use of systemic insecticides to control the mealybug vectors of swollen shoot disease of cocoa. Phytopharmacology. 1954:425-432

[37] Acknonor JB. Preliminary studies on breeding and predation on *Scymnus* (*pullus*) sp. and *Hyperaspis egregia* Mader on *Plannococcus njalensis* (Laing) In: Ollennu LAA, Owusu GK, Padi B, editors. Proceedings of the First International Cocoa Pests and Diseases Seminar; 6-10 November 1995; Accra, Ghana; pp. 238-241

[38] Legg JT, Lockwood G. Resistance of cocoa to swollen shoot virus in Ghana. I. Field trials. The Annals of Applied Biology. 1981;**97**:75-89

[39] Adu-Ampomah Y. The cocoa breeding program in Ghana: Achievements and prospects for the future. Cocoa Growers' Bulletin. 1996;**50**:17-21

[40] Legg J, Owusu GK, Ollennu LAA, Lovi NK. The Problems of Controlling Cocoa Swollen Shoot Disease in Ghana. In: Proceedings of 6th International Cocoa Research Conference; Caracas, Venezuela; Lagos, Nigeria: Cocoa Producers' Alliance (COPAL); 1981. pp. 267-278

[41] Adomako B, Adu-Ampomah Y, Ollennu LAA, Dzahini-Obiatey H, Takrama JF. Breeding for cocoa varieties resistant/tolerant to cocoa swollen shoot virus. Annual Report; Cocoa Research Institute of Ghana; 2003. pp. 201-203

[42] Ameyaw GA, Dzahini-Obiatey HK, Domfeh O, Ollennu LAA, Owusu G. Appraisal of cocoa swollen shoot virus mild isolates for cross protection of cocoa against severe strains in Ghana. Plant Disease. 2016;**100**(4):810-815

[43] Domfeh O, Ameyaw GA, Dzahini-Obiatey HK. The effects of mild cacao swollen shoot virus strains N1 and SS365B on growth and yield of cacao. Journal of General Plant Pathology. 2018;**84**:369-375. DOI: 10.1007/s10327-018-0794-3

[44] Owusu GK, Ollennu LAA, Dzahini-Obiatey HK. The prospects for mild strain cross-protection to control cocoa swollen shoot disease in Ghana. In: Proceedings of 12th International Cocoa Research Conference; Salvador, Bahia, Brazil; Lagos, Nigeria: Cocoa Producers' Alliance (COPAL); 1996. pp. 121-127

[45] Hughes JA, LAA O. Mild strain protection of cocoa in Ghana against cocoa swollen shoot virus—A review. Plant Pathology. 1994;**43**:442-457

[46] Ollennu LAA, Owusu GK, Dzahini-Obiatey HK. Recent studies of mild strain cross protection with cocoa swollen shoot virus. Journal of the Ghana Science Association. 1999;**2**:5-11

[47] Muller E. Cacao Swollen Shoot Virus (CSSV) History, Biology, and Genome. In: Bailey BA, Meinhard LW, editors. Cacao Diseases—A History of Old Enemies and New Encounters. Switzerland: Springer International Publishing AG; 2016

[48] INCOPED. Proceedings of 5th International Seminar on Cocoa Pests and Diseases (INCOPED); 15-17 October 2006; San Jose, Costa Rica

Chapter 11

# Emergence of Benzimidazole- and Strobilurin-Quinone Outside Inhibitor-Resistant Strains of *Colletotrichum gloeosporioides* sensu lato, the Causal Fungus of Japanese Pear Anthracnose, and Alternative Fungicides to Resistant Strains

*Nobuya Tashiro, Youichi Ide, Mayumi Noguchi, Hisayoshi Watanabe and Mizuho Nita*

## Abstract

Japanese pear anthracnose (JPA) can cause severe tree defoliation during the growing season. Infected trees become weak and produce fewer flower buds the following spring. This economically serious fungal plant disease has affected cultivated pears in Japan since 1910. Initially, JPA was controlled by benzimidazole fungicides. However, benzimidazole-resistant pathogen strains emerged in the late 1990s, and the range of JPA has expanded in Japan. Since then strobilurin-quinone outside inhibitors (ST-QoIs) such as azoxystrobin and kresoxim-methyl became popular, but ST-QoI-resistant pathogen strains appeared. By 2005, JPA control became difficult once again. In this chapter, we outline the history of JPA fungicide resistance problems, assess advantages and disadvantages of available fungicide options, and develop JPA management strategies based on evidences we obtained from a series of field and lab studies.

**Keywords:** anthracnose, benzimidazole, deciduous disease, Japanese pear, *Pyrus pyrifolia*, ST-QoI

## 1. Introduction

A sudden and severe outbreak of Japanese pear anthracnose (JPA) occurred in July 1999 on the Japanese pear cultivars "Housui" and "Niitaka" (*Pyrus pyrifolia* Nakai var. culta Nakai) in Saga prefecture on Kyushu Island, which is one of the major Japanese pear-producing regions located in southwestern Japan [1, 2].

At first, phytotoxicity was suspected owing to extensive and rapid symptom development throughout the orchard. Subsequent investigation revealed that it was JPA caused by *Colletotrichum gloeosporioides* sensu lato (Cgsl) [1, 2].

JPA was first reported in Japan by Kurosawa in 1910 [3]. He observed JPA in Fukuoka prefecture which is adjacent to Saga prefecture in June 1910. The infection caused black spots on the leaves and severe defoliation. Disease incidence and severity differed among varieties. It was severe on "Doitsu," moderate on "Nijusseiki," and mild on "Chojuro." Morphological analyses indicated that the causal organism was *C. gloeosporioides*. Kurosawa stated that Bordeaux mixture could be an effective treatment and damaged leaves should be incinerated to prevent the spread of the disease. Based on Kurosawa's research, Hara introduced JPA in his textbook entitled *Fruit Tree Disease Theory* [4]. Ikata reported that JPA was uncommon and caused no severe damage except for an outbreak in Fukuoka prefecture in 1910 [5]. There were no further reports on JPA until 1974.

In 1974, severe JPA infestations on the "Yakumo" cultivar were reported in Fukushima prefecture of the Tohoku region, which is located in northeastern Japan. The outbreak caused severe defoliation. Ochiai et al. monitored the progress of the outbreak and isolated the causal organism [6]. Ochiai and Hayashi discussed the pathogenicity of isolated *Colletotrichum* sp. and indicated that disease severity differed among host cultivars [7]. They also mentioned the effect of the infection timing (the number of days elapsed after leaf expansion) [8], temperature and leaf wetness on infection and disease incidence [9], and growth medium and temperature on pathogen growth [10]. However, there were no published reports on pathogen control methods.

In 1987 and 1998, severe incidences of JPA were reported in Kochi prefecture in Shikoku Island, located in southwestern Japan. Morita et al. reported the symptoms and transition of the outbreak. They documented the efficacy of thiophanate-methyl/maneb wettable powder (WP), maneb WP, and benomyl WP at controlling this disease [11]. There was also a report of an outbreak of moderately benzimidazole-resistant strains in 1998 [12].

Probably because JPA happened sporadically over a long time period and in small and isolated geographical areas, there was a very limited effort to identify fungicides that are effective against JPA. Therefore, no registered fungicides were available for JPA when the major JPA outbreak occurred in Saga prefecture in 1999.

## 2. JPA symptoms and causal organism

### 2.1 Symptoms

In JPA-affected orchards in Saga prefecture, Japanese pear cultivars "Housui" and "Niitaka" developed minute black spots formed on the leaf laminae and petioles starting in mid-June. The leaves appear as though they have been stabbed with a fine needle. The perforations are visible when the leaves are held up to the sunlight. Since the lesions are very small, it is difficult for the grower to notice the initial disease symptoms unless the leaves are inspected very closely. The initially tiny black dots then expand into small curved black spots 0.5–1 mm in diameter. Certain lesions may develop into large blackish-brown spots ~2 cm in diameter. By that time, the leaves rapidly turn yellow and abscise (**Figure 1**).

When the JPA outbreaks were observed in 1999, JPA caused a severe defoliation by mid-July and markedly reduced tree vigor. The intense defoliation caused new leaves to emerge soon after the event; however, these new leaves were quickly and fatally infested with JPA. In addition, defoliation triggered flowering in autumn

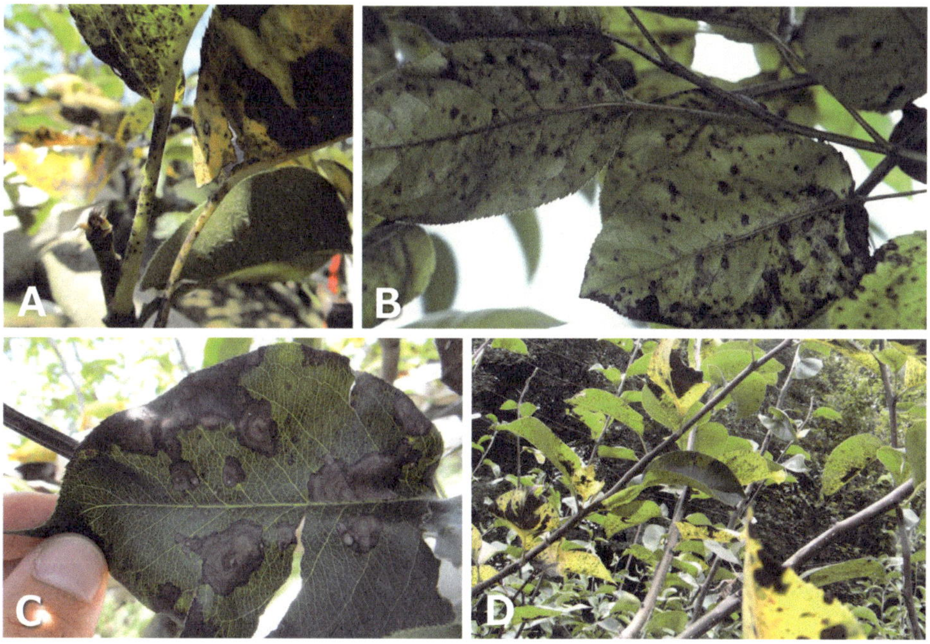

**Figure 1.**
*Black spots on anthracnose-infected petioles and leaves caused by* Colletotrichum gloeosporioides *sensu lato observed in Japanese pear cv. Housui* (Pyrus pyrifolia *Nakai var.* culta *Nakai) in the field. (A) Very minute black spots symptoms on the petioles, (B) leaf symptoms showing numerous black spots of various sizes, (C) large blackish brown spots with a diameter of about 1–2 cm, (D) yellowing leaves with large blackish brown spots.*

which leads to a fewer number of flowers in the next spring, which caused serious yield loss in the following year (**Figure 2**).

### 2.2 Causal organism

Fungal cultures were isolated from the large dark brown lesions on leaves and smaller lesions on petioles of the 'Housui' and "Niitaka" Japanese pear cultivars. Morphologically, these isolates were identical. The isolates formed light salmon flesh-colored conidial masses on spore-inducing media ($K_2HPO_4$ 1 g, $MgSO_4$ 0.5 g, peptone 5 g, lactose 10 g, agar 30 g, and distilled water 1000 mL) (**Figure 3**). Foliar spray inoculation of a conidial suspension (105 $mL^{-1}$) on 'Housui' reproduced disease symptoms similar to those observed in the orchards (**Figure 3**). The inoculated fungi were re-isolated to confirm Koch's postulates [1, 2].

The conidia are cylindrical with an average size of 15.8 μm × 5.0 μm (**Figure 3**). The mycelia from these isolates grow at 10–35°C with an optimum at 28°C. PCR using primer CgInt [13] to detect Cgsl disclosed a band at ~450 bp similar to that obtained by using Cgsl as a control.

Based on its morphological characteristics, a similar foliar disease observed on "Kousui" in Akita prefecture in the Tohoku region of Japan was thought to be anthracnose caused by *Colletotrichum acutatum* sensu lato [14]. However, DNA-based identification failed to establish *C. acutatum* sensu lato as the cause of JPA in the pear orchards of other regions of Japan [12, 15]. Therefore, most of the JPA pathogens in Japan are probably caused by Cgsl.

In China, *C. fructicola* was reported as an anthracnose pathogen causing leaf black spot in sandy pear (*Pyrus pyrifolia* Nakai) in 2015 [16]. In 2019, 12 species of *Colletotrichum* spp. including *C. fructicola* and *C. gloeosporioides* were reported as

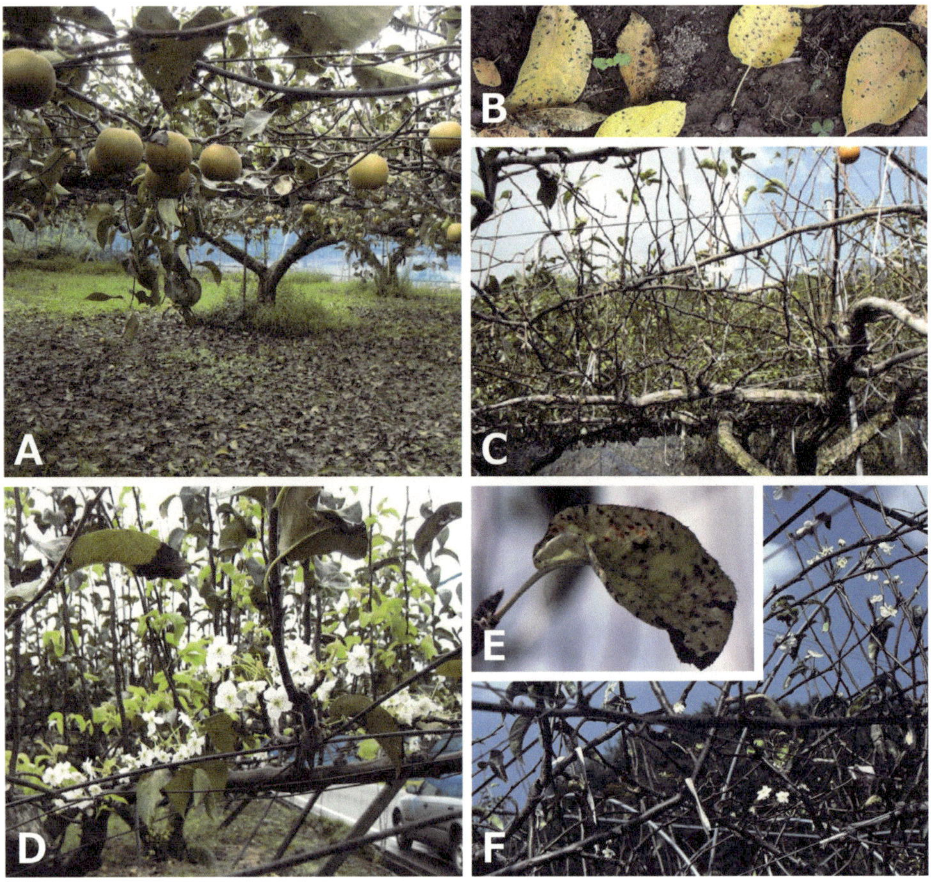


**Figure 2.**
*Defoliation in summer and flowering in autumn caused by* Colletotrichum gloeosporioides *sensu lato observed in Japanese pear cv. Housui (*Pyrus pyrifolia *Nakai var.* culta *Nakai) in the fields. (A) Severe defoliation in the field of Japanese pear cv. Housui (*Pyrus pyrifolia *Nakai var.* culta *Nakai) (courtesy M. Suzuki); (B) yellowish discolored fallen leaves with a lot of black spots; (C) twigs with no leaves in summer; (D) emerging of new leaves and flowers soon after intense defoliation, the number of flowers in the next spring was dramatically decreased to cause great yield loss in the following year (courtesy M. Suzuki); (E) black spots symptoms on newly emerged leaves after defoliation, these new leaves quickly withered; (F) defoliation of almost all of the leaves in the summer, leading to the reduced vigor of the trees.*

pathogens causing anthracnose on pear leaves and fruit [17]. In Japan, we did not confirm anthracnose symptoms on Japanese pear fruit caused by Cgsl. A report of JPA outbreak from Akita prefecture, where they suspected *C. acutatum* sensu lato to be the causal agent, did not include anthracnose on fruits. However, *C. fioriniae* destroyed "Niitaka" fruit in Oita prefecture in 2013 [18]. In Korea, two species of *C. gloeosporioides* sensu lato [19] and *C. acutatum* sensu lato [20] were reported as the causal organisms of Asian pear fruit rot.

The *Compendium of Apple and Pear Diseases and Pests* describes apple and pear bitter rot as a common disease and mentions that apple anthracnose causes speckle spots followed by defoliation [21]. In 1988, Leite et al. [22] described a new apple leaf spot disease on the Gala and Golden Delicious cultivars in Brazil and demonstrated that it was caused by *G. cingulata* which is the sexual stage of *C. gloeosporioides*. This disease was named *Glomerella* leaf spot (GLS). This report was the first to cite any *Colletotrichum* sp. as the causative agent of leaf spot in the apple orchard. Under favorable conditions, a GLS infestation may result in 75% defoliation by harvest time. It can weaken trees and reducing yield [23, 24]. GLS was first reported in the United States in 1998 as a severe leaf spot on Gala apples [25].

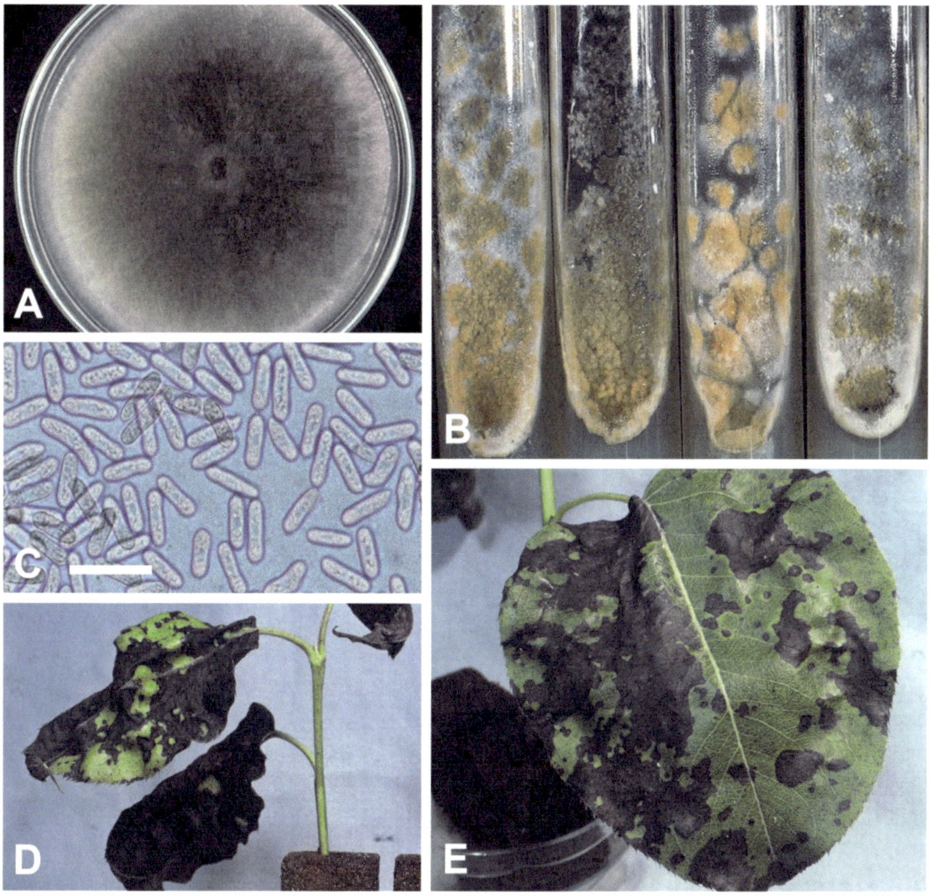


**Figure 3.**
*Causal pathogen of Japanese pear (*Pyrus pyrifolia *Nakai var.* culta *Nakai) anthracnose and representative symptoms induced by inoculation of conidial suspension under unwounded condition. (A) A 7-day-old colony of strain C-17 grown on potato dextrose agar medium at 25°C, (B) salmon pink spore mass produced on spore-inducing medium ($K_2HPO_4$ 1 g, $MgSO_4$ 0.5 g, peptone 5 g, lactose 10 g, agar 30 g, distilled water 1000 mL), (C) conidia of strain C-17 produced on spore-inducing medium (scale bar = 20 μm), (D) shoots of Japanese pear cv. Housui that showed severe symptoms by inoculation of conidial suspensions of strain C-15 under unwounded condition, (E) black spot lesions of different sizes reproduced by unwounded inoculation of spore suspension.*

*Colletotrichum karstii* has been reported as a new GLS pathogen [26]. Apple GLS caused by *Glomerella cingulata* was reported in China in 2012 [27].

On the other hand, the compendium makes no reference to foliar anthracnose in pear or Asian pear [21], which occurs on leaves and causes severe defoliation. Since this disease may be unique to Asian and Japanese pear, further investigations of its causal pathogens using molecular diagnostic tools are required.

## 3. Development of fungicide control technology for JPA (until 2004)

Our aim was to select efficacious fungicides at the Fruit Tree Experiment Station in Saga prefecture [1, 28]. The JPA fungicide spray timing was the same as that for Japanese pear ring rot caused by *Botryosphaeria berengeriana* De Notaris f. sp. piricola (Nose) in Koganezawa and Sakuma. Thus, these diseases had to be addressed simultaneously, and fungicide efficacy on ring rot was also evaluated [2].

### 3.1 Selection of effective fungicides

#### *3.1.1 Benzimidazoles, benomyl, and thiophanate-methyl*

Benzimidazole fungicides, which inhibit β-tubulin assembly during mitosis, were introduced ca. 1970. This group includes thiophanate-methyl, carbendazim, and benomyl. Benomyl (methyl [1-(butylcarbamoyl)benzimidazole-2-yl]carbamate) was registered under the brand name Benlate (50% wettable powder) by DuPont in Japan in 1971. Sumitomo Chemical Co., Ltd. (Tokyo, Japan) acquired the business in 2002. Thiophanate-methyl, dimethyl 4,4′-(o-phenylene) bis(3-thioallophanate), was registered in Japan in 1971 under the brand name Topsin-M (70% wettable powder; Nippon Soda Co., Ltd., Tokyo, Japan).

Initially, benomyl and thiophanate-methyl were considered as broad-spectrum fungicides with low phytotoxicity, and these materials controlled the diseases caused by *Ascomycetes*, *Deuteromycetes*, and *Basidiomycetes*. Thus, benzimidazoles were frequently used on a wide range of crop groups. However, the pathogens rapidly developed field resistance; then, the usage of these fungicides decreased over time. They are still widely used on certain crops as they are broad-spectrum antifungal agents. In Japan, they are often applied to fruit trees.

Benomyl WP and thiophanate-methyl WP have been used since 1975 to prevent Asian pear scab (APS) caused by *Venturia nashicola*. These benzimidazoles were initially highly efficacious [29]. Therefore, their usage increased in frequency. APS fungus resistant to benzimidazoles were first detected in 1980 [30–33]; then the efficacy of benzimidazoles at suppressing APS diminished. In 1985, a demethylation inhibitor (DMI) with significant efficacy against the APS pathogen was introduced [34–37]; then, the use of benzimidazoles against APS was discontinued.

Benzimidazoles are very effective at suppressing ring rot [38] and powdery mildew [39] caused by *Phyllactinia mali* (Duby) U. Braun. Instead of targeting scab disease from April to June, growers applied benzimidazoles three to four times from mid-June until harvest to prevent ring rot and powdery mildew. This time window is also the main JPA infection period. Since benzimidazoles were effective against anthracnose caused by *C. gloeosporioides* sensu lato [11, 40–43], these materials were used often to prevent JPA.

#### *3.1.2 Fungicide screening against the JPA pathogen*

We conducted preventive application screening using "Housui" leaves and using fungicides registered for Japanese pears in Japan. Fungicide suspensions were diluted to predetermine concentrations and sprayed onto the leaves on branches excised from the "Housui" tree. The leaves were air-dried and sprayed with a Cgsl spore suspension ($\sim$105 $mL^{-1}$). The inoculated leaves were maintained in humid conditions at 25°C for 2 days. The lesions on the leaves were counted 7 days after inoculation.

Propyneb WP, dithianon FL, fluazinam FL, organic copper FL, azoxystrobin FL, kresoxim-methyl DF, captan WP, and mancozeb WP had excellent preventive efficacies (**Table 1**). In contrast, the benzimidazoles, benomyl, and thiophanate-methyl which were previously considered effective against anthracnose caused by Cgsl [11] were significantly less efficacious against both strains than the best treatment (**Table 1**), indicating the presence of benzimidazole-resistant strains.

| Generic name | Trade name in Japan | FRAC code | Active ingredient (%) | Rate applied ($mg\ L^{-1}$)[1] | Control (%)[2] | |
|---|---|---|---|---|---|---|
| | | | | | Strain C-17 | Strain C-25 |
| Benomyl | Benlate WP | 1 | 50.0 | 250 | 0 | 90.2 |
| Thiophanate-methyl | Topsin-M WP | 1 | 70.0 | 700 | 6.8 | 93.6 |
| Fluazinam | Frowncide SC | 29 | 39.5 | 198 | 100 | 100 |
| Dithianon | Delan FL | M9 | 42.0 | 420 | 98.9 | 99.1 |
| Propineb | Antracol WG | M3 | 70.0 | 1400 | 100 | 100 |
| Kresoxim-methyl | Storoby DF | 11 | 50.0 | 250 | 100 | 98.6 |
| Azoxystrobin | Amistar 10 FL | 11 | 10.0 | 100 | 99.6 | 99.8 |
| Oxyquinoline copper | Quinondo FL | — | 35.0 | 350 | 98.5 | 96.8 |
| Captan | Orthocide WP 80 | M4 | 80.0 | 1000 | 93.8 | 94.3 |
| Captan/oxyquinoline copper | Oxyrane WP | M4/– | 20.0/30.0 | 400/600 | 74.1 | 70.1 |
| Captan/benomyl | Caplate WP | M4/1 | 60.0/10.0 | 1000/167 | 86.8 | 91.6 |
| Iminoctadine tris(albesilate) | Bellkute WP | M7 | 40.0 | 400 | 53.1 | 46.4 |
| Mancozeb | Zimandithane WP | M3 | 80.0 | 2000 | 95.1 | 96.1 |
| Hexaconazole | Anvil FL | 3 | 2.0 | 20 | 33.8 | 28.6 |
| Difenoconazole | Score WG | 3 | 10.0 | 25 | 36.3 | 40.0 |
| Fosetyl | Aliette WP | P7 | 80.0 | 1000 | 7.4 | 8.1 |
| Mepanipyrim | Frupica FL | 9 | 40.0 | 200 | 0 | 0 |

[1]*Standards on the use of pesticide in agricultural chemical regulation law of Japan.*
[2]*Control (%) = (1 – average lesion number per leaf with fungicide application/average lesion number per control leaf)* × *100.*

**Table 1.**
*Preventive effect of various fungicides for anthracnose on Japanese pear.*

### *3.1.3 Confirming the lack of susceptibility to benzimidazoles among the JPA pathogen strains*

Based on the results of the previous study (**Table 1**), we investigated the susceptibility of 122 Cgsl strains to benomyl. The strains were isolated from infected leaves collected in 1999 from nine orchards known to have frequent outbreaks of this disease. Before the experiment, the pathogenicity of these strains was confirmed by inoculation tests. The strains were divided into those with minimum inhibitory concentration (MIC) $\leq 0.39$ mg $L^{-1}$ and those with MIC $\geq 1600$ mg $L^{-1}$ (**Table 2**). The former were deemed susceptible. The latter were considered highly resistant and were prevalent at all nine orchards investigated (**Table 2**). These highly resistant strains were also highly resistant to thiophanate-methyl, which are very similar to benomyl in the mode of action (**Table 3**). When "Housui" leaves were sprayed with benomyl (250 mg $L^{-1}$) and then inoculated with the highly

| Source orchard | Variety | Number of strains | Number of strains for each MIC (mg $L^{-1}$) range | | |
|---|---|---|---|---|---|
| | | | 0.78 | 25–100 | >1600 |
| Minamihata-1 | Housui | 13 | 0 | 0 | 13 |
| Minamihata-2 | Housui | 15 | 4 | 0 | 11 |
| Minamihata-3 | Housui | 14 | 0 | 0 | 14 |
| Minamihata-4 | Niitaka | 13 | 0 | 0 | 13 |
| Okawa-1 | Housui | 10 | 0 | 0 | 10 |
| Okawa-2 | Housui | 10 | 1 | 0 | 9 |
| Okawa-3 | Housui | 12 | 0 | 0 | 12 |
| Okawa-4 | Housui | 22 | 4 | 0 | 18 |
| Okawa-5 | Niitaka | 13 | 3 | 0 | 10 |
| Total | | 122 | 12 (9.8)[1] | 0 (0.0) | 110 (90.2) |

[1]*Values in parentheses are the percentage of the total for each category.*

**Table 2.**
*Benomyl sensitivity of* C. gloeosporioides *sensu lato, the causal organism of anthracnose in Japanese pear varieties "Housui" and "Niitaka" at Imari district in Saga Prefecture in 1999.*

| Strain | Location of isolation[1] | Year of isolation | $EC_{50}$ (mg $L^{-1}$) values of | |
|---|---|---|---|---|
| | | | Benomyl | Thiophanate-methyl |
| SCG-25 | Minamihata town | 1999 | 0.151 | 0.151 |
| SCG-30 | Ohkawa town | 1999 | 0.166 | 0.206 |
| SCG-64 | Ohkawa town | 1999 | 0.155 | 0.186 |
| SCG-08 | Minamihata town | 1999 | 485 | 2856 |
| SCG-17 | Minamihata town | 1999 | 481 | 2386 |
| SCG-72 | Ohkawa town | 1999 | 491 | 3211 |

[1]*Minamihata town and Ohkawa town are both in the Imari area of Saga prefecture.*

**Table 3.**
*Effect of benomyl and thiophanate-methyl on the mycelial growth of benzimidazole-sensitive (SCG-25, SCG-30, and SCG-64) strains and highly benzimidazole-resistant (SCG-08, SCG-17, and SCG-72) strains of C. gloeosporioides obtained from lesions of Japanese pear anthracnose.*

| Strain | Benomyl (250 mg $L^{-1}$) sprayed trees | | Control trees | | Control (%)[2] |
|---|---|---|---|---|---|
| | Tested leaves | Lesions/leaf | Tested leaves | Lesions/leaf | |
| SCG-25 | 27 | 14.6[a] | 26 | 126.8[a] | 88.5[a] |
| SCG-30 | 28 | 6.3[a] | 24 | 98.6[a] | 93.6[a] |
| SCG-17 | 26 | 152.5[b] | 21 | 142.3[a] | 0[b] |
| SCG-72 | 22 | 96.5[b] | 24 | 106.8[a] | 9.6[b] |

[1]*The Japanese pear variety "Housui" (2-year-old trees) was sprayed with wettable powder of benomyl and thoroughly dried. Conidial suspensions (approx. $10^5$ $mL^{-1}$) of each strain (benzimidazole-sensitive strains, SCG-25 and SCG-30; highly benzimidazole-resistant strains, SCG-17, SCG-72) were then inoculated. Seven days after inoculation, the development of symptoms was assessed. Values followed by different letter differ significantly in a multiple comparison based on the Tukey–Kramer HSD test ($P < 0.05$).*
[2]*Control (%) = (1 – average lesion number per leaf on the trees with benomyl application/average lesion number per leaf on the control trees) × 100.*

**Table 4.**
*Control efficacy of benomyl against benzimidazole-sensitive (SCG-25 and SCG-30) strains and highly benzimidazole-resistant (SCG-17 and SCG-72) strains of* C. gloeosporioides *sensu lato on the leaves of the Japanese pear variety "Housui".*[1]

resistant Cgsl strains, the treated leaves became severely diseased, i.e., benomyl did not suppress JPA (**Table 4**).

Benzimidazole-resistant Cgsl that occurred at a high frequency over a wide range in the Japanese pear-growing areas of Saga prefecture caused benzimidazoles to be no longer effective against JPA. In addition, benzimidazole-resistant Cgsl was also confirmed in Chiba, Oita, and Kochi prefectures. Only highly resistant strains were observed in Chiba prefecture [44], a mixture of highly and moderately resistant strains was detected in Oita prefecture [45], and only moderately resistant strains were confirmed for Kochi prefecture [12].

### 3.2 Change in detection frequency of highly benzimidazole-resistant strains after discontinuing benzimidazoles

To determine the changes in detection frequency of benzimidazole-resistant strains, Cgsl strains from orchards where benzimidazoles were discontinued were challenged with benomyl in 1999, 2000, 2001, and 2004. The discontinuation of benzimidazole fungicides in each orchard was confirmed from fungicide spray records. The frequency of benzimidazole-resistant strain ranged from 81 to 88% during the study, and there was no indication of a reduction over time (**Figure 4**). Therefore, reintroduction of benzimidazoles to the pear-producing areas of this region was not recommended.

The proportion of benzimidazole-resistant Cgsl strains causing JPA did not decrease even 4 years after discontinuation. Pathogen populations in abscised leaves may be carried over to the following year, and pathogen latently infected with twigs may remain viable for several years [46]. Also, both the resistant and sensitive strains may have similar levels of competitiveness or fitness.

Impacts on the detection frequency of benzimidazole-resistant isolates after the discontinuation were highly variable for other crops and pathogens. The discontinuation of benzimidazole immediately reduced the ratios of highly resistant *Botrytis cinerea* strains causing grape gray mold [47] and *Gloeosporium theae-sinensis* causing tea anthracnose [48]. The ratio of highly resistant *Venturia nashicola* strains causing Japanese pear scab was immediately reduced upon benzimidazole discontinuation; however, the overall ratio of resistant strains did not decline as moderately and weakly resistant strains emerged [49]. As with JPA, the frequency of highly

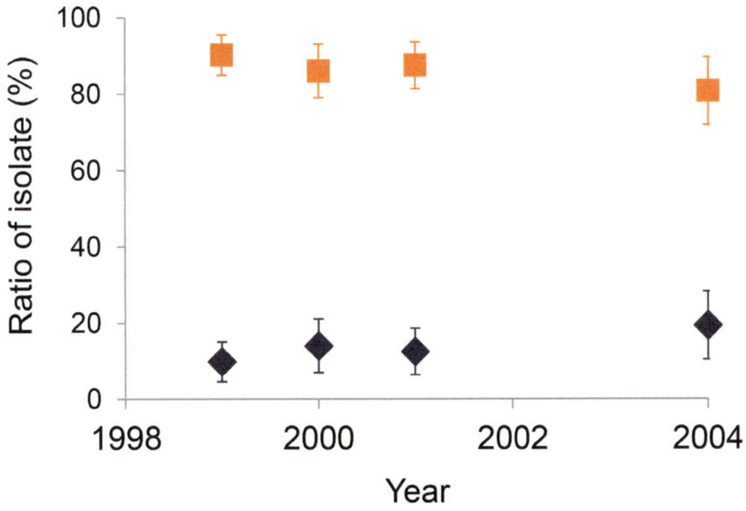


**Figure 4.**
*Change in detection frequency of highly benzimidazole-resistant strains after discontinuing benzimidazoles.*

resistant strains did not change for *V. nashicola* [50–52] and *V. inaequalis* which cause pear and apple scab, respectively [53].

### 3.3 Residual efficacy and rainfastness of fungicides effective against benzimidazole-resistant strains of *Colletotrichum gloeosporioides* sensu lato

#### *3.3.1 Residual efficacy of the sprayed fungicides*

To ensure effective pathogen control, it is important to know the length of time fungicidal efficacy persists after product application. Experiments were conducted to determine the period of residual fungicidal activity against JPA. Each fungicide was sprayed onto "Housui" trees in Japanese pear orchards where JPA had never been previously detected. Branches with their leaves intact were excised and brought to the laboratory. A conidial suspension (~105 mL$^{-1}$) was sprayed onto the leaves. Relative product efficacy was scored based on the number of foliar lesions. Duration of efficacy after product application was also evaluated. Two experiments, where each had different sets of treatments, were conducted in late July and mid-September 2002. In each treatment, 100 leaves from new branches were examined.

For the late July experiment, a mean % disease control (=% suppression of the mean disease incidence relative to the mean disease incidence of the positive control) of >70% was taken as the threshold of satisfactory disease control. The disease control sustainability was measured as days post-application. Dithianon FL and azoxystrobin FL continued to suppress disease onset for 14 days after application (**Table 5**). Satisfactory disease control was observed for fluazinam FL, kresoxim-methyl DF, and captan/benomyl WP until 7 days after application. However, at 14 days after the application, the disease control effect (%) dropped to 69 and 68% for fluazinam FL and captan/benomyl WP, respectively, and 15% for kresoxim-methyl DF. Thus, these fungicides, especially kresoxim-methyl DF, had comparatively shorter disease control durations.

In the mid-September experiment, dithianon FL presented with satisfactory disease control efficacy until 14 days after application as in the previous experiment (**Table 6**). The efficacies of the other fungicides were inferior to that of dithianon FL, and none of the treatment achieved the mean % disease control of >70%. Propineb WG showed no disease control efficacy whatsoever.

| Generic name | Trade name in Japan | FRAC code | Active ingredient (%) | Rate applied (mg L$^{-1}$) | Changes of control (%)[1] | | |
|---|---|---|---|---|---|---|---|
| | | | | | 7 days after | 14 days after | 21 days after |
| Azoxystrobin | Amistar 10 FL | 11 | 10.0 | 100 | 84 | 78 | 45 |
| Kresoxim-methyl | Storobi DF | 11 | 50.0 | 250 | 75 | 15 | 20 |
| Dithianon | Delan FL | M9 | 42.0 | 420 | 83 | 90 | 50 |
| Fluazinam | Frowncide SC | 29 | 39.5 | 198 | 77 | 69 | 39 |
| Captan/benomyl | Caplate WP | M4/1 | 60.0/10.0 | 1000/167 | 98 | 68 | 46 |

[1]*Control (%) = (1 – mean ratio of diseased leaves of trees with fungicide application/mean ratio of diseased leaves of trees without fungicide application) × 100.*

**Table 5.**
*Residence period of sprayed fungicides against anthracnose on the Japanese pear "Housui" (1).*

| Generic name | Trade name in Japan | FRAC code | Active ingredient (%) | Rate applied (mg L$^{-1}$) | Changes of control (%)[1] | | |
|---|---|---|---|---|---|---|---|
| | | | | | 7 days after | 14 days after | 21 days after |
| Dithianon | Delan FL | M9 | 42.0 | 420 | 92 | 83 | 41 |
| Fluazinam | Frowncide SC | 29 | 39.5 | 198 | 59 | 0 | 0 |
| Captan/oxyquinoline copper | Oxyrane WP | M4/– | 20.0/30.0 | 400/600 | 67 | 57 | 0 |
| Copper (II) sulfate | IC Bordeaux 48Q | M1 | 31.2 | 10,400 | 69 | 70 | 0 |
| Propineb | Antracol WG | M3 | 70.0 | 1400 | 0 | 0 | — |

[1]*See* ***Table 5****.*

**Table 6.**
*Residence period of sprayed fungicides against anthracnose on the Japanese pear "Housui" (2).*

### *3.3.2 Rainfastness of the sprayed fungicides*

The JPA pathogen propagates and infects during rainfall. The amount of rain determines the degree of attenuation of the fungicide spray on the pear leaves. Thus, the establishment of the rainfastness of various fungicides helps develop an efficient and successful disease control program.

Several fungicide treatments were tested on pot-grown "Housui" trees in 2002. One day after fungicide application, a rainfall treatment of 17 mm h$^{-1}$ and 50 mm d$^{-1}$ was conducted using an artificial rainfall machine (DIK-6000; Daiki Rika Kogyo Co., Ltd., Tokyo, Japan). The leaves were excised from each tree and inoculated with a pathogen conidial suspension (2 × 105 conidia mL$^{-1}$ and 4.0 mL leaf$^{-1}$) before treatment application, at 100, 200, 300, and 400 mm cumulative rain. The efficacy of the fungicide was visually assessed to estimate % disease control.

The level of JPA suppression was high when the leaves received no rainfall, resulting in 100% disease control (=no disease development). As expected, disease control efficacy decreased with increasing cumulative rainfall. For azoxystrobin FL and dithianon FL, the disease control was ≥70% at 200 mm cumulative rainfall after fungicide application (**Figure 5**). Fluazinam FL and kresoxim-methyl DF achieved ≥70% disease control at 100 mm cumulative rainfall, but the disease control efficacy fell to <70% at 200 mm cumulative rainfall. For captan/oxyquinoline-copper WP and captan/benomyl WP, the mean disease control efficacy was 90% and >60% at 100 mm cumulative rainfall but sharply declined to 0 and 23%, respectively, at 200 mm cumulative rainfall (**Figure 5**).

### *3.3.3 Preventive efficacy of fungicide treatments against JPA in Japanese pear orchards*

In the "Housui" orchard, an experiment was conducted over three seasons to determine the efficacy of preventive fungicide application against JPA. Two experiments were conducted in late June 2000. Trees were sprayed at 10- to 14-day intervals. When the cumulative rainfall after the previous application was

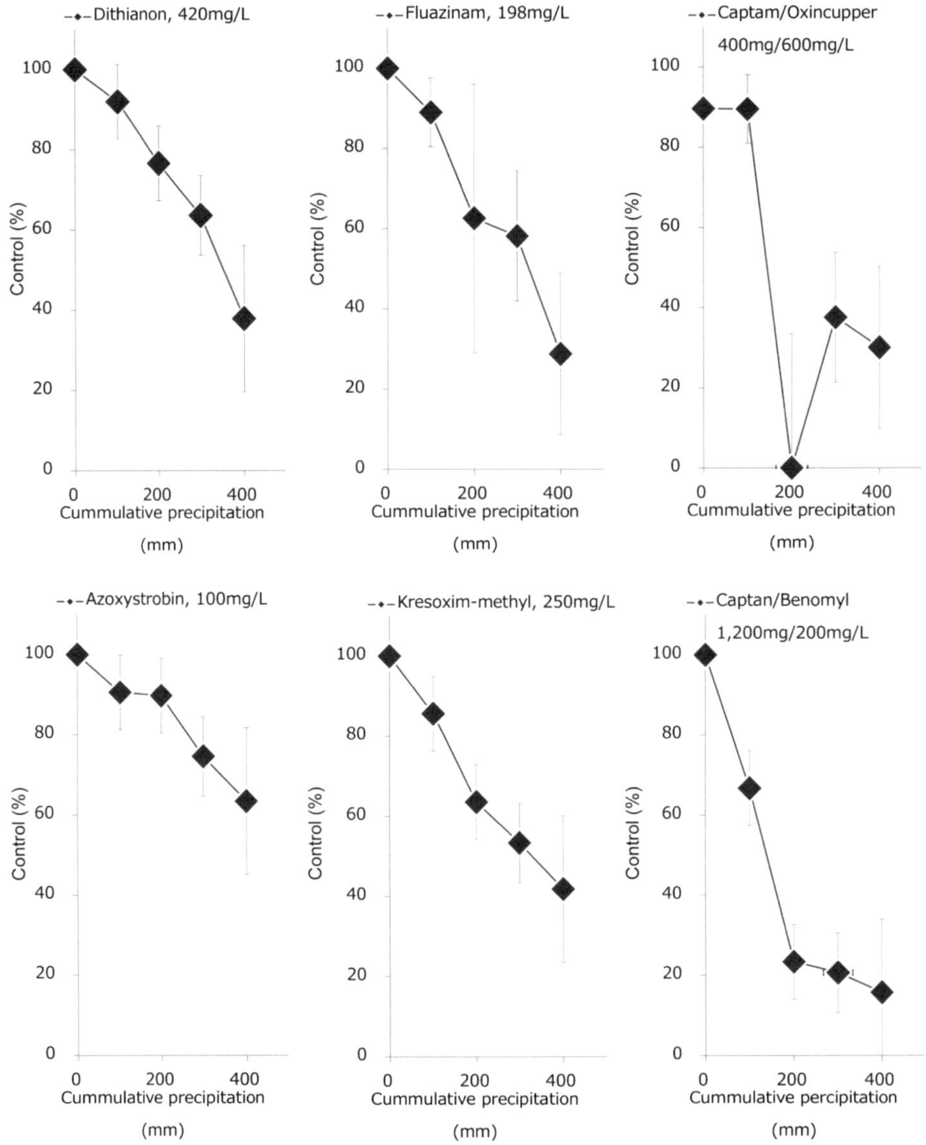


**Figure 5.**
*Reduction of the control effect of various fungicides on Japanese pear anthracnose associated with artificial rainfall after spraying; error bar, 95% confidence interval.*

>200 mm, the trees were immediately resprayed to compensate for the product washed off by the rain. Experiments were conducted in mid-June 2001 and mid-May 2002 using a slightly modified spray guideline. The treatments were applied either 20 days after the previous treatment or when the post-application cumulative rainfall was 200 mm. Several heavy rain events increased the cumulative rainfall to >200 mm, but all fungicide treatments were applied before the cumulative rainfall reached 300 mm.

As with the previous experiments, 70% control was set as the efficacy threshold. For all 3 years, preventive azoxystrobin FL and dithianon FL application provided >70% disease control (**Table 7**). Both treatments resulted in consistently high disease control efficacy as they did in the residual efficacy and rainfastness tests (**Tables 5** and **6**).

Kresoxim-methyl DF demonstrated >80% disease control efficacy in one of the residual activity experimental runs in 2000 and 2002, but the results were not consistent among three trials (**Table 7**). In the other trials, the mean % disease control of kresoxim-methyl DF varied from 15 to 75% in the residual efficacy test (**Table 5**), and the mean % disease control efficacy dropped very sharply to below 70% in the rainfastness test at 200 mm cumulative rain fall (**Figure 5**). Thus, the environmental conditions, especially the amount of precipitations, may negatively impact kresoxim-methyl DF to be effective.

Fluazinam showed good levels of disease control (75%) in this experiment (**Table 7**), but it did not perform well with the residual tests (**Tables 5** and **6**), and the mean % disease control dropped at 200 mm cumulative rainfall (**Figure 5**). A trend with propineb was similar where 80% mean disease control was observed in this experiment, but it did not provide any level of control in the residual efficacy test (**Table 6**). We need to investigate more to determine what created these differences.

The lack of disease prevention efficacy for benomyl WP was expected as benzimidazole-resistant strains were detected in this orchard (**Table 7**). The disease prevention efficacy of captan/benomyl WP was ~70% in all 3 years, possibly because of benzimidazole-resistant strains and low rainfastness of captan, which is also shown in the rainfastness test (**Figure 5**). Thus, captan probably needs to be applied with a non-benzimidazole material, and if sprayed with captan alone, it should be applied using a 100 mm cumulative rainfall threshold.

Fungicide application on a 10- to 14-day schedule from the first cover until harvest is the main disease control method that growers use. JPA is very difficult to control after the leaves have been infected with it. Dithianon, fluazinam, strobilurin-quinone outside inhibitor (ST-QoI) fungicides, and captan/benomyl WP provide good disease control when they are applied preventively.

#### *3.3.4 Use of fungicides effective to JPA against ring rot of Japanese pear*

We evaluated fungicide efficacy against Japanese pear ring rot because spray application timing was the same as that for JPA [2]. The ST-QoIs azoxystrobin and kresoxim-methyl were highly efficacious against ring rot (**Table 8**). Captan/benomyl also showed high efficacy. In contrast, the efficacy of dithianon against ring rot was highly variable (from 100 to 0% control) during the years it was tested. Fluazinam provided unsatisfactory disease control efficacy against ring rot.

| Generic name | Trade name in Japan | FRAC code | Active ingredient (%) | Rate applied (mg $L^{-1}$) | Control (%)[2] | | | |
|---|---|---|---|---|---|---|---|---|
| | | | | | In 2000 | | In 2001 | In 2002 |
| | | | | | Experiment 1 | Experiment 2 | | |
| Benomyl | Benlate WP | 1 | 50.0 | 250 | 3 | — | — | — |
| Fluazinam | Frowncide SC | 29 | 39.5 | 198 | 75 | — | 85 | |
| Dithianon | Delan FL | M9 | 42.0 | 420 | 82 | 99 | 93 | 95 |
| Propineb | Antracol WG | M3 | 70.0 | 1400 | 80 | — | — | — |
| Kresoxim-methyl | Storobi DF | 11 | 50.0 | 250 | 61 | 79 | 69 | 87 |
| Azoxystrobin | Amistar 10 FL | 11 | 10.0 | 100 | 81 | 87 | 91 | 88 |
| Oxyquinoline copper | Quinondo FL | — | 35.0 | 350 | 26 | | — | — |
| Captan/benomyl | Caplate WP | M4/1 | 60.0/10.0 | 1000/167 | 65 | — | 72 | 67 |
| Hexaconazole | Anvil FL | 3 | 2.0 | 20 | 29 | — | — | — |
| | | | Ratio of diseased leaves in control | | 67.0% | 70.5% | 38.3% | 63.0% |

[1]*Sprays have been done in May to August each year.*
[2]*See* ***Table 5****.*

**Table 7.**
*Control effect of several fungicides against anthracnose on the Japanese pear "Housui".*[1]

| Generic name | Trade name in Japan | FRAC code | Active ingredient (%) | Rate applied (mg $L^{-1}$) | Control (%)[2] | | |
|---|---|---|---|---|---|---|---|
| | | | | | **In 2000** | **In 2001** | **In 2002** |
| Benomyl | Benlate WP | 1 | 50.0 | 250 | 32 | — | — |
| Fluazinam | Frowncide SC | 29 | 39.5 | 198 | 30 | 37 | — |
| Dithianon | Delan FL | M9 | 42.0 | 420 | 19 | 0 | 100 |
| Kresoxim-methyl | Storobi DF | 11 | 50.0 | 250 | 39 | 70 | 54 |
| Azoxystrobin | Amistar 10 FL | 11 | 10.0 | 100 | 47 | 73 | 100 |
| Oxyquinoline copper | Quinondo FL | — | 35.0 | 350 | 0 | — | — |
| Captan/benomyl | Caplate WP | M4/1 | 60.0/10.0 | 1000/167 | 17 | 69 | 78 |
| | | | Ratio of diseased leaves in control | | 45.0% | 40.6% | 10.9% |

[1]*Sprays have been done in May to August each year.*
[2]*See **Table 5**.*

**Table 8.**
*Control effect of several fungicides against ring rot on the Japanese pear "Housui".*[1]

### 3.4 Temporary suspension of the 1999 JPA outbreak

Before the 1999 JPA outbreak, the main disease to control in Japanese pear cultivation was Asian pear scab (APS). Sterol demethylation inhibitor (DMI), belonging to sterol biosynthesis inhibitors (SBIs), was the product most frequently used to control this disease. Iminoctadine tris(albesilate), captan/oxyquinoline copper, and captan were applied for APS a few times. Benzimidazoles were applied three to four times to control ring rot and powdery mildew. However, by 2000, benzimidazoles were no longer recommended in Japanese pear production due to its resistance issue. In their place, local systemic fungicides such as strobilurins (azoxystrobin and kresoxim-methyl) and protective fungicides such as dithianon and fluazinam were applied.

Dithianon FL, fluazinam FL, ST-QoI fungicides (azoxystrobin FL, kresoxim-methyl DF), captan/oxyquinoline copper WP, and captan/benomyl WP were effective against JPA, APS, and ring spot, and all except dithianon were efficacious against powdery mildew. Therefore, these materials were incorporated into the spray calendar with heavy reliance on DMIs, which were popular at that time. As a result, JPA incidence was drastically reduced.

Although Dithianon FL has high JPA control efficacy, it has a 60-day pre-harvest interval (PHI) in Japan. Thus, it cannot be used after mid-June which is a critical JPA control period. The PHI of fluazinam SC was 30 days, so it could be applied until mid-July. Captan/oxyquinoline copper WP has a very short PHI of only 3 days. On the other hand, it leaves visible residues on the fruit and may not be sprayed too soon before harvest.

In contrast, the ST-QoIs (azoxystrobin FL, kresoxim-methyl DF, and pyraclostrobin with boscalid WP in a pre-mix) showed excellent anti-JPA efficacy [28, 44, 54]. These fungicides have a 1-day PHI and can, therefore, be applied up until the day before harvest. Moreover, they leave no visible residues on the fruit. Consequently, the application frequency of ST-QoIs against JPA increased.

## 4. Emergence of strobilurin (ST)-QoI fungicide-resistant strains and new treatment recommendations after 2011

### 4.1 ST-QoIs

ST-QoIs or strobilurins were first used in the 1990s and became one of the most important fungicides of the past 25 years. They inhibit ubiquinol oxidation at the quinone outside (Qo) binding site on the cytochrome bc1 complex in the inner mitochondrial membranes of fungi [55]. At the time of introduction, ST-QoIs showed very high efficacy against many different pathogen-crop combinations; however, ST-QoI fungicides are highly prone to inducing resistance in target pathogens that can lead to reduced field efficacy. The ST-QoI resistance risk has been rated high by the Fungicide Resistance Action Committee (FRAC) [56]. ST-QoI-resistant strains have been detected in ~60 fungal and oomycete pathogen species worldwide including powdery and downy mildews, gray mold, *Alternaria* disease, scab, and anthracnose [57]. Currently, disease control strategies that are overly reliant on ST-QoIs are considered undesirable [57]. A major source of ST-QoI resistance is a point mutation in the cytochrome b gene that substitutes alanine for glycine at amino acid position 143. This site may be associated with the pathogen binding affinity of the fungicide [58].

In Japan, ST-QoI resistance has emerged in cucumber powdery mildew (*Podosphaera xanthii*), downy mildew (*Pseudoperonospora cubensis*) [59, 60], eggplant leaf mold (*Mycovellosiella nattrassii*) [61], *Corynespora* cucumber leaf spot (*Corynespora cassicola*) [62], citrus gray mold (*Botrytis cinerea*) [63], European pear black spot (*Alternaria alternata*) [64], *Alternaria* apple blotch (*Alternaria alternata* apple pathotype) [65], grapevine leaf blight (*Pseudocercospora vitis*) [66], strawberry anthracnose (*Colletotrichum gloeosporioides*) [67, 68], tea gray blight (*Pestalotiopsis longiseta*) [69], apple bitter rot (*Colletotrichum gloeosporioides*) [70], rice blast (*Magnaporthe oryzae*) [71], mango anthracnose (*Colletotrichum gloeosporioides*) [72], apple scab (*Venturia inaequalis*) [73], grapevine downy mildew (*Plasmopara viticola*) [74], cucurbits gummy stem blight (*Didymella bryoniae*) [75], chrysanthemum white rust (*Puccinia horiana*) [76], wheat powdery mildew (*Erysiphe* (Blumeria) *graminis f.sp. tritici*), and strawberry powdery mildew (*Sphaerotheca aphanis* var. aphanis) [77].

### 4.2 Emergence of strains of *Colletotrichum gloeosporioides* sensu lato resistant to ST-QoIs

Over nearly a decade in the Saga and Oita prefectures, ST-QoIs were sprayed three to four times annually between June and early August as countermeasures against JPA and APS. That is, many growers heavily depended on ST-QoIs, especially late in the season because ST-QoIs are phytotoxic to Japanese pear leaves at their early growth stage. In addition, ST-QoIs were also highly efficacious against APS [78, 79].

The alternative material, thiuram FL, has a 30-day PHI; therefore, it cannot be used after mid-July. The other options, such as iminoctadine tris(albesilate)/captan WP, have a relatively shorter PHI (14 days), and captan WP has a 3-day PHI. Captan/oxyquinoline copper WP (3-day PHI), captan WP (3-day PHI), and iminoctadine tris(albesilate)/captan WP (14-day PHI) showed adequate efficacy against JPA [28, 44, 54, 80]. However, the ST-QoIs were preferred over these choices by growers as they were more effective than these; in addition, the common component of these materials, captan, tends to cause stains on the fruit.

As JPA became very prevalent in 2010–2011 in the Oita and Saga prefectures where above-mentioned spraying system. We assessed ST-QoI sensitivity in Cgsl isolates by placing mycelial discs on potato dextrose agar (PDA) containing 100 μg $mL^{-1}$ azoxystrobin and 1000 μg $mL^{-1}$ salicylhydroxamic acid (SHAM). Mycelial elongation was measured 4 days post-inoculation [81]. Isolates from Saga [80] and Oita [45] prefecture grew on the PDA containing azoxystrobin (**Table 9, Figure 6**).

To determine the effect of ST-QoI pretreatment on JPA development, conidial suspensions were sprayed on "Housui" leaves previously exposed to azoxystrobin FL. The appearance of JPA lesions caused by the sensitive strain was nearly zero

| Source orchard | Number of tested strains | Number of resistant strains[1] |
|---|---|---|
| Imari district in Saga prefecture | 61 | 20 (32.8%)[2] |
| Hita district in Oita prefecture | 254 | 49 (16.2%) |

[1]*Number of strains that grew on PDA with 1000 μg $mL^{-1}$ SHAM and 100 μg $mL^{-1}$ azoxystrobin cultured 4 days at 25°C.*
[2]*Values in parentheses are the percentage of the resistant strains.*

**Table 9.**
*Azoxystrobin sensitivity of* C. gloeosporioides *sensu lato, the causal organism of anthracnose in Japanese pear varieties "Housui" and "Niitaka" at Imari district in Saga prefecture and Hita district in Oita prefecture both Kyushyu island in 2011.*

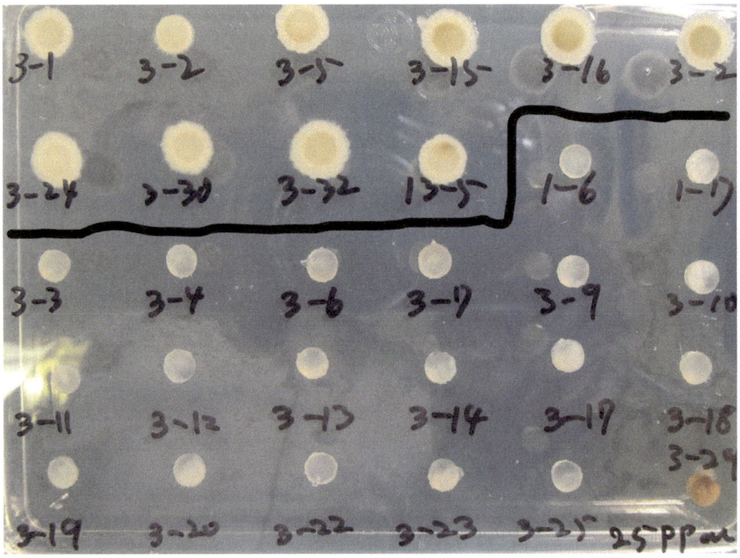


**Figure 6.**
*Effect of azoxystrobin on the mycelial growth of azoxystrobin-resistant and azoxystrobin-sensitive strains of* Colletotrichum gloeosporioides *sensu lato, the causal fungus of Japanese pear anthracnose, 4 days after inoculation of mycelial disks (4 mm) at 25°C; medium, potato dextrose agar medium with 25 μg mL$^{-1}$ azoxystrobin and 1000 μg mL$^{-1}$ SHAM; strains above the line, azoxystrobin-resistant strains; strains under the line, azoxystrobin-sensitive strains.*

(99.6% control). In contrast, the two resistant strains induced many lesions, and there was a very low rate of disease control (**Table 10**).

## 4.3 Effective spraying program in the presence of benzimidazole- and ST-QoI-resistant strains

### *4.3.1 Use of the adjuvant to reduce the risk of phytotoxicity caused by captan*

Products containing captan provide a sufficient level of disease control, but they blemish the fruit to reduce its quality. We investigated the application of spreaders such as Makupika (polyoxyethylene methylpolysiloxane 93.0%; Ishihara Bio-Science Co., Ltd., Tokyo, Japan) and Santokuten 80 (polyoxyethylene dodecyl ether 80.0%; Sumitomo Chemical Co., Ltd., Tokyo, Japan). We also tested the adjuvant

| Strain[2] | Azoxystrobin (100 mg L$^{-1}$) sprayed trees | | Control trees | | Control (%)[3] |
|---|---|---|---|---|---|
| | Tested leaves | Lesions/leaf | Tested leaves | Lesions/leaf | |
| 1–7 | 5 | 0.2 | 5 | 56.8 | 99.6 |
| 3–1 | 5 | 24.8 | 5 | 26.8 | 7.6 |
| 3–2 | 4 | 5.6 | 4 | 16.3 | 65.5 |

[1]*The Japanese pear variety "Housui" (2-year-old trees) were sprayed with wettable powder of azoxystrobin and thoroughly dried. Conidial suspensions (approx. $10^5$ mL$^{-1}$) of each strain (azoxystrobin-sensitive strains, 1–7; azoxystrobin-resistant strains, 3–1, 3–2) were then inoculated. Seven days after inoculation, the development of symptoms was assessed.*
[2]*All strains was isolataed at Hita city of Oita prefecture in 2011.*
[3]*Control (%) = (1 – average lesion number per leaf on the trees with azoxystrobin application/average lesion number per leaf on the control trees) × 100.*

**Table 10.**
*Control efficacy of azoxystorobin against azoxystrobin-sensitive (1–7) strains and azoxystrobin-resistant (3–1 and 3–2) strains of* C. gloeosporioides *sensu lato on the leaves of the Japanese pear variety "Housui".*[1]

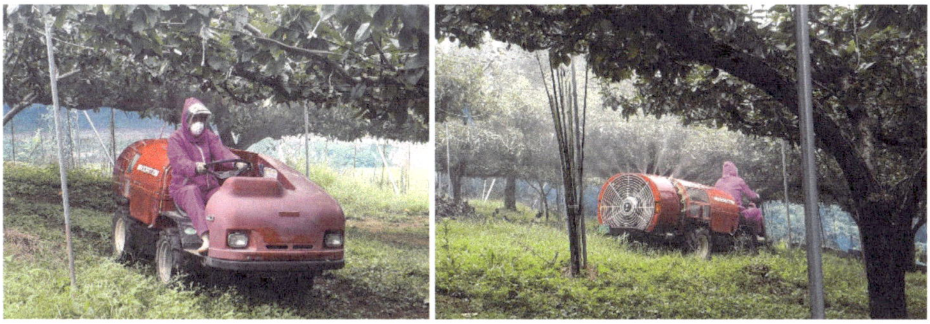

**Figure 7.**
*Fungicide application by air-blast sprayer in the Japanese pear orchard.*

squash (sorbitan fatty acid ester 70.0% and polyoxyethylene resin acid ester 5.5%; Maruwa Biochemical Co., Ltd., Tokyo, Japan). These agents render the spray spots inconspicuous by lowering droplet surface tension. All the three agents reduced the visibility of the captan residues on the plant surfaces. There is a concern that the addition of the spreader can decrease the amount of fungicide that attached to the host plant [82, 83]. However, the mixture had nearly the same efficacy levels as captan alone in the field trial [80].

#### *4.3.2 Current recommendation against JPA*

By 2014, pear producers had fully recognized the presence of benzimidazole- and ST-QoI-resistant pathogen strains and stopped relying on ST-QoI to manage JPA. The current recommended JPA management protocol for Japanese pear is dithianon FL in early June; thiuram FL, captan/oxyquinoline copper, and iminoctadine tris(albesilate)/captan WP from mid-June to early July; and captan WP with a spreader several times after mid-July. The occurrence of JPA has abated as growers are now comparatively less dependent on ST-QoI fungicides [80].

We also advocate proper spray coverage. For example, we recommend every-row spray over alternate-row spray with an air-blast sprayer (**Figure 7**), because of better fungicide coverage achieved by the former. It has been shown in one of our studies that JPA is more effectively controlled when fungicides are sprayed onto all rows [84]. Moreover, infected and abscised leaves should be promptly removed from orchards to reduce the inoculum pool [85].

## 5. Potential options for JPA management in the future

Our test results of 1999 and the data obtained at the experiment stations in other prefectures promoted the registration of additional fungicides to control this disease. In 2019, 11 products were registered for use against JPA in Japan (**Table 11**). This step provides a wider selection of fungicides to control or manage this disease.

### 5.1 Benzylcarbamate (BC)-QoI and pyribencarb

Pyribencarb (methyl{2-chloro-5-[(1E)-1-(6-methyl-2-pyridylmethoxyimino) ethyl]benzyl} carbamate) was formulated by Kumiai Chemical Industry Co., Ltd. and Ihara Chemical Industry Co., Ltd. in Japan. It is a novel benzylcarbamate-type QoI fungicide (BC-QoI) and is active against a wide range of fungal plant pathogens [86]. Pyribencarb is both preventive and curative [87], and its chemical structure

| Generic name | Trade name in Japan | FRAC code | Active ingredient (%) | LPHI[2,4] | MNAPS[3,4] | Rate applied (mg $L^{-1}$)[4] | Resistered year in Japan | References |
|---|---|---|---|---|---|---|---|---|
| Dithianon | Delan FL | M9 | 42.0 | 60 | 4 | 420 | 2003 | [28, 44, 54, 80] |
| Kresoxim-methyl | Storoby DF | 11 | 50.0 | 1 | 3 | 250 | 2003 | [28, 54] |
| Azoxystrobin | Amistar 10 FL | 11 | 10.0 | 1 | 5 | 100 | 2006 | [28, 54] |
| Thiuram | Thionoc FL | M3 | 40.0 | 30 | 5 | 800 | 2008 | [44, 80] |
| Thiuram | Trenox FL | M3 | 40.0 | 30 | 5 | 800 | 2008 | [44, 80] |
| Pyraclostrobin/boscalid | Naria WDG | 11/7 | 6.8/13.6 | 1 | 3 | 34/68 | 2008 | [44] |
| Captan/oxyquinoline copper | Oxyrane WP | M4/M1 | 20.0/30.0 | 3 | 9 | 400/600 | 2009 | [44, 54, 80] |
| Captan | Orthocide WP 80 | M4 | 80.0 | 3 | 9 | 1000 | 2011 | [44, 80] |
| Iminoctadine tris(albesilate)/captan | Dyepower WP | M7/M4 | 20.0/45.0 | 14 | 5 | 200/450 | 2012 | [44] |
| Pyribencarb | Fantasista WDG | 11 | 40.0 | 1 | 3 | 133.3 | 2013 | [44] |
| Captan/penthiopyrad | Fruitguard WDG | M4/7 | 70.0/7.5 | 3 | 3 | 700/75 | 2019 | — |

*[1]2019 confirmed on September 1, 2019.*
*[2]Legal pre-harvest interval.*
*[3]The maximum number of application per season.*
*[4]Standards on the use of pesticide in agricultural chemical regulation law of Japan.*

**Table 11.**
*Registered fungicides for Japanese pear anthracnose in Japan.*[1]

resembles that of ST-QoIs such as kresoxim-methyl and azoxystrobin. However, it has a substitution of the carbonyl moiety on the benzene ring [88]. The binding site of pyribencarb on cytochrome b may be slightly different from that of the ST-QoIs [89].

Pyribencarb more effectively controlled ST-QoI-resistant gray mold isolates than other ST-QoI fungicides [90]. It also had relatively higher efficacy against ST-QoI-resistant *Pestalotiopsis longiseta* which causes tea gray blight [69]. Pyribencarb shows differential cross-resistance patterns to ST-QoI [89].

Since pyribencarb has an excellent effect on JPA [44], it has been recommended to use it in orchards where ST-QoI-resistant strains are present or ST-QoI effects are reduced. However, there have been no reports of the effects of pyribencarb in an orchard where ST-QoI-resistant strains exist. Moreover, the risk of fungal pathogen resistance development of pyribencarb is high [91]. Therefore, it is necessary to take careful approaches to prevent the similar mistake we made with ST-QoIs. The number of pyribencarb application must be limited, and the application should be mixed with another broad-spectrum protective fungicide with a different mode of action.

Pyribencarb may be used less than three times per season on Japanese pear (**Table 11**). The Japan Fungicide Resistance Action Committee (Japan FRAC) guidelines recommend that QoIs be used up to twice annually on Japanese pear [92]. But we believe that it should be used only once between mid-June and early July which is the most critical disease control period of JPA and JPS for proper fungicide resistance management. In addition, pyribencarb must always be co-applied with the protective (multisite) fungicide such as captan, thiuram, iminoctadine tris (albesilate), and iminoctadine tris(albesilate)/captan to reduce the resistant risk. This treatment protocol may enhance disease control efficacy, lower pathogen density, and delay resistant strain development. In the future, comparative field trials would help validate the efficacy of the current treatment recommendations.

### 5.2 Benzodioxoles and fludioxonil

Fludioxonil is a benzodioxole that affects the signal transduction in the target fungal pathogen. These agents are also known as phenylpyrroles or PP-fungicides. According to the FRAC, the risk of pathogen resistance to this chemical class is low to medium [91]. Fludioxonil had extremely strong efficacy against JPA [93]. As of 2019, however, it has not yet been registered for use on Japanese pear in Japan. Data from field trials are being compiled for fludioxonil registration, and it is hoped that products containing fludioxonil will soon be available so that they may be integrated into our JPA management strategies.

## 6. Conclusions

Highly efficacious fungicides tend to be used the most. At the same time, the risks of fungicide-resistant fungal pathogen strains against the heavily used fungicide increase with the usage in the field. Fungicides that are prone to inducing pathogen resistance must be used properly by targeting the correct pathogens, applying the agents only at the appropriate times during the season, reducing application frequency, and mixing with other fungicides that are at low risk of inducing pathogen resistance. A mathematical model-based study suggested that the efficacy of high-risk fungicides may be substantially extended if they are mixed with low-risk fungicides [94]. This hypothesis should be validated by field trials, which are costly, time-consuming, and labor-intensive. On the other hand, these field-based data are invaluable in the development of effective measures against fungicide-resistant plant pathogens.

We conceptualized a series of efforts to develop the best plant disease control practice at agricultural sites as an evidence-based control (EBC) [95–103]. The management of plant diseases needs to be developed based on the accumulated evidences, but not anecdotal observations. To gather useful evidence, the data need to be collected from the combination of field, controlled environment, and lab experiments, and then these data must be statistically validated to come up with repeatable and reliable information.

In this chapter, we demonstrated the use of EBC using the development of JPA management strategies against recent outbreaks as an example. JPA outbreak in 1999 and a detection of benzimidazole-resistant Cgsl strains [1, 28] triggered us to investigate alternatives such as fungicides ST-QoI, dithianon, and fluazinam, which were registered for use on Japanese pear [1, 2, 28, 54]. We also established the residual efficacy and rainfastness of these alternative fungicides [54]. We also obtained the evidence of long-term retention of benzimidazole-resistant strains in the field. Based on these results, an effective fungicide spray program without the use of benzimidazoles was established, and JPA was effectively controlled 2 years after the outbreak [1, 28].

However, JPA became conspicuous in 2006 and 2007 in two geographically distant regions, Kyushu (southeast) and Kanto (central). Outbreaks were reported in Oita prefecture in the Kyushu region in 2006 [45] and in Chiba and Kanagawa prefectures in the Kanto region in 2007 [44, 104]. Also a resurgence of JPA was reported around 2011 in Saga prefecture where the 1999 outbreak occurred [80]. Excessive dependence on ST-QoI fungicides induced ST-QoI-resistant Cgsl strains in Oita and Saga prefecture, which contributed to these new outbreaks [45, 80]. In Chiba and Kanagawa prefecture, the occurrence of QoI-resistant strains has not been investigated, but we suspect that the situation is very similar to Oita and Saga prefectures.

In order to increase the number of options to be used in late-season JPA management, we tested the efficacy of adjuvants to reducing visible chemical residues on fruits. Information from these experiments enabled us to determine appropriate and effective combinations of fungicides against JPA without relying on either the benzimidazole or ST-QoI. We intend to keep conducting similar holistic evidence-based approaches to develop effective management strategies for other pathosystems.

## Acknowledgements

We appreciate the collaboration and information exchange with Dr. Yohei Kaneko of the CAFRC. In addition, we sincerely thank Dr. Kayo Manabe of Nippon Steel Eco-tech Corporation for assisting in the collection of references and Ms. Noriko Orihara and Mr. Makoto Suzuki of the Kanagawa Agricultural Technology Center for providing photos of JPA outbreak. Moreover, for implementation of the study, we sincerely thank the staff members of the Plant Protection Laboratory of Saga Prefectural Fruit Tree Experiment Station including Ms. Hisako Fukumoto, Setsumi Morinaga, and Hatsumi Nakayama and students of Saga Prefectural Agricultural College Fruit Tree Branch School.

## Author details

Nobuya Tashiro[1]*, Youichi Ide[2], Mayumi Noguchi[3], Hisayoshi Watanabe[4] and Mizuho Nita[5]

1 Saga Prefectural Upland Farming Research and Extension Center, Karatsu, Saga, Japan

2 Saga Prefectural Agricultural Research Center, Saga, Japan

3 Saga Prefectural Nishimatsuura Agricultural Extension Center, Imari, Saga, Japan

4 Oita Prefectural Agriculture, Forestry and Fisheries Research Center, Usa, Oita, Japan

5 Alson H. Smith Jr. Agricultural Research and Extension Center, Virginia Polytechnic Institute and State University, Winchester, VA, USA

*Address all correspondence to: tashirongreen12@gmail.com

## References

[1] Tashiro N, Ide Y, Etho T. Occurrence of benzimidazole tolerant isolate of *Colletotrichum gloeosporioides*, a causal fungus of anthracnose of Japanese pear and its effective fungicides. Kyushu Agricultural Research. 2001;**63**:81 (in Japanese)

[2] Tashiro N, Ide Y. Occurrence of anthracnose of Japanese pear caused by *Colletotrichum gloeosporioides*, and its effective fungicides. Plant Protection. 2003;**57**:111-115 (in Japanese)

[3] Kurosawa R. Anthracnose of Japanese pear (short communication). Syokubutugaku-Zasshi. 1912;**26**:359-360 (in Japanese)

[4] Hara K. Anthracnose on Japanese pear. In: Kazyubyougairon. Nippon Kankitsukai, Tokyo. 1916. pp. 107-110 (in Japanese)

[5] Ikata S. Anthracnose on Leaves in Japanese Pear. Tokyo: Zikkennkazyubyougaihen. Yokendo; 1927. pp. 54-55 (in Japanese)

[6] Ochiai M, Inomata M, Hayashi S. Study on Japanese pear leaf anthracnose like disease (1). Progress of outbreak and isolation of causal organism. Annual Report of the Society of Plant Protection of North Japan. 1976;**27**:81 (in Japanese)

[7] Ochiai M, Hayashi S. Study on Japanese pear leaf anthracnose like disease (2). Pathogenicity of isolated *Colletotrichum* sp. Annual Report of the Society of Plant Protection of North Japan. 1977;**28**:73 (in Japanese)

[8] Ochiai M, Hayashi S. Study on Japanese pear leaf anthracnose like disease (3). Influence of the elapsed days after expand of leaf and the back and forth of the leaves at the inoculation on the disease development. Annual Report of the Society of Plant Protection of North Japan. 1977;**28**:74 (in Japanese)

[9] Ochiai M, Hayashi S. Study on Japanese pear leaf anthracnose like disease (4). Effects of temperature and leaf wetness period on infection and disease incidence. Annual Report of the Society of Plant Protection of North Japan. 1977;**28**:75 (in Japanese)

[10] Ochiai M, Hayashi S. Study on Japanese pear leaf anthracnose like disease (5). Effects of medium and temperature on the growth of pathogen. Annual Report of the Society of Plant Protection of North Japan. 1978;**29**:58 (in Japanese)

[11] Morita Y, Yano K, Matsumoto K, Kotani S, Kurata M. Occurrence and control of anthracnose on leaves of Japanese pear. Bulletin of the Kochi Agricultural Research Center. 1994;**3**: 1-10 (in Japanese)

[12] Yano K, Ishii H, Fukaya M, Kawada Y, Sato T. Anthracnose on Japanese pear caused by intermediately benzimidazole-resistant strains of *Colletotrichum gloeosporioides* (*Glomerella cingulata*). Japanese Journal of Phytopathology. 2004;**70**:314-319 (in Japanese with English summary)

[13] Adaskaveg JE, Hartin RJ. Characterization of *Colletotrichum acutatum* isolates causing anthracnose of almond and peach in California. Phytopathology. 1997;**87**:979-989

[14] Fukaya M. First report of Japanese pear anthracnose disease caused by *Colletotrichum acutatum* and its chemical control. Japanese Journal of Phytopathology. 2004;**70**:184-189 (in Japanese with English summary)

[15] Chung WH, Ishii H, Nishimura K, Fukaya M, Yano K, Kajitani Y. Fungicide sensitivity and phylogenetic relationship of anthracnose fungi isolated from various fruit crops in Japan. Plant Disease. 2006;**90**:506-512

[16] Zhang PF, Zhai LF, Zhang XK, Huang XZ, Hong N, Xu WX, et al. Characterization of *Colletotrichum fructicola*, a new causal agent of leaf black spot disease of sandy pear (*Pyrus pyrifolia*). European Journal of Plant Pathology. 2015;**143**:651-662

[17] Fu M, Crous PW, Bai Q, Zhang PF, Xiang J, Guo YS, et al. *Colletotrichum* species associated with anthracnose of *Pyrus* spp. in China. Persoonia. 2019;**42**: 1-35

[18] Oita Prefecture. Anthracnose of Japanese pear caused by *Colletotrichum fioriniae* (Marcelino & R.G. Shivas & Y.P. Tan). In: Temporary Pest Outbreak Forecast Information. Vol. 3. 2013. pp. 1-2 (in Japanese)

[19] Cho WD, Shin HD. List of Plant Disease in Korea (edition 4). Seoul, Korea Republic: Korean Society of Plant Pathology; 2004. 348 p

[20] Kim WG, Hong SK, Park YS. Occurrence of anthracnose on fruits of Asian pear tree caused by *Colletotrichum acutatum*. Mycrobiology. 2007;**35**:238-240

[21] Sutton TB, Aldwinckle HS, Agnello AM, Walgenbach JF, editors. Compendium of Apple and Pear Diseases and Pests. 2nd ed. St. Paul, MN: APS Publications; 2014

[22] Leite RP Jr, Tsuneta M, Kishino AY. Ocorrência de mancha foliar de Glomerella em macieira no Estado do Paraná. Londrina; Fundação Instituto Agronômico do Paraná. Informe de Pesquisa. 1988;**81**:6 (in Portuguese)

[23] Cerezine PC, Leite RP, Tsuneta M. Efeito de tratamentos químicos no controle da mancha foliar de Glomerella en macieira. No Estado de Paraná. Fitopatologia Brasileira. 1992;**17**:258-267 (in Portuguese)

[24] Sutton TB, Sanhueza RM. Necrotic leaf blotch of Golden delicious-Glomerella leaf spot: A resolution of common names. Plant Disease. 1998;**82**:267-268

[25] González E, Sutton TB. First report of Glomerella leaf spot (*Glomerella cingulata*) of apple in the United States. Plant Disease. 1999;**83**:1074

[26] Velho AC, Stadnik MJ, Casanova L, Mondino P, Alaniz S. First report of *Colletotrichum karstii* causing Glomerella leaf spot on apple in Santa Catarina State, Brazil. Plant Disease. 2014;**98**:157

[27] Wang CX, Zhang ZF, Li BH, Wang HY, Dong XL. First report of Glomerella leaf spot of apple caused by *Glomerella cingulata* in China. Plant Disease. 2012;**96**:912

[28] Tashiro N, Manabe K, Ide Y. Emergence and frequency of highly benzimidazole-resistant *Colletotrichum gloeosporioides*, pathogen of Japanese pear anthracnose, after discontinued use of *benzimidazole*. Journal of General Plant Pathology. 2012;**78**:221-226

[29] Misonou T, Fukatsu R. Effect of benomyl spraying on the infesting of pear scab. Proceedings of the Kanto-Tosan Plant Protection Society. 1970;**17**: 59-60 (in Japanese)

[30] Umemoto S, Nagai Y. Decline of sensitivity of *Venturia nashicola* against benomyl and thiophanate-methyl in Chiba prefecture. Proceedings of the Kanto-Tosan Plant Protection Society. 1976;**23**:56-57 (in Japanese)

[31] Ishii H, Yamaguchi A. Tolerance of *Venturia nashicola* to thiophanate-methyl and benomyl in Japan. Annals of the Phytopathological Society of Japan. 1977;**43**:557-561

[32] Sato S, Fujikawa T, Tomiku T, Ando S, Goto D, Mino T. Occurrence of benomyl tolerant *Venturia nashicola* causing Japanese pear scab. Proceedings of Association of Plant Protection Kyushu. 1978;**24**:74-76 (in Japanese)

[33] Ishizaki H, Kohno M, Tsuchida M, Umino M, Hazumi Y, Katoh S, et al. Yearly fluctuation in the occurrence of thiophanatemethyl-resistant strains of the pear scab fungus in pear orchards at Karasu town, Mie Prefecture. Japanese Journal of Phytopathology. 1983;**49**: 347-351 (in Japanese with English summary)

[34] Hashimoto S, Sano S, Murakami A, Mizuno M, Nishikawa H, Yasuda Y. Fungitoxic properties of triflumizole. Annals of the Phytopathological Society of Japan. 1986;**52**:599-609

[35] Umemoto S, Murata A. Effects of the different spraying time of some fungicides on Japanese pear scab. Proceedings of the Kanto-Tosan Plant Protection Society. 1988;**35**:99-102 (in Japanese)

[36] Tomita Y, Ogawara S, Nagatsuka H. Control of pear scab by sterol demethylation inhibitors (DMIs). Annual Report of the Kanto-Tosan Plant Protection Society. 2003;**50**:75-77 (in Japanese)

[37] Umemoto S, Kaneko Y, Kameda K, Yamamoto A, Suzuki J, Fukuda H, et al. Fungicidal effect and effective duration period of sterol demethylation inhibitor (DMI) fungicides in Japanese pear scab control. Annual Report of the Kanto-Tosan Plant Protection Society. 2012;**59**: 115-118 (in Japanese with English summary)

[38] Nitta H, Ogasawara S. Chemical control of Physalospora canker to Japanese pear's current shoots. Annual Report of the Kansai Plant Protection Society. 1997;**39**:57-58 (in Japanese)

[39] Imamura S, Saito Y. Application timing and effects of some fungicides against powdery mildew of pear. Annual Report of the Kanto-Tosan Plant Protection Society. 1979;**26**:73 (in Japanese)

[40] Ohnuma T, Hirasawa H, Tanaka T, Shibahashi T. Studies on the ecology and control of anthracnose of cherry caused by *Glomerella cingulate* Spaulding et Schrenk. Bulletin of the Yamagata Prefectural Horticultural Experiment Station. 1986;**5**:9-27 (in Japanese with English summary)

[41] Adaskaveg JE, Forster H. Occurrence and management of anthracnose epidemics caused by *Colletotrichum* species on tree fruit crops in California. In: Prusky D, Freeman S, Dickman MB, editors. Colletotrichum: Host Specificity, Pathology, and Host-Pathogen Interaction. St. Paul: APS Press; 2000. pp. 317-336

[42] Timmer LW, Brown GE. Biology and control of anthracnose disease of citrus. In: Prusky D, Freeman S, Dickman MB, editors. Colletotrichum: Host Specifity, Pathology, and Host-Pathogen Interaction. St. Paul: APS Press; 2000. pp. 300-316

[43] Om P, Misra AK, Pandey BK. Anthracnose disease of tropical and subtropical fruits. In: Agnihotri VP, Prakash O, Kishun R, Misa AK, editors. Disease Scenario in Crop Plants, Vol. 1. Fruits and Vegetables. Pitampura, New Delhi: International Books and Periodicals Supply Service; 1996. pp. 1-27

[44] Kaneko Y, Suzuki T, Takeuchi T. Occurrence and control of anthracnose of Japanese pear caused by *Glomellera cingulate*. CAFRC Research Bulletin. 2010;**2**:7-16 (in Japanese with English summary)

[45] Watanabe H. Strobilurin & benzimidazole resistant in *Colletotrichum gloeosporioides*, the anthracnose fungus of Japanese pear in Oita prefecture. Bulletin of Oita Prefectural Agriculture, Forestry and Fisheries Research Center. 2013;**3**: 23-30 (in Japanese)

[46] Kaneko Y, Umemoto S, Takeuchi T. Investigation of the primary inoculum source for anthracnose caused by *Glomerella cingulata* on Japanese pear.

Japanese Journal of Phytopathology. 2010;**76**:282-285 (in Japanese with English summary)

[47] Fukaya M, Katoh S, Satoh H. Studies on the tolerance of grape gray mold (*Botrytis cinerea* Persoon) 1. Tolerance of grape gray mold (*Botrytis cinerea*) for thiophanate-methyl and some of its characteristics. Bulletin of Akita Fruit-Tree Experiment Station. 1979;**11**:33-38 (in Japanese with English summary)

[48] Nonaka T. Tolerance of tea anthracnose fungus, *Gloeosporium theae-sinensis*, to thiophanate-methyl and benomyl fungicides. (4) Fluctuation in the occurrence of resistant fungi under restricted use of fungicides. Proceedings of Association of Plant Protection Kyushu. 1984;**30**:73-76 (in Japanese)

[49] Ishii H, Udagawa H, Yanase H, Yamaguchi A. Resistance of *Venturia nashicola* to thiophanate-methyl and benomyl: Build-up and decline of resistance in the field. Plant Pathology. 1985;**34**:363-368

[50] Tomikawa A, Nagae S. Studies on resistance of the pear scab fungus (*Venturia nashicola*) to thiophanate-methyl (1). Pear scab fungus in Mie Pref. and yearly fluctuation in the occurrence of thiophanate-methyl resistant-strains of the pear scab fungus in pear orchards. Bulletin of Mie Agricultural Research Center. 1984;**12**: 21-28 (in Japanese)

[51] Umemoto S, Murata A. Change of benzimidazole-resistant populations of *Venturia nashicola* (Japanese pear scab fungus) in pear orchards. Bulletin of Chiba Agricultural Experiment Station. 1988;**29**:137-147 (in Japanese with English summary)

[52] Osada S. Yearly fluctuation in the occurrence of benomyl-resistant strain of Japanese pear scab fungus in Miyagi Prefecture. Annual Report of the Society of Plant Protection of North Japan. 1990;**41**:86-88 (in Japanese with English summary)

[53] Schwabe WTS. Resistance of the apple scab fungus (*Venturia inaequalis*) to benzimidazole fungicides. Deciduous Fruit Grower. 1979;**29**:418-422

[54] Ide Y, Tashiro N. Evaluation of fungicides about residue, rainfastness and efficacy of disease inhibition for the purpose of efficient control to the anthracnose with *Colletotrichum gloeosporioides* on Japanese pear. Japanese Journal of Phytopathology. 2004;**70**:1-6 (in Japanese with English summary)

[55] Ishii H. QoI fungicide resistance: Current status and the problems associated with DNA-based monitoring. In: Gisi U, Chet I, Gullino ML, editors. Recent Developments in Management of Plant Diseases, Plant Pathology in the 21st. Dordrecht, Heidelberg: Springer Science + Business Media B.V; 2010. pp. 37-45

[56] Brent KJ, Hollomon DW. QoIs (quinone outside inhibitors). In: Fungicide Resistance in Crop Pathogens: How Can it be Managed?. FRAC Monograph No. 1. 2nd revised ed. Brussels: The Fungicide Resistance Action Committee; 2007. pp. 42-43

[57] Hirooka T, Ishii H. Chemical control of plant diseases. Journal of General Plant Pathology. 2013;**79**:390-401

[58] Knight SC, Anthony VM, Brady AM, Greenland AJ, Heaney SP, Murray DC, et al. Rationale and perspectives on the development of fungicides. Annual Review of Phytopathology. 1997;**35**:349-372

[59] Ogasawara K, Enoyoshi T, Miyahara T, Kojiguchi, Kadota G, Takamatsu S, et al. Cucurbit powdery mildew resistant to strobilurins. Japanese Journal of Phytopathology. 1999;**65**:655 (Japanese abstract)

[60] Ishii H, Fraaije BA, Sugiyama T, Noguchi K, Nishimura K, Takeda T, et al. Occurrence and molecular characterization of strobilurin resistance in cucumber powdery mildew and downy mildew. Phytopathology. 2001; **91**:1166-1171

[61] Yano K, Kawada Y. Occurrence of strobilurin-resistant strains of *Mycovellosiella nattrassii*, causal fungus of leaf mold of eggplants. Japanese Journal of Phytopathology. 2003;**69**: 220-223 (in Japanese with English summary)

[62] Fuji M, Yamaguchi J, Furuta A, So K. Sensitivity of *Corynespora* leaf spot on cucumber fungus isolated from Saga Prefecture to strobilurin fungicides and methods for testing the sensitivity. Japanese Journal of Phytopathology. 2003;**69**:299-300 (Japanese abstract)

[63] Kansako M, Yoneda Y, Shimadu K, Ishii H. Occurrence of strobilurin-resistant *Botrytis cinerea*, pathogen of citrus gray mold. Japanese Journal of Phytopathology. 2005;**71**:249 (Japanese abstract)

[64] Tanahashi M, Nakano T, Ishii H, Kodama M, Otani H. Possible occurrence of strobilurin resistant strains in *Alternaria alternata* causing black spot of European pear. Japanese Journal of Phytopathology. 2006;**72**:275 (Japanese abstract)

[65] Tsushima Y, Yukita K, Fukushi Y, Akahira T. Resistance to strobilurin fungicides of *Alternaria alternata* apple pathotype and simplified test method. Japanese Journal of Phytopathology. 2007;**73**:51-52 (Japanese abstract)

[66] Koya N, Inoue K, Kawaguchi A. Occurrence of strobilurin resistant isolates of *Pseudocercospora vitis*, grapevine leaf blight fungus. Japanese Journal of Phytopathology. 2008;**74**: 73-74 (Japanese abstract)

[67] Inada M, Ishii H, Chung W-H, Chung WH, Yamada T, Yamaguchi J, et al. Occurrence of strobilurin-resistant strains of *Colletotrichum gloeosporioides* (*Glomerella cingulata*), the causal fungus of strawberry anthracnose. Japanese Journal of Phytopathology. 2008;**74**: 114-117 (in Japanese with English summary)

[68] Hirayama Y, Kawamoto Y, Matsutani S, Nishizaki M, Okayama K. Occurrence of fungicides resistant isolates of *Glomerella cingulata* causing the strawberry anthracnose in Nara Prefecture. Annual Report Kansai Plant Protection. 2008;**50**:93-94 (in Japanese)

[69] Tomihama T, Nonaka T, Omatsu N, Nishi Y. Occurrence of QoI resistance in *Pestalotiopsis longiseta*, the pathogen causing gray blight disease in tea plants. Kyushu Plant Protection Research. 2009;**55**:83-88 (in Japanese with English summary)

[70] Akahira T, Hanaoka T. Occurrence of trifloxystrobin resistant strains of *Colletotrichum gloeosporioides* (*Glomerella cingulata*), the causal fungus of apple bitter rot in Aomori Prefecture. Japanese Journal of Phytopathology. 2013;**79**:197-198 (Japanese abstract)

[71] Miyagawa N, Fuji M. Occuurrence of QoI-fungicide-resistant strains of *Magnaporthe oryzae* on rice and fungicidal effective. In: Abstracts of the 23rd Symposium of PSJ Research Committee on Fungicide Resistance, Gifu, Japan. 2013. pp. 25-35 (in Japanese with English summary)

[72] Takushi T, Kadekaru K, Arasaki C, Taba S. Occurrence of strobilurin-resistant strains of *Colletotrichum gloeosporioides*, the causal fungus of mango anthracnose. Japanese Journal of Phytopathology. 2014;**80**:119-123 (in Japanese with English summary)

[73] Hirayama K, Akahira T, Hanaoka T. QoI-resistant strains of *Venturia*

*inaequalis* causing apple scab in Aomori Prefecture, Japan. Annual Report of the Society of Plant Protection of North Japan. 2017;**68**:115-119 (in Japanese with English summary)

[74] Furuya S, Mochizuki M, Saito S, Kobayashi H, Takayanagi T, Suzuki S. Monitoring of QoI fungicide resistance in *Plasmopara viticola* populations in Japan. Pest Management Science. 2010; **66**:1268-1272

[75] Orihara N, Uekusa H, Miyakawa K, Okamoto M, Kobatashi N. Occurrence of QoI-resistant strains of *Didymella bryoniae*, causal fungus of gummy stem blight of cucurbits in Kanagawa prefecture. Annual Report of the Kanto-Tosan Plant Protection Society. 2013;**60**: 31-33 (in Japanese)

[76] Matsuura S. Current status of QoI (strobilurin) fungicides sensitivity in isolates of *Puccinia horiana*, the causal agent of chrysanthemum white rust, occur in western Japan. Plant Protection. 2019;**73**:370-373 (in Japanese)

[77] Ishii H. Current status of QoI fungicide resistance. Plant Protecton. 2015;**69**:469-474 (in Japanese)

[78] Ogata T, Kanno E. Application period and selection of effective chemicals for the Japanese pear scab control in autumn. Annual Report of the Society of Plant Protection of North Japan. 2000;**51**:141-143 (in Japanese)

[79] Tomita Y, Ogawara T, Miyamoto T. Fungicidal control of Japanese pear scab caused by *Venturia nashicola* in Ibaraki Prefecture. Plant Protection. 2011;**65**: 131-133 (in Japanese)

[80] Noguchi M. Occurrence of QoI-resistance to *Glomerella cingulate* on Japanese pear and countermeasures in Saga Prefecture. Plant Protection. 2015; **69**:494-497 (in Japanese)

[81] Watanebe H. Methods for detecting QoI fungicide resistance in *Colletotrichum gloeosporioides* (Japanese pear anthracnose). Plant Protection. 2017;**71**:327-330 (in Japanese)

[82] Tashiro N, Sadamatsu M. The effect of additional wetting spreaders on the effect of fungicides for control of Japanese pear black spot caused by *Alternaria alternata* Japanese pear pathotype. Bulletin of Saga Prefectural Fruit Tree Experiment Station. 1996;**13**:104-113 (in Japanese with English summary)

[83] Tashiro N. The effective use of the spreading agent in the disease control of fruit trees. Plant Protection. 2009;**63**: 212-217 (in Japanese)

[84] Ide Y, Tashiro N. Effect of row-passage styles by speed sprayer on the efficacy against the scab by *Venturia nashicola* and anthracnose by *Colletotrichum gloeosporioides* and chemical adhesion on Japanese pear leaves. Japanese Journal of Phytopathology. 2007;**73**:289-294 (in Japanese with English summary)

[85] Kaneko Y, Fukuta H. Use of 'Makupika' spreader for the purpose of reducing fruit stains with captan wettable powder just before the pear harvest period in Chiba Prefecture. CAFRC. Research Bulletin. 2010;**9**:49-55 (in Japanese)

[86] Ozaki M, Fukumoto S, Tamai R, Yonekura N, Ikegaya K, Kawashima T, et al. Kumiai Chemical Industry Co, Ltd. and Ihara Chemical Industry Co. Ltd.; 2001. WO 01/10825 A1

[87] Takagaki M, Kawata M, Fukumoto S, Miura I. Efficacy and in vitro activity of new fungicide KUF-1204 on *Botrytis cinerea*. Japanese Journal of Phytopathology. 2005;**71**:256 (Japanese abstract)

[88] Kataoka S, Takagaki M, Kaku K, Shimizu T. Mechanism of action and

selectivity of a novel fungicide, pyribencarb. Journal of Pesticide Science. 2010;**35**:99-106

[89] Ishii H. Fungicide research in Japan —An overview. In: Dehne HW, Deising HB, Gisi U, Kuck KH, Russell PE, Lyr H, editors. Modern Fungicides and Antifungal Compounds V. 15th International Reinhardsbrunn Symposium May 06–10, 2007, Friedrichroda, Germany. DPG Selbstverlag, Braunschweig. 2008. pp. 11-17

[90] Takagaki M, Kataoka S, Fukumoto S, Ishii H, Yamaguchi J, Inada M, et al. The efficacy of the novel fungicide pyribencarb to the several QoI resistant fungal strains. Japanese Journal of Phytopathology. 2006;**72**:274-275 (Japanese abstract)

[91] Fungicide Resistance Action Committee. FRAC Code List 2019: Fungal control agents sorted by cross resistance pattern and mode of action (including FRAC Code numbering). Available at: https://www.frac.info/docs/default-source/publications/frac-code-list/frac-code-list-2019.pdf?sfvrsn=98ff4b9a_2 [Accessed: 14 October 2019]

[92] Japan Fungicide Resistance Action Committee. Guide line of QoIs in Japan. Available at: https://www.jcpa.or.jp/labo/jfrac/guidelines.html [Accessed: 14 October 2019]

[93] Kaneko Y. Screening of substitutes for quinone outside inhibitor fungicides for control of Japanese pear anthracnose caused by *Glomerella cingulata* and their effects on several Japanese pear diseases. CAFRC Research Bulletin. 2016;**8**:1-7 (in Japanese with English summary)

[94] Hobbelen PHF, Paveley ND, van den Bosch F. Delaying selection for fungicide insensitivity by mixing fungicides at a low and high risk of resistance development: S modeling analysis. Phytopathology. 2011;**101**: 1224-1233

[95] Tashiro N. New concept of disease and pest management: Construction of a control system with less frequent spray by EBC (evidence-based control). In: Proceedings of the 9th Forum of MAFF on Disease and Pest Management for Agricultural Product. Tokyo, Japan. 2003. pp. 18-27 (in Japanese)

[96] Tashiro N. Evidence-based control: The new concept of pest management. Journal of Evidence-Based Control. 2011;**7**:26-29 (in Japanese)

[97] Tashiro N. Evidence-based control: The new concept of pest management. Plant Protection. 2005;**59**:69-73 (in Japanese)

[98] Tashiro N. EBC (evidence-based control) is necessary for development of plant protection in the future. Annual Report of the Society of Plant Protection of North Japan. 2007;**58**:1-15 (in Japanese)

[99] Kawaguchi A. Concept for study of plant disease control at research committee for the EBC (evidence-based control), on the 7th workshop. Journal of Evidence-based Control. 2011;**7**:26-29 (in Japanese with English summary)

[100] Kawaguchi A. Concept and practice of EBC (evidence-based control) for on-farm research. Plant Protection. 2012;**66**:450-455 (in Japanese)

[101] Ide Y. Evidence of the chemical control to the disease on fruit trees. Plant Protection. 2012;**66**:456-459 (in Japanese)

[102] Tashiro N. Study on the improvement of fruit tree disease management using evidence-based control. Journal of General Plant Pathology. 2015;**81**:470-475

[103] Tashiro N, Yamaguchi S, Nakashima K, Syouji K, Matsuo Y, Yamaguchi M. Evidence-based control (EBC) to greenhouse mandarin sooty mold caused by *Cladosporium cladosporioides*. Japanese Journal of Phytopathology. 2016;**82**:79 (Japanese abstract)

[104] Kanagawa Prefecture. Anthracnose of Japanese pear (in Japanese). In: Temporary Pest Outbreak Forecast Information. Vol. 3. 2007. pp. 1-2 (in Japanese)

Chapter 12

# Biological Control of Citrus Canker: New Approach for Disease Control

*Sonia Villamizar and Juan Carlos Caicedo*


## Abstract

Citrus canker is a disease that affects the major types of commercial citrus crops. *Xanthomonas citri* subsp. *citri*, the etiological agent, reaches to mesophyll tissue through the stomata and afterward induces cell hyperplasia. Disease management has been based on both tree eradication and copper spray treatment. Overuse of copper for control of bacterial citrus canker has led to the development and prevalence of copper-resistant strains of Xcc. Several genera of both soil- and plant-associated bacteria became powerful tools in sustainable agriculture for control of Xcc and reduction of citrus canker disease severity. In this chapter we present bacteria able to interfere with quorum sensing as well to display antibacterial activity against *Xcc* by production of secondary metabolite. These bacteria may represent a highly valuable tool in the process of biological control and offer an alternative to the traditional copper treatment currently used for the treatment of citrus canker disease, with significant environmental, economic, and health implications worldwide.


**Keywords:** quorum quenching, *Pseudomonas*, biofilm, secondary metabolites, *Bacillus*

## 1. Introduction

The steady increase in global overpopulation has forced the agricultural producer to introduce environmentally aggressive practices (e.g., undiscriminating use of pesticides and chemical fertilizers), in order to respond to the rising request of cultivated crops for food. The growing breach between supply and request and the negative impact on the environment have stimulated researchers to develop alternative strategies, pursuing to promote a sustainable agriculture.

The interactions between plants and their associated microorganisms have generated a huge interest. A deep understanding of these processes allows the implementation of innovative agricultural applications. Plants produce an extensive collection of organic compounds comprising sugars, organic acids, and vitamins, which can be served as nutrients or signals for microbial communities. On the other hand, microorganisms release phytohormones, small molecules, or volatile compounds, which may act directly or indirectly reducing disease severity caused by phytopathogenic agents. Some of these actions are nutrient competition, antibiotic activity, plant immunity activation or plant growth, and morphogenesis activation [1].

Prokaryotes and mainly the bacterial domain are the numerically dominant component of most microbial communities in plants. Numerous genera of both soil- and plant-associated bacteria turn out to be powerful tools in sustainable agriculture, because these bacteria display extremely versatile secondary metabolisms with valuable biological activities, including quorum quenching and antibiotic activity. The aim of this chapter is to present two different approaches for biological control of bacterial citrus canker. This antagonism specifically focus in a quorum quenching of DSF pathway and antibacterial activity by *Pseudomonas* bacteria against *Xanthomonas citri* subsp. *citri* ethological agent of citrus canker disease.

## 2. Citrus canker disease

One of the most important diseases of citrus is citrus canker, affecting almost all commercial varieties. Bacterium *Xanthomonas citri* subsp. *citri* (*Xcc*) is the etiological agent of citrus canker. In the last decade, citrus canker disease rise as one of the main threats to citrus industry, because of the rise of copper-resistant Xcc strains. Factors such as bacterial species and weather conditions determine the disease severity. The geographical origin of the disease is not clear; some researchers report that the first disease cases appeared at Southern China [2]. However, according to Fawcett and Jenkins in 1933, the disease originated in regions of India and Java [3]. These reports suggest, therefore, that the origin of the disease occurred in tropical areas of Asia, where it is assumed that citrus species originated and has been distributed to other areas through grafting [4]. In America, the first report of the disease occurred in the United States in 1915 [5]. Currently, citrus canker is present in more than 30 countries in Asia, the Indian Ocean and Pacific Islands, South America, and the Southeastern United States [4].

Traditional control of citrus canker disease centered on the application of copper-based products seeks the reduction of bacterial population in leaf surfaces. However, multiple applications are needed in order to obtain a significant reduction in bacterial burden on phyllosphere. Weather conditions, i.e., wind and rain, decrease drastically the effectiveness of copper applications. The drawbacks of the long-term use of copper compounds to control plant pathogens in the field include selection of copper resistance and horizontal transfer in bacterial populations [6].

### 2.1 Disease cycle and transmission mechanisms

Invasion and colonization of the citrus host by *Xcc* occur by stomata and wounds in plant tissues, infecting leaves, fruits, and stems. The bacterium *Xcc* multiplies within the intercellular spaces in the mesophilic tissue, inducing cellular hyperplasia, leading to rupture of the leaf epidermis and resulting in high and spongy lesions surrounded by a margin soaked in water. Upon leaf epidermis eruption, a great number of bacteria are released to the environment to reach other leaves and plants. Rain, wind, and agriculture tools are the main agents of natural dispersion of disease; the insect larvae of the citrus tree cause extensive wounds in the foliar tissues and greatly increase the spread of the disease. Rainwater collected from foliage with lesions contains between $10^5$ and $10^8$ cfu/ml [4].

### 2.2 Types of disease

There are three different types of citrus canker caused by two species of *Xanthomonas*, citrus canker type: A, B, and C. The differentiation of these types is mainly based on the geographical distribution and pathogen host range [7].

The Asian type of canker (canker A) is caused by *Xanthomonas citri* subsp. *citri*. Canker A is the most common and widespread disease, and its geographical distribution continues increasing. The disease is endemic in more than 30 countries: Asia, in the Pacific of India, Pakistan, the Indian Ocean islands, Southeast Asia, South America, Southeast China, and Japan. The bacterium Xcc has a wide range of host and produces the disease in the great majority of the citrus species as *C. paradisi*, *C. aurantifoli*, *C. sinensis*, and *C. reticulata* [8]. Type B canker is caused by the bacterium *Xanthomonas fuscans* subsp. *aurantifolii* type B (*XauB*) [9]. Type B canker has similar symptoms to type A canker; however, the symptoms take longer to appear as a consequence of the slower growth rate of XauB, and the host range is restricted to *C. limon* but has also been sporadically isolated from *C. sinensis and C. paradisi* [10]. C-type canker has only been identified in the state of São Paulo, Brazil [11], and has the same symptoms as type A citrus canker, caused by *Xanthomonas fuscans* subsp. *aurantifolii* type C (XauC) and only infects *C. aurantifolii* [9].

### 2.3 Symptomatology

The diseased plants are characterized by the occurrence of conspicuous raised necrotic lesions that develop on leaves, branches, and fruits. In the leaves, the first appearance is circular patches of 2–10 mm in diameter; their appearance is oily and usually appears on the abaxial surface reflecting stomatal entrance. The lesions are often similar in shape and size. Subsequently, both epidermal surfaces may become ruptured by pathogen-induced tissue hyperplasia. In the leaves, stems, thorns, and fruits, circular lesions became like a raised boil, growing in spongy white or yellow pustules. These pustules then darken and thicken brown cork type, which is rough to the touch. Often, a watery swell develops around the necrotic tissue and is easily visualized with transmitted light (**Figure 1**).

### 2.4 Management and treatment

Bacterial citrus canker management involves different approaches ranging from strict quarantine measures to chemical control. Quarantining is a practical usually used in Brazil and United States of America. Extinction of infected and adjacent

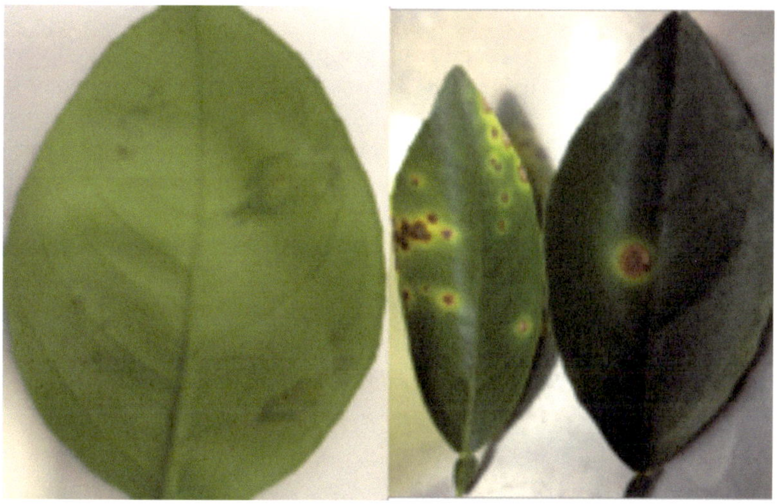

**Figure 1.**
*Symptoms of citrus canker. Left, early stage of the disease. Right, hyperplasia and rupture of the foliar tissue.*

trees is one of the major prophylactic measures against citrus canker in commercial citrus crops. Once a symptomatic tree is identified, it is uprooted, stacked, and burned, as prophylactic measure surrounding trees is destroyed as mentioned before [12].

Prevention of primary infection in the new sprouts perhaps is the major effective approach to reduce citrus canker spread. The eradication methodology comprises conducting periodic surveys of the orchard, identifying and eliminating the outbreaks of the disease before its proliferation. Brazilian regulation stipulates that any field that has a number of diseased trees greater than 0.5% of the total orchard must be eliminated. After eradication, the contaminated field should be sprayed with copper fungicide based on 1.5 kg of metallic copper per 1 mL of water (0.15% of metallic copper). The contaminated plantations are prohibited and are forbidden from marketing the production until eradication works are completed.

The use of bactericidal products based on copper by spray application is a practice widely used for more than two decades for the bacterial citrus canker control. The prolonged exposure of bacterial strains to copper has led to the rise of resistant strains in endemic areas. Behlau et al. reported that the genes *copAB* and *cohAB* may encode copper-binding proteins responsible for the copper resistance in *Xanthomonas citri* subsp. *citri* [13].

## 3. *Xanthomonas citri* subsp. *citri*

The genus *Xanthomonas* includes a vast group of phytopathogenic bacteria belonging to the group of γ proteobacteria. *Xanthomonas* infects 124 species of monocotyledonous and 268 dicotyledonous plants [14]. *Xanthomonas* are Gram-negative bacillus endowed with a sole polar flagellum. After 24-hour incubation at 29°C, yellow and shiny colonies appear in a culture media. Xanthomonadin is an unique pigment, and it is responsible for the yellow color of bacterial colonies; the biological role is explained in detail below. The exopolysaccharide known as xanthan gum gives the shiny appearance to colonies [15]. Although the genus itself has a very broad host range, individual members are often specialized to cause disease in a limited number of taxonomically related hosts as mentioned above.

### 3.1 Isolation and identification

The bacterium *Xcc* can be isolated from symptomatic plants and its diverse infected tissues. Xcc grows easily in regular microbiological culture media. In order to isolate Xcc, infected tissues must be excised and washed, and subsequently the surface must be sterilized for 3 minutes in a 10% NaClO solution. The water-soaked tissue at the lesion margin is streaked across agar medium containing 50 ppm kasugamycin. *X. citri* strains grow easily on regular nutrient agar media containing 0.5% tryptone, 0.3% yeast extract, 0.09% $CaCl_2$, 0.05% $K_2HPO_4$, and 1.5% agar in tap water, pH 7.2 [16]. After 48 hours of incubation at 29°C, mucoid yellow colonies begin to appear in microbiological medium.

### 3.2 Determinants of virulence in *Xanthomonas citri* subsp. *citri*

#### *3.2.1 Adhesins*

An essential stage in bacterial host colonization is its attachment ability. Adhesins are bacterial surface structures that facilitate the attachment to host tissues. The nature of these structures is mainly polysaccharidic, e.g., lipopolysaccharides and exopolysaccharides. However, some of these structures share a proteinaceous nature (type IV pili, chaperone/usher pili, two-partner secretion) [17].

### *3.2.2 Protein secretion systems and their effectors*

Bacteria inside in *Xanthomonas* genus exhibit at least six different types of protein secretion system (i.e., T1SS to T6SS), which vary in their arrangement, function, and in a recognition of secretion substrates [18]. Like many other Gram-negative phytopathogenic bacteria, *Xcc* employs mainly secretion systems T3SS, T4SS, and T5SS and their effectors as effective tools in an attempt to invade and to multiply in a susceptible host.

Protein transport from bacterial periplasm to the extracellular environment occurs mainly by T2SS secretion system. Extracellular enzymes as lipases, proteases, and cell wall-degrading enzymes are translocated using this secretion system. Possibly the major enzymes responsible for the degradation of the plant cell wall are secreted by T2SS. T2SS translocator apparatus is composed of up to 12–15 constituents, most of which are linked to the bacterial inner membrane [19].

The T3SS secretion system also known as "needle" delivers effectors directly into host cells. These act as virulence factors influencing cell host activities [20]. In the Xcc genome, 24 effectors have been identified [21]. One of the main effectors delivered by the T3SS in *Xcc* belongs to the AvrBs3/PthA family. Xcc contains four PthA genes that encode transcription activator-like effector (TALE); of these four genes, pthA4 is responsible for the formation of citrus canker lesions. In citrus host the gene known as CsLOB is targeted by the TALE encoded by the Xcc gene pthA4; this gene was assessed in two susceptible host to Xcc infection, i.e., grape fruit and sweet orange [22]. CsLOB1-specific function still remains unclear; some previous studies suggest that CsLOB1 is involved in the regulation of development of lateral organ and metabolism of nitrogen and anthocyanin. Some plant hormones such as auxin, gibberellin, and cytokines also have proven to exert an effect on CsLOB1 gene [23].

T4SS secretion system is an important virulence factor in a wide range of bacterial pathogens. This secretion system involves the secretion of protein or DNA into the host cells [24]. Xcc harbors two gene arrays encoding for T4SS components [25]; one of them has chromosomal location, and the other one is located at the plasmid pXAC64. Proteins VirB1–VirB11 and VirD4 make up the T4SS translocator apparatus. Nowadays, the structural disposition is well established:

(i). Three ATPases (VirB4, VirB11, and VirD4) located at the cytoplasm. These enzymes have been involved in the process of providing the necessary energy for the secretion process.

(ii). Fourteen repetitions of VirB7-VirB9-virB10 trimer. These repetitions form the periplasmic core. It is noteworthy that VirB10 is anchored on both inner and outer membranes; on the other hand, VirB7 is a lipoprotein located at the outer membrane.

(iii). An inner membrane complex formed by VirB3, VirB6, and VirB8.

(iv). An extracellular pili formed by VirB2 and VirB5.

(v). VirB1 which is a periplasmic transglycosylase [26].

A recent study has shown that T4SS in Xcc displays the ability to secrete toxins; these toxins are known as VirD4-interacting proteins (XVIPs), and they are recruited by VirD4. The biological role of XVIPs is targeting and destabilizing the peptidoglycan layer in the cell wall of bacterial contenders in the ecological niche. This feature is distinctive in *Xcc*, and the protein VirD4XAC2623 endows the bacterium with an extra ability to compete in the phyllosphere [27].

## 4. Biological control of Xcc approaches

### 4.1 Biological control based on DSF quorum quencher pathway

A wide majority of bacterial genera have developed a cell-to-cell communication system known as quorum sensing (QS). This communication system is based on a signal translation mechanism whose objective is to coordinate the expression of genes at the population level in order to respond and fit to environmental changes. The cell-to-cell communication system is based on the production, secretion, and perception of small molecules known as autoinducers. A basal quantity of autoinducers are produced by every single cell, subsequently, which is secreted to extracellular milieu reflecting the bacterial population density. At high population density, the autoinducers reach a critical concentration and enable to cognate receptor to sense them. Consequently, this biological event results in triggering a cascade of diverse cell functions [28]. In the *Xanthomonas* genus, the bacteria display a quorum sensing system in which the autoinducer molecule is a short acid fat called diffusible signal factor (DSF). The DSF autoinducer family is cis-2-unsaturated fatty acids. In Xcc this DSF was characterized as cis-11-methyl-2-dodecenoic acid. The gene cluster that encodes element of quorum sensing system in *Xanthomonas* genus is the *rpf* cluster [29].

Since quorum sensing helps to coordinate community-based bacterial behavior, it is not essential for bacterial survival; therefore, the inhibition of QS interrupts only the desired phenotype, i.e., virulence, biofilm formation, and bacterial resistance to different antibiotics. Interference with QS can provide a route for disease control. This interference may involve signal degradation (quorum quenching) or excess signal production (pathogen confusion) [30]. Quorum quenching is a mechanism adopted by a number of bacteria to break the QS signaling of competitors, giving these organisms an advantage within a particular habitat [31]. It is rational that microorganisms can develop mechanisms to disarm the QS systems of competing organisms in order to increase their competitive strength in an ecosystem [32].

We have conducted a recent study that allows the isolation and identification of bacteria isolated from citrus leaves belonging to plant of field crops with and without citrus canker symptoms. From a total of 114 isolates recovered, 7 bacteria able to disrupt DSF quorum sensing pathway in *Xac* (quorum quencher bacteria) were identified. These bacteria were identified by API kits (bioMérieux's API®) and sequencing of PCR-mediated amplification products of the 16S rRNA genes as *Bacillus amyloliquefaciens*, *Bacillus vallismortis*, *Pseudomonas oryzihabitans, Pseudomonas aeruginosa, Raoultella planticola*, *Kosakonia cowanii*, and *Citrobacter freundii* [33].

Virulence assays were conducted under controlled growth conditions, and canker lesions were quantified at 21 days post inoculation. These assays demonstrated that, when citrus leaves were inoculated with mixtures of Xcc and quorum quencher bacteria, the number of cancer lesions decreased significantly reducing the severity disease (**Figure 2**).

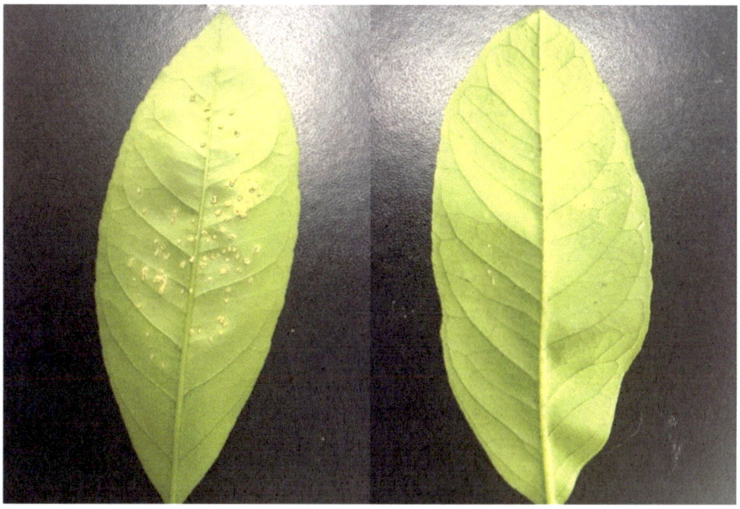

**Figure 2.**
*Virulence assay. Leaves infected by spray method at the same concentration 1 × 10$^6$ UFC/mL. Left, Xcc wild type. Right, Xcc plus Pseudomonas oryzihabitans. Picture was taken after 21 days of infection.*

Quorum quencher bacteria impaired the attachment and biofilm formation of Xcc to leave the surface. These are essential steps in the maintenance, survival, and initial establishment of tissue pathogenicity in citrus canker. In fact, it is completely accepted that QS plays an important, if not an essential, role in the formation of bacterial biofilm [34]. Studies of scanning electron microscopy SEM confirmed the substantial reduction in the adherence ability of Xcc after 10 hours when it was co-infected with quorum quencher bacteria relative to the control used, i.e., the leaves infected with Xcc alone. After 7 days post-infection with Xcc and the inhibitory bacteria of DSF, SEM has shown the absence of biofilm formation on the surface of leaves co-inoculated with *P. oryzihabitans* and *B. amyloliquefaciens*, relative to the control used, i.e., the infected leaves just with *Xcc*.

A possible mechanism for explaining the modification or degradation of DSF molecule produced by Xcc could be the quorum quencher bacteria using the DSF molecule as a possible substrate for the UDP-sugar transferase enzyme. The addition of one unit of sugar (from UDP-sugars, i.e., UDP-glucose or UDP-galactose to the short chain of fatty acid impossible the recognition of this version of modified DSF molecule by sensor RpfC. These UDP-sugar pools are produced by the activity of carbamoyl phosphate synthetase enzyme, which is encoded by *carA* and *carB* genes. The nucleotide sequence of the *carAB* locus in the DSF inhibitory bacteria *Pseudomonas oryzihabitans* and *Bacillus amyloliquefaciens* has a strong similarity to the sequences of *carAB* genes present in the *Pseudomonas* G strain isolated and identified as efficient quorum quencher bacteria in *Xanthomonas campestris* [35].

### 4.2 Biological control based on antibacterial activity of *Pseudomonas* strains

*Pseudomonas* species show traits that allow them to act as effective biological control agents (BCAs) against several phytopathogens. Among these traits the most common shared by a broad range of *Pseudomonas* strains are (a) pronounced colonizing ability of plant surfaces, internal plant tissues, and phytopathogen structures [36]; (b) the ability for production of numerous kinds of antibiotic providing additional advantage in antagonism with local microbiota and phytopathogens [37]; and (c) the ability to trigger resistance responses in host plants [38]. Thus, mechanisms of direct antagonism as antibiosis or indirect mechanisms such as competition for nutrients (e.g., siderophore production), besides induction of systemic resistance responses, actively participate in phytopathogenic disease suppression by the pseudomonads [39]. The *Pseudomonas* strains most usually recognized for their biocontrol activity against both eukaryotic and prokaryotic phytopathogenic microorganisms are *P. fluorescens*, *P. protegens*, *P. chlororaphis*, and *P. putida* [40].

In recent study (in press), we have isolated and identified from soil samples added with a compost five *Pseudomonas* strains which displayed a strong activity against Xcc. Virulence assays in very susceptible citrus host using these strains result in a deep decrease of canker lesions, which suggest a great reduction in citrus canker severity. This effect could be attributed to the great production of secondary metabolites by the *Pseudomonas* strains isolated.

## 5. Conclusions

Quorum sensing is an important target for prophylactic and therapeutic interventions. Identification of new bacteria species as ABC could be a new alternative for the treatment of copper traditionally used for the treatment of citrus canker disease, thus reducing selection pressure for copper resistance. We believe that the search for microorganisms that act as inhibitors of quorum sensing in phytopathogenic bacteria also as antagonist agent could be an effective strategy in a broader context. Since the organisms characterized here were originally isolated from the citrus phylloplane, the present study also contributes to an understanding of the potential interactions of bacteria on leaf surfaces.

## Acknowledgements

The authors thank Professor Jesus A Ferro from the Technology Department, Faculdade de Ciencias Agrarias e Veterinarias, Universidade estadual Paulista, UNESP, Jaboticabal, SP, Brasil, and to CREBIO Centro de Recursos Biologicos e Biologia Genomica Univ. Estadual Paulista, Jaboticabal SP, Brazil, for the DNA sequencing.

## Conflict of interest

The authors declare no conflict of interest.

## Author details

Sonia Villamizar[1] and Juan Carlos Caicedo[2]*

1 School of Agricultural and Veterinarian Sciences, São Paulo State University (UNESP), Jaboticabal, Brazil

2 Faculty of Exact, Natural and Agricultural Sciences, Research Group CIBAS, Universidad de Santander, Bucaramanga, Colombia

*Address all correspondence to: caicedocepeda@gmail.com

## References


[1] Ortiz-Castro R, Contreras-Cornejo HA, Macías-Rodríguez L, López-Bucio J. The role of microbial signals in plant growth and development. Plant Signaling and Behavior. 2009;**4**:701-712

[2] Lee HA. Further data on the susceptibility of rutaceous plants to citrus-canker. Journal of Agricultural Research. 1918;**15**:661-665

[3] Fawcett HS, Jenkins AE. Records of citrus canker from herbarium specimens of the genus Citrus in England and the United States. Phytopathology. 1933;**23**:820-824

[4] Das AK. Pathogenic variability in *Xanthomonas axonopodis* pv. citri, causal agent of citrus canker. Journal of Mycology and Plant Pathology. 2002;**54**:274-279

[5] Dopson RN. The eradication of citrus canker. The Plant Disease Reporter. 1964;**48**:30-31

[6] Civerolo EL. Bacterial canker disease of citrus. Journal of the Rio Grande Valley Horticultural Society. 1984;**37**:127-145

[7] Stall RE, Seymour CP. Canker: A threat to citrus in the Gulf Coast states. Plant Disease. 1983;**67**:581-585

[8] Schaad NW, Postnikova E, Lacy GH, Sechler A, Agarkova I, Stromberg PE, et al. Reclassification of *Xanthomonas campestris* pv. citri (ex Hasse 1915) dye 1978 forms A, B/C/D, and E as *X. smithii* subsp. *citri* (ex Hasse) sp. nov. nom. rev. comb. nov., *X. fuscans* subsp. *aurantifolii* (ex Gabriel 1989) sp. nov. nom. rev. comb. nov., and *X. alfalfae* subsp. *citrumelo* (ex Riker and Jones) Gabriel et al., 1989 sp. nov. nom. rev. comb. nov.; *X. campestris* pv. *malvacearum* (ex smith 1901) dye 1978 as *X. smithii* subsp. *smithii* nov. comb. nov. nom. nov.; *X. campestris* pv. *alfalfae* (ex Riker and Jones, 1935) dye 1978 as *X. alfalfae* subsp. *alfalfae* (ex Riker et al., 1935) sp. nov. nom. rev.; and "var. fuscans" of *X. campestris* pv. *phaseoli* (ex Smith, 1987) dye 1978 as *X. fuscans* subsp. *fuscans* sp. nov. Systematic and Applied Microbiology. 2005;**28**:494-518

[9] Moreira LM, Almeida NF Jr., Potnis N, Digiampietri LA, Adi SS, Bortolossi JC, et al. Novel insights into the genomic basis of citrus canker based on the genome sequences of two strains of *Xanthomonas fuscans* subsp. *aurantifolii*. BMC Genomics. 2010;**11**:238

[10] Namekata T, Balmer E, University of São Paulo. Estudos comparativos entre *Xanthomonas citri* (Hasse) Dow., agente causal do cancro cítrico e *Xanthomonas citri* (Hasse) Dow., n.f.sp. aurantifolia, agente causal da cancrose do limoeiro Galego. Piracicaba; 1971

[11] Malavolta Júnior VA, Yamashiro T, Nogueira EMC, Feichtenberger E. Distribuição do tipo C de *Xanthomonas campestris* pv. citri no Estado de São Paulo. Summa Phytopathologica. 1984;**10**:11

[12] Sharma SK, Sharma RR. Citrus canker approaching century: A review. Tree and Forestry Science and Biotechnology. 2009;**2**(Special Issue):54-56

[13] Behlau F, Canteros BI, Minsavage GV, Jones JB, Graham JH. Molecular characterization of copper resistance genes from *Xanthomonas citri* subsp. *citri* and *Xanthomonas alfalfae* subsp. *citrumelonis*. Applied and Environmental Microbiology. 2011;**77**:4089-4096

[14] Chan JWYF, Goodwin PH. The molecular genetics of virulence of *Xanthomonas campestris*. Biotechnology Advances. 1999;**17**:489-508

[15] Swings J, Vauterin L, Kersters K. The bacterium *Xanthomonas*. In: Swings JG, Civerolo EL, editors. Xanthomonas. 1st ed. Dordrecht: Springer; 1993. pp. 121-146

[16] Gabriel DW, Kingsley MT, Hunter JE, Gottwald TR. Reinstatement of *Xanthomonas citri* (ex Hasse) and *X. phaseoli* (ex Smith) and reclassification of all *X. campestris* pv. *citri* strains. International Journal of Systematic Bacteriology. 1989;**39**:14-22

[17] Soto GE, Hultgren SJ. Bacterial adhesins: Common themes and variations in architecture and assembly. Journal of Bacteriology. 1999;**181**:1059-1071

[18] Gerlach RG, Hensel M. Protein secretion systems and adhesins: The molecular armory of Gram-negative pathogens. International Journal of Medical Microbiology. 2007;**297**:401-415

[19] Sandkvist M. Biology of type II secretion. Molecular Microbiology. 2001;**40**:271-283

[20] Büttner D, Bonas U. Regulation and secretion of *Xanthomonas* virulence factors. FEMS Microbiology Reviews. 2010;**34**:107-133

[21] Moreira LM, de Souza RF, Almeida NF Jr, Setubal JC, Oliveira JC, Furlan LR, et al. Comparative genomics analyses of citrus-associated bacteria. Annual Review of Phytopathology. 2004;**42**:163-184

[22] Yang H, Junli Z, Hongge J, Davide S, Ting L, Wolf BF, et al. Lateral organ boundaries 1 is a disease susceptibility gene for citrus bacterial canker disease. Proceedings of the National Academy of Sciences of the United States of America. 2014;**111**:E521-E529

[23] Majer C, Hochholdinger F. Defining the boundaries: Structure and function of LOB domain proteins. Trends in Plant Science. 2011;**16**(1):47-52. DOI: 10.1016/j.tplants.2010.09.009

[24] Cascales E, Christie PJ. The versatile bacterial type IV secretion systems. Nature Reviews. Microbiology. 2003;**1**:137-150

[25] da Silva AC, Ferro JA, Reinach FC, Farah CS, Furlan LR, Quaggio RB, et al. Comparison of the genomes of two *Xanthomonas* pathogens with differing host specificities. Nature. 2002;**417**:459-463

[26] Low HH, Gubellini F, Rivera-Calzada A, Braun N, Connery S, Dujeancourt A, et al. Structure of a type IV secretion system. Nature. 2014;**508**:550-553

[27] Souza DP, Oka GU, Alvarez-Martinez CE, Bisson-Filho AW, Dunger G, Hobeika L, et al. Bacterial killing via a type IV secretion system. Nature Communications. 2015. Article number: 6453

[28] Federle MJ, Bassler BL. Interspecies communication in bacteria. Journal of Clinical Investigation. 2003;**112**:1291-1299

[29] Tang JL, Liu YN, Barber CE, Dow JM, Wootton JC, Daniels MJ. Genetic and molecular analysis of a cluster of rpf genes involved in positive regulation of synthesis of extracellular enzymes and polysaccharide in *Xanthomonas campestris* pathovar campestris. Molecular Genetics and Genomics. 1991;**226**:409-417

[30] Uroz S, Dessaux Y, Oger P. Quorum sensing and quorum quenching: The yin and yang of bacterial communication. Chembiochem. 2009;**10**(2):205-216

[31] Zhang LH, Dong YH. Quorum sensing and signal interference: Diverse implications. Molecular Microbiology. 2004;**53**:1563-1571

[32] Frederix M, Downey AJ. Quorum sensing: Regulating the regulators.